# TRIBAL HEALTH AND MEDICINES

---

**About the Editors**

**A.K. Kalla,** Currently Professor and Head of the Department of Anthropology, University of Delhi, he has worked in the area of demography, population genetics, clinical genetics and molecular anthropology. He has been a visiting scientist to the Institute of Human Genetics, University of Heidelberg and the past president of Indian Anthropological Association.

**P.C. Joshi,** Currently Professor of Social Anthropology in the Department of Anthropology, University of Delhi, he received his M.Phil. and doctorate in Anthropology from the same department. He has been the past president of Society for Indian Medical Anthropology and has served the Department of Anthropology, HNB Garhwal University, Srinagar as well as Department of Medical Anthropology, Institute of Human Behaviour and Allied Sciences. He has been the visiting Lecturer, School of Tropical Hygiene and Public Health, Heidelberg University and visiting faculty, Global Forum for Health, Geneva.

# TRIBAL HEALTH AND MEDICINES

*Edited by*

**A.K. Kalla**

and

**P.C. JOSHI**

Department of Anthropology,
Delhi University, Delhi

**CONCEPT PUBLISHING COMPANY, NEW DELHI-110059**

**Declaration**: This book is the outcome of papers received for the National Workshop on 'Emerging Issues in Tribal Health and Medicines' supported by The Ministry of Tribal Affairs, Government of India, Indian Council of Medical Research and University Grants Commission. The view expressed in the articles are the responsibilities of the authors concerned.

ISBN 81-8069-139-X

First Published 2004



*Published and Printed by*
Ashok Kumar Mittal
**Concept Publishing Company**
A/15-16, Commercial Block, Mohan Garden
New Delhi-110059 (INDIA)

*Phones* : 25351460, 25351794
*Fax* : 091-11-25357103
*Email* : publishing@conceptpub.com

# Contents

## Part II
## DEMOGRAPHIC AND ECOLOGICAL ASPECTS OF TRIBAL HEALTH



## Part III
## SOCIAL AND CULTURAL ASPECTS OF TRIBAL HEALTH

## Part V
## POLICY ASPECTS IN TRIBAL HEALTH AND MEDICINES

# List of Contributors

**Banerjee, B.G.**, Currently Professor of Social Anthropology, Department of Anthropology, Panjab University, Chandigarh. He has obtained his doctorate from Delhi University and has been teaching in Panjab University for more than two decades. He has worked with Prof. Charles Leslie and has contributed in the fields of medical anthropology, socialization and Tibetan medicines.

**Bhasin, Veena,** Currently UGC research scientist C in the Department of Anthropology, Delhi University. She has obtained her doctorate from Delhi University and has written many books and research articles on Himalayan communities, ecological anthropology and medical anthropology.

**Bhat, H.K.,** Currently Professor in the Department of Studies in Anthropolgy, Mysore University, he has served the Anthropological Survey of India and NEHU, Shillong. He is the president of Society for Indian Medical Anthropology and had received his doctorate from Karnataka University, Dharwad.

**Chadda, R.K.,** Currently Professor of Psychiatry at Institute of Human Behaviour and Allied Sciences, Delhi, he is an alumnus of the prestigious PGIMER, Chandigarh. He is a recipient of 8 National Awards in the field of Psychiatry including the ICMR's Tilak Venkoba Rao Award, Dr. Vimla Virmani Award, and Tilak Venkoba Rao Oration Award and Bhagwat Award of Indian Psychiatric Society. He is currently the Member Secretary, State Mental Health Authority, Delhi, Secretary General, Indian Association for Social Psychiatry, Chairperson, Geriatric Psychiatry Section. He is also Member of the Transcultural Psychiatry Section of the World Psychiatric Association and Member, National Academy of Medical Sciences (India).

**Chadha, N.K.**, Currently Professor of Psychology, Department of Psychology, University of Delhi. He has been doing research in the area of organizational behaviour, gerontology and quantitative methods in social sciences.

**Chandra, Ramesh,** Currently Director, Ministry of Tribal Affairs, Government of India, he has served the Anthropological Survey of India, Space Application Centre and National Wasteland Development Board in past.

**Chao, D.**, Currently a doctoral student in the Department of Psychology, University of Delhi, Delhi.

**Chaudhuri, Buddhadeb,** Currently Ambedkar Professor of Anthropology at the Department of Anthropology, Calcutta University, he is the coordinator of International Post Graduate Course on Human Rights. His area of interest includes environment and development, indigenous people, traditional knowledge and human rights.

**Chowdhary, R.,** Doctoral student in the Department of Anthropology, University of Delhi.

**Das, Mitoo,** Doctoral student in the Department of Anthropology, University of Delhi.

**Dash Sharma, P.,** Recently retired as Professor of Physical Anthropology, Ranchi University, Ranchi, Jharkhand, he obtained his doctorate from the University of Delhi and served initially in the Anthropological Survey of India and later joined the Department of Anthropology, Ranchi University. He is editor of South Asian Anthropologist and has extensively worked among the tribes of Chotanagpur and Manipur.

**Elizabeth, A.M.,** Former doctoral student in the Department of Anthropology, University of Delhi, she is currently working as research assistant in the National Institute of Health and Family Welfare, New Delhi.

**Ganguly, K.K.,** Currently Assistant Director General in the Indian Council of Medical Research, New Delhi, he has served as Assistant Professor of Medical Anthropology in the Institute of Human Behaviour and Allied Sciences. He has doctorate from Centre for Social Medicines and Community Health, Jawaharlal Nehru University, New Delhi.

**Gupta, Meena,** Currently the Director of the Institute of Human Behaviour and Allied Sciences, Delhi, she has served in the Department of Neurology, GB Pant Hospital, New Delhi as Professor and Head. She holds MD in medicines and DM in Neurology and has been the President of The Indian Epilepsy Association, Delhi.

**Gusain, Suman Singh,** Currently Lecturer in the Department of

Anthropology, HNB Garhwal University, Tehri, he received his doctorate in anthropology on childhood illness in a high altitude village from the HNB Garhwal University.

**Ibata, Atsuko,** Currently research student in Centre for Social Medicine and Community Health, JNU, she has also studied at Vishwabharti Shantiniketan.

**Joshi, P.C.,** Currently Professor of Social Anthropology in the Department of Anthropology, University of Delhi, he received his M.Phil. and doctorate in Anthropology from the same department. He has been the past president of Society for Indian Medical Anthropology and has served the Department of Anthropology, HNB Garhwal University, Srinagar as well as Department of Medical Anthropology, Institute of Human Behaviour and Allied Sciences. He has been the visiting lecturer, School of Tropical Hygiene and Public Health, Heidelberg University and visiting faculty, Global Forum for Health, Geneva.

**Kalla, A.K.,** Currently Professor and Head of the Department of Anthropology, University of Delhi, he has worked in the area of demography, population genetics, clinical genetics and molecular anthropology. He has been a visiting scientist to the Institute of Human Genetics, University of Heidelberg and the past president of Indian Anthropological Association.

**Kapoor, A.K.,** Currently Professor in the Department of Anthropology, University of Delhi, he received doctorate in Anthropology from the same department. He has extensively worked on the high altitude Himalayan populations.

**Kar, R.K.,** Currently Professor of Anthropology, Dibrugarh University, he has been the past president of the section on Anthropology and Archaeology, Indian Science Congress Association. He has extensively worked on the tea garden populations and the tribes of North-east.

**Kaushal, Sonia,** Doctoral student in the Department of Anthropology, University of Delhi.

**Kshatriya, G.K.,** Currently Reader in the Department of Anthropology, he has worked in the National Institute of Health and Family Welfare on various projects concerning tribal health. He received his doctorate from Department of Anthropology, University of Delhi.

**Moyon, L.N,** She has done her M.Phil. in Social Anthropology from the Department of Anthropology, University of Delhi.

**Murmu, Dolly Florence,** Doctoral student in the Department of Anthropology, University of Delhi.

**Paliwal, Mridula,** Doctoral student in the Department of Anthropology, University of Delhi.

**Rath, Swetansu Sekhar,** Currently Lecturer in the Department of Anthropology, B.J.B. College, Bhubaneswar, he received his doctorate from the Department of Anthropology, University of Delhi.

**Sachdeva, M.P.,** Currently Reader in the Department of Anthropology, University of Delhi, he received his doctorate from the Department of Anthropology, Panjab University, Chandigarh.

**Saraswathy, K.N.,** Currently Lecturer in the Department of Anthropology, University of Delhi, she received her doctorate from the same department. She has worked in the Amity Institute of Biotechnology in past.

**Sharma, Anima,** Currently a free lance Social Scientist and Consultant in social sector, she has received her doctorate from Department of Anthropology, University of Delhi in Social Anthropology. She has worked extensively among the Gond tribe of Madhya Pradesh.

**Singh, A.P.,** Currently a Reader at the Department of Anthropology, Lucknow University, he has served as Professor in the Department of Anthropology, HNB Garhwal University. He obtained his doctorate in Anthropology, Lucknow University.

**Sinha, A.K.,** Currently a Reader in the Department of Anthropology, Panjab University, Chandigarh, he has served the Department of Social Anthropology, Guru Ghasi Das University, Bilaspur.

**Srivastava, A.K.,** Currently Dean and Coordinator, Amity Institute of Biotechnology, he has been actively associated with the PUC, Ludhiana and RAU, Pusa where he was the Director Research and Vice Chancellor. His area of interest includes environmental physiology and biotechnology.

**Subramanyam, V.,** Currently Associate Professor of Anthropology in the Department of Anthropology, Andhra University, Visakhapatnam, he has undertaken studies for WHO, India CLEN and NACO.

**Tewari, Disha,** Currently a Research Student in the Centre for the study of Regional Development, Jawaharlal Nehru University, New Delhi.

**Vijayendra, B.R.,** Currently Research Associate in the Anthropological Survey of India, Mysore

# Introduction

India is an enigma to the world at large. This sea of humanity, whether we call it a melting pot, salad bowl or else bunch of flowers, carries forward a legacy of civilized existence of at least five thousand years. These five thousand years are also testimony to the existence of various shades of cultures, races, political systems, subsistence patterns, dietary habits, dress, dances and ethnomedicines. The dialogues between cultures have been explained by anthropologists through the processes such as universalization, parochialization and sanskritization. The formation of caste system in itself bears testimony to the assimilation of distinct cultures into hierarchical order with technologically, militarily, politically and educationally advanced cultures occupying the positions of influence in the caste system. Some cultures which were either away from the agrarian plain lands or did not prefer assimilation were pushed back to wilderness which they made their abode. The tribal societies therefore have more of less remained relatively isolated but there has been considerable exchange between the state and the tribal societies. In fact, in many parts there existed largely tribal states.

The independence of India from the British dominance however has been a turning point in India's destiny and consequently of its tribal inhabitants. The tribal for the first time became a political entity and were incorporated as sections of society needing special provision in matters concerning education, employment and political representation. The planned development made special provision for the tribal regions and this was closely monitored through the constitutional bodies. Where are we after more than five decades of planned development? Has there been an equal distribution of planned development across all areas? How much have been the progress on the three principal domains of development, namely education, health and poverty eradication? The present workshop is primarily concerned with the examination of progress at the level of health. The idea behind is not to find faults but to diagnose the problems and churn out some suitable strategy.

The theme of the workshop "Emerging Issues in Tribal Health and Medicines" is chosen to cover both the clinical as well as social science perspectives in examining the health care issues. The clinical side of tribal health care concerns itself with examination of 'disease' domain, issues of prevalence of diseases, bio-genetic morbidity patterns, and demographic trends influencing morbidity, nutritional deficiencies and associated environmental and cultural correlates. The picture that emerges from this primarily 'etic' and biomedicinal enquiry tells us about the gaps that exist in the health care coverage helping thereby in formulating appropriate programmes for interventions. In other perspective, the 'disease' is seen as 'illness', in the framework of social and cultural experience of people who suffer and seek health. This perspective is 'emic' and ethnographic. This domain of enquiry concerns itself with tribal systems of medicines, tribal healers, rituals, ethnomedicines, culture-specific patterns of health seeking and reactions to public health care programmes. Both perspectives compliment each other and help us in understanding better the real issues that lie behind failures in covering the tribal communities which have been lagging behind. Besides these two dominant paradigms, it has also been considered appropriate to examine special issues that have become very pertinent in the present context, namely the issue of tribal medicines and the policy perspective of tribal health and medicines,

The theme of the workshop therefore has been subdivided into five sections. The first section is titled "Clinical and bio-genetic aspects of tribal health" which has adopted the paradigm of biomedicines in order to examine the tribal health problems. The first paper is by a clinician on the subject of neurological disorders. Taking stock of very limited studies that have been attempted in the Indian tribal context, Meena Gupta informs us of the burden of neurological disorders. In a plethora of neurological disorders, the status of epilepsy is shrouded in great mystery. This disease, due to seizures is attributed to supernatural forces and effects of ancestral or evil spirits. She strongly advocates for a community based approach to deal with the problems of neurological disorders in general and epilepsy in particular.

Mental health of the tribals is the focus of discussion for R.K. Chadha in his paper. He raises his concern about very little information being available about the mental health issues and prevalence of psychiatric morbidity among them, although he observes that the nature of illness among the tribals is not much different from that of the general population and that the tribals frequently resort to various medico-religious methods and some indigenous herbs for the psychiatric problems.

Gautam Kumar Kshatriya having discussed the demographic nuances and their health implications among tribals adds that the prevalence rates of genetic disorders like sickle cell haemoglobin and Glucose-6-Phosphate Dehydrogenaes defficiency plays important role in the health status of many Indian tribal populations because of which they need special health care programmes; he seems to propagate the "Healthcare Delivery Model" proposed by National Institute of Health and Family Welfare (2004) as appended to his article.

The health problems of tribal communities have been dichotomized as urgent health need problems and emerging health problems by Svetansu Sekhar Rath. He includes maternal health, nutritional status, sexually transmitted diseases, genetic disorders, malaria and impact of family welfare programmes into urgent health need problems while socio-demographic indicators which contribute to health status under emerging health need problems. Thus, status of women, sex ratio, literacy, marriage pattern and age at marriage, fertility and mortality and life expectancy at birth are covered by the author under emerging health problems. Rath found that there is variability in health problems of the tribal, some being built in while others imposed upon them. He advocates for a focused approach through community based health care delivery system as a real solution to the health problems of the tribal.

The nutrition deficiencies that characterize the tribal communities in most parts have been the principal focus of paper by Das Sharma. Das Sharma presents a panoramic view of the studies done using anthropometric surveys among the primitive tribes of Jharkhand, Orissa, Madya Pradesh, Chatisgarh and West Bengal. He finds that most of the tribes, with exception of Toto of West Bengal had considerable nutritional deficiencies. He therefore calls our attention to the alarming situation of the tribal communities, specially the primitive tribal groups with respect to nutritional deficiencies. In some part, such as Orissa hinterlands, food supply itself is the main cause of mal-nutrition but, in other parts, there is a need to intensify vigorous health education drive and identification of locally available food items to cover up the deficiencies.

A sex-wise comparison of growth in age group 5 to 14 has been presented by Suman Singh Gusain on the basis of anthropometric measurements covering the Tharu tribal children of Uttaranchal. Anthropometric studies, as stressed by Das Sharma are required to be taken up on a longitudinal basis in order to monitor the nutritional health of the tribal commumities as most tribal children known to be showing nutritional deficiencies. Mridula Paliwal has touched upon a very important but neglected dimension of the tribal health issues. She argues that the prevalence of sexually transmitted diseases and reproductive tract infections is very alarming among some selected tribal populations. It is very well correlated with the practices such as multiple marriages, premarital sex, consanguinity, youth dormitory, divorce, out migration and above all poor health coverage and low literacy. Such a situation, coupled with the fact that there are doubts over the way estimates are being made from the hospital going populations, is indeed very serious. The tribal community may be sitting over a dormant volcano of HIV. Then there are the primitive tribal communities which are already endangered.

The second section titled "Demographic and Ecological aspects of Tribal Health' brings to focus the demographic and environmental indicators that greatly contribute to the specific morbidity profile which the tribal communities exhibit.

Dealing with ecology of malnutrition in the agency area of Visakhapatnam, V. Subramanyam brings out the fact that in several cases, tribal ecology is not meeting the subsistence of its entire population. He points out that the influence of myth, food taboos and (surprisingly) modernization process seems to add miseries to the tribals, which are reflected in nutritional deficiencies and health disorders among them. He suggests that a clear-cut food policy, with reinforced nutritional rehabilitation centres with people's participation is the need of the time for safe guarding these tribals.

In discussing the issue of health and ecology among the tribes of Ladakh, Veena Bhasin found this multi-religious and multi-ethnic landmass subscribing to medical pluralism. In her view, "the status, growth and evaluation of co-existing therapy systems have been influenced by cultural ideology, ecology, political patronage, changing social institutions, disenchantment with and romaticization of values represented therapy sytems". The multiple therapy system of the Ladakhi includes allopathy, shamanism or Lhawaism, Lamaism and scholarly amchi medicine. The choice of therapy among Ladakhi is basically eclectic following no fixed pattern as is largely dependent upon the illness specific patterns of resort.

Reproductive health among two primitive tribes inhabiting Andhra Pradesh has been the theme of the paper presented by M.P. Sachdeva *et al.* Kolam and Thoti are the two tribal groups where demographic data on 350 and 246 ever-married women, respectively was collected along with reproductive details. A comparative study of both the tribes the Thotis show higher prenatal mortality while the Kolam high infant mortality. But the prenatal mortality among Thotis is attributed to the poor health care coverage, especially lack of antenatal mother and child health care programmes. The reason for high infant mortality among the Kolams, despite relatively better health care coverage than the Thotis is because of biogenetic factors, especially the high incidence of thalassaemia which is observed among the Kolams.

Disha Tiwari, using the secondary data, highlights the dismal state of health of the tribals living in BIMARU states, as indicated by their infant and child mortality and like others suggests elevating their educational and nutritional levels to meet the challenges. Langlom Naomi Moyon brings to focus the health situation confronting the women of the Moyon tribe of Manipur. The Moyon women, like other women of the north-east are hard working contributing immensely to the family income by means of doing multiple domestic and income generating tasks. Although, they are the backbone of the Moyon economy, they tend to neglect their health and thus suffer from adverse health consequences. The difference between the main land and the remote resident Moyon is brought out by the author which contributes to the drastic variation in the morbidity and mortality. The Moyons, according to Langlom mostly prefer Allopathic treatment with some usage of homeopathy. They are also helped by NGOs and visionaries, in cases of supernatural causation.

The third section deals with the social and cultural aspects of tribal health and medicines. It brings to focus the issues of cultural beliefs and values, social relations, health seeking, healing traditions from myriad tribal communities.

A.K. Sinha and B.G. Banerjee present a critical and scholarly appraisal of the magico-religious dimension of the tribal systems of medicines. The authors have discussed the issue of anthropological discourse on witchcraft, sorcery, evil eye, personalistic system and have then looked at the comtemporary tribal causative theories. They finally conclude that the beliefs in witchcraft and magic are deeply rooted in the traditional customary ideas whereby the societies categorize and order the universe around them. They make a passionate plea that such systems should not merely be discarded as mere superstitions and should be understood in the framework of context and meaning. In the paper World of Tribal Healers, P.C. Joshi presents ethnographic account of the Jaunsari healer which range from baman, mali, jariyara, female specialist to doctor. He presents intimate details of the practice and cultural features of the healer's role. The account, presented from an 'emic' perspective gives some ideas regarding why people visit these healers, at times when the doctor is available within easy reach.

A.P. Singh presents the scenario of Uttaranchal tribal ethnomedicines highlighting the role of 'witch doctors' or traditional healers. He advocates that there is a need to train witch doctors into scientific use of indigenous pharmacopoeia. The paper by D. Chao, N.K. Chadha and P.C. Joshi covers the psychosocial well-being of the elderly belonging to Naga tribe. Gerontological studies in India have largely confined themselves to the urban and rural areas and no study of any consequence has been reported from the tribal perspective. The study, which is based on quantitative and qualitative study of 200 elderly Naga has touched upon indicators such as deprivation, loneliness, happiness, health awareness, disability in daily activities, adjustment, leisure activities, self-rated quality of life and social network in order to cover the sex differences. The commonly held belief among the scholars has been that the elderly are living a better quality of life as tribal subscribe to traditional values. The impact of changing trends when the tribal culture is in flux, required to be studied in respect of tribal areas.

Health care practices of various tribes inhabiting Manipur have been the concern of Hemlata and Krishna Kumari's paper. The authors have found that the tribal system of medicines in Manipur is largely magico-religious under which the tribal subscribe to myriad supernatural agencies through the healers and perform a wide variety of rituals and sacrifices in order to propitiate the angry spirits. The excessive dependence on the supernatural form of treatment, according to authors is primarily due to its easy accessibility and in absent of any alternative.

The Rathwas inhabit western coastal region of India and are agriculturist subscribing to traditional healers and folk medicines besides the government run Primary Health Centre. According to Mitoo Das, they classify the disease causation into supernatural, magical and natural factors. Besides the doctors working in the health centre which is nearly six kilometres away, they consult local shaman Bhua and the herbalist for various problems. The health of women was found to be very poor and most of the women were found to be suffering from reproductive tract infections, dysfunctional uterine bleeding, pelvic inflammatory disease and anaemia. Their usual complaint of white discharge, menstrual cramp, irregular menses and heavy menstrual flow is symptomatic of poor genital hygiene, chronic and severe infections needing concerted health care efforts on part of the government and civil society. The wealth of herbal medicines that the Rathwas use in treatment of various symptoms related to reproductive tract also needs thorough pharmacological investigations for ascertaining medicinal properties.

The Gaddi of Himachal Pradesh are transhumance criss-crossing the Himachal mountains with their animals in different seasons. Their healing practices have been highlighted by Sonia Kaushal which rely very heavily on supernatural theory of disease causation and treatment. The Gaddi worldview is full of different benevolent and malevolent supernatural forces such as Kailung, Gunga, Jogni, Rakshanis, Banasat, Chungu, Naags, Sidhas, Devis, Birs, etc. The author hold generalized apathy of public health care personnel and inaccessibility responsible for the current state of affairs in Gaddi tribe. Anima Sharma touches upon an important dimension of the changing Gonds. She looks at the emergence of stress among the Gonds in view of the new work patterns.

Atsuko Ibata presents the concept of illness and craft of bonpo from an emic perspective. She reveals the complex interplay of spirits, supernatural agencies and bonpo craft in the cognitive framework of Bon philosophy. The remarkable similarity in the conceptualization of *bis* among Jaunsari and poisoning among the Monpas of Arunachal Pradesh is reflective of the cultural exchange that occurs so smoothly in the medical domain.

The fourth section concerns the issue of medicines which includes plant medicines and ethnomedicines. A.K. Srivastava in his article "Road map for tribal Medicines" points out that of the 1500 medicinal plants, Indian systems of medicine have identified use of over 7500 species of plants for preservative, primitive and curative application and that the tribals specifically have vast knowledge about the medicinal characteristics of plants in and around dense forests in their adjoining areas. He argues than there is a pressing need for protective fencing of the herbal in the forests, especially the tribal belts, particularly because of callous exploitation of the tribal herbal wealth in India.

Dolly Florence Murmu offers a insider's view of medicinal plants being used in the tribal hinterlands of Jharkhand. She stresses upon the fact that the tribal worldview of plants connotes deep meaning that the people attach to the medicinal plants that they use. However, the effectiveness of the plant medicines needs to be experimentally validated and useful herbal preparations should be promoted and marketed for income generation. She suggests formation of tribal markets with the stackholdership of the community as cooperatives so that the benefits could come back to the tribal.

Buddhadeb Chaudhary has examined traditional tribal medicine and treatment in India in the context of globalization process; because of important implications of traditional knowledge and wisdom in this context he fears that over the years traditional knowledge and skills have been neglected and a prejudice has been engineered and encouraged by powerful nationals and multinationals. He puts forth a sixfold strategy to meet this challenge so that good health may be delivered to the tribals, being fully conscious of the limitations of traditional knowledge and wisdom in this regard.

R.K. Kar presents the case of ethnomedicines in the context of northeastern tribes of India which is bestowed with around eight per cent of world's total biodiversity is perceived as a hotspot and therefore the 7,500 medicinal plant species that India has are very precious resources. The north-east wet forested area with its rich biodiversity and traditional knowledge of medicinal plant use is going to play a very important role in the field of herbal medicines. Taking example of Mishings, Kar presents a panoramic view of the plant use for various diseases by the tribal community.

Vijayendra and Bhat present the system of ethnomedicines among the Jenu Kuruba of Karnataka. This tribe classifies illness into four major categories and has immense knowledge of the plant medicines. The general pattern of mistrust and suspicion, according to authors, is also reflected in the ethnomedicines.

The last section has focused on the policy issues with special reference to the tribal health and medicines. In his article on "Issues in Tribal Health and Medicines", P.C. Joshi brings out the significance of medico-religious rituals in maintenance of health of the tribals, particularly because tribals, as a group, are involved in the therapy. If such a group involvement could be ensured for different alternative therapies, the health scenario of the tribals could be considerably improved, and this, as he suggests, could be achieved by not only educating the tribals in this regard, but also by gearing and upgrading clinical infrastructure along with improvement of the human resources involved

Ramesh Chandra highlights the contributory factors responsible for the tirbal health. He lists need for correct approach, lack of faith and awareness as well as hesitancy as the main reasons for poor medical attendance in tribal areas. He advocates for a multi-pronged approach to deal with tribal health delivery challenges.

Dr. K.K. Ganguly offers a critical appraisal of social science perspective in tribal health as well as the development model. His paper assumes significance in the light of structural adjustment compulsions and globalization which has totally left the tribal at the mercy of dominant forces. In the times when the state is shrinking away to take up the task of preventive and public health services leaving the curative health to private players, the state of tribal health is further doomed. It is a big challenge confronting us and alternative funding for tribal health requires to be looked into.

While advocating for Public-Private Partnership (PPP) for improvement of health in scheduled tribes, Khanna and Kapoor point out in their paper the uses as well as the risks involved in this strategy. However, they believe that with the involvement of committed NGOs and local governments, there seems a possibility of delivering the results in this regard.

# PART I

# CLINICAL AND BIO-GENETIC ASPECTS

# 1

# Neurological Disorders among Tribals

MEENA GUPTA

India is a large country, measuring approximately 3,300,000 km$^2$ with a population of 1,027,015,247 (census 2001), 70 per cent of India lives in villages, 70 per cent of the medical manpower in urban and 100 per cent of the facilities for investigations located in metropolitan or similar cities. According to the census of 1991, the tribals constitute 8.08 per cent of the population of India. Nearly, three fourth of the tribal population lives in the 7 states of our country. They occupy around 15 per cent of the geographical area of India, which is the most inaccessible and underdeveloped area.

The health status of the tribals is marked by poverty, illiteracy, malnutrition, lack of personal hygiene, poor sanitation, poor mother and child health services, absence of health education, lack of national preventive programmes, lack of available health services is responsible for the poor health of the tribals.

The tribal health in India, unfortunately was never taken seriously. Though some intensive field work has been done by social scientists but some of the studies treated the problem of tribal health in peripheral and casual manner. For a meaningful understanding of the tribal health, it is important to understand the people themselves their indigenous medicines and understand how under the existing social, economic and cultural setting these needs can be best met to the satisfaction of people themselves.

The problems of tribal health cannot be studied in isolation from the general population of India. Tribal people suffer from the same diseases as others with marked preponderance of infective over degenerative diseases. The tribals who have remained isolated will soon be exposed to the rapid pace of development and industrialization in our country[1].

The general health problems of the tribals resemble those of the rural and other underprivileged sections of our society. These comprise malnutrition, anaemia, parasitic infestations and infections like diarrhoeal and respiratory disorders. The life of the tribal is so beset with these disorders right from birth that the average life expectancy is much lower in contrast with the national average of 58-60 years[2].

There are 635 tribes located in five major belts in India. Each tribe is not only geographical area specific but also culture specific. Hence, what is true in one case may not be true in the other case. The tribal belief of causation of disease can be broadly categorized into two areas. They are strong believers of natural theory of diseases. According to them when man falls out of harmony with nature suffers from illnesses and becomes susceptible to diseases and accidents. Hence the rituals to restore balance and harmony with nature.

Treatment is influenced by the cause of sickness perceived by the group. The tribals have some scientific knowledge, learnt through traditional experience. This knowledge is a part of their socio-cultural religious system. The treatment procedure amongst the tribals can be broadly divided into preventive and curative methods.

The preventive procedures include use of charms, amulets, animal sacrifice propitiations of disease seeking spirits, worship of God-belief in protective function of rituals.

The curative practices include first worship of deities and spirits. To the tribals religion and medicine are not separate. It has also been found that some tribals practice their traditional system along with western system of medicine, if available.

While reviewing the literature, it is observed that there is hardly any mention of neurological disorders among the tribal population.

In a study conducted in Phulbani (funded by ICMR, 1986) regarding health and morbidity status of tribals. Population under study was 2325 and 1614 (69.24%) person were found sick. This study mentions that the cardiovascular and diseases relating to nervous system were relatively less[3].

Unfortunately, in India, being the second most populous country in the world, there are very few neuroepidemiological studies on rural population except from Bangalore, Rural Kashmir and Rural Bengal.

The community studies provide a basic data for formulating health policy, a guidance to focus attention on priority sectors and also to take preventive measures wherever possible.

A neuroepidemiological survey was carried at Malda district, 350 km away from Calcutta, exactly at midpoint between Siliguri and Calcutta on a rural population of 37,286 (M18,507;F19,229; 1981 Census) under three Gram Panchayat areas with the help of nonprofessionals like Gram members, ICDS workers, multipurpose health workers and motivated local youths, based on WHO protocol (1981). House to house survey was carried out. Sensitivity reached 90 per cent and specificity 86 per cent. Total 961 individuals with neurological problems were screened and classified according to simple, but well defined criteria. Single disease was seen in 857 patients and 104 patients had double diseases. Crude prevalence rate stands at 2856.29 per 100,000; 2.85 per cent of population. The commonest diseases were headache (1858 per 1,00,000), epilepsy (305 per 1,00,000), vertigo (249 per 1,00,000), stroke (126 per 1,00,000), degenerative vertebral diseases with radiculopathy (160 per 1,00,000) and peripheral neuropthy (75 per 1,00,000), Cerebral palsy (21.45 per 1,00,000), mental retardation (42.90 per 1,00,000), paralytic poliomyelitis (53.63 per 1,00,000), movement disorder (26.81 per 1,00,000), spinal cord disorders (21 per 1,00,000), motor neurone disease (2.7 per 1,00,000), development of speech and language (34 per 1,00,000). Age specific prevalence of disease showed progressive increase in rate with advancing age upto 4th decade followed by a slightly decrease plateau upto 60 years of age and then sharp decline. Age and sex specific disease prevalence shows female dominance with maximum cases in 4th decade[4].

Community studies on major neurological disorders are very few in our country. Some of the diseases with subjective bias show widely ranging values, but in other cases, the values are comparable. Certainly, India is a country of heterogeneity; hence it is possible, that the prevalence data will differ.

Epilepsy with its unpredictable, episodic and varied manifestations has been shrouded in mysticism and superstition since the ancient times. The ancient Ayurvedic system of medicine classifies epilepsies into 6 types and is believed to be caused by the vitiation and imbalance of bodily humors. Management is holistic and includes a strict dietary regimen, change in life style to follow the middle path and medication to restore the balance of humors. "Apasmara (epilepsy) bahu gorun' expresses the grotesque nature of the disorder in the charak samhita (circa 4th century BC)-the treatise on Ayurvedic medicine. Other Indian systems of medicine are also practiced. Epilepsy is thought to be due to supernatural forces, effects of ancestral spirits or bad spirits. It is also thought to be due to witchcraft, poisoning and/or contagious. Exorcism to drive away the evil spirits, incantations and herbal remedies are practiced for epilepsy control in various parts of India[5]. This socio-cultural environment leads to an important treatment gap. Closures of this situation remain a high priority. Important aspects to consider are: literacy, cultural beliefs, distance from modern health care facilities and completing threats to the health of the community. It has been shown that primary health care workers can achieve a reasonable level of seizure treatment, however, given the objection to vertical programs, sufficient back-up for the primary health care workers should be available in order to give epilepsy care its proper place among their many other duties.

The Indian Epilepsy Association, Bangalore chapter joined hands with the Karuna Trust in Yelandur in 1990 to study epilepsy in the area. Yelandur is a taluk in south Karnataka, the abode of the tribals called Soligas. The people in the plains are of India-Aryan-Dravidian stock, while the soligas have Negroid characteristics. The tribals grow millet, but live mainly on jungle produce. Of the total population, 64963 persons were surveyed. The prevalence for epilepsy was 5.97/thousand. Sridharan and Murthy carried metaanalysis of the prevalence of epilepsy in India. They estimated a general prevalence rate of 5.59 with urban areas at 6.34 and rural areas at 4.94.

In the Yelandur series 1051 seizure suspects were seen in one year (April 1990 to March 1991). Some of them residing in neighboring taluks. On perusal it was seen that 62 cases did not have a seizure phenomena e.g. Breath holding attacks, syncope, mental retardation, vertigo, neurosis, psychosis, tremors tics etc. 421 of 989 (42.6%) had seizures but not epilepsy, 355 had febrile seizures, 28 pseudoseizures; 20 single seizure, while eclampsia 8 acute symptomatic seizures and 1 had alcohol abuse. The remaining 568 (54%) were suffering from genuine epilepsy.

Out of 568 who had genuine epilepsy 239 subjects refused long term treatment, either because they did not consider – their illness a disability or because they were willing to accept treatment only if a quick cure was promised. A total of 157 patients accepted treatment with antiepileptic drugs supplied free (Phenobarbitone/Phenytoin)[6].

The Yelandur model teaches us that with the existing resources epilepsy can be controlled to a large extent by peripheral decentralized care from trained primary care physicians and para medical workers.

A knowledge attitude Practice (KAP) survey of 372 patients or relatives was also conducted. This showed that 76 per cent of people surveyed knew about epilepsy, only 9 per cent could relate it to the brain. Regarding modern drugs 72 per cent felt they could cure the illness, and 66 per cent had tried such medicines in the past but seldom on a long term basis and without any benefits. Rejection by family, society or both was reported by only 20 per cent patients. Poor rural families look after relatives with epilepsy as best as they can, just as they care for those with mental retardation, leprosy, stroke or dementia. The treatment gap in this community-based study was 78 per cent.

The Global Campaign Against Epilepsy (GCAE) is a joint program of the WHO, the International League Against Epilepsy (ILAE) and the International Bureau of Epilepsy (IBE). The campaign was launched in 1997 to bring epilepsy 'out of the shadows'. Its mission statement is 'to improve the acceptability of treatment services and prevention of epilepsy in people with epilepsy, and to diminish the treatment gap in the developing regions of the world[7].

The GCAE provides a platform for general awareness and assist department of health in developing National Epilepsy Programmes. The concept of Regional Declarations on Epilepsy has been elaborated with the goal of identifying problems and proposing solutions for ministries of health and other health care organizations.

In 1999, WHO raised the GCAE to cabinet level, waking it one of its highest priority projects. Every regional office of WHO has pledged to commit personnel and resources to this campaign.

The GCAE has demonstration projects that have been designed to identify people with epilepsy and offer them appropriate treatment. The specific objectives are: to develop a model for promotion of epilepsy control world-wide, to reduce the treatment gap, to reduce the social and physical burden: stigma: to prevent epilepsy determined causes and to integrate epilepsy care in national health systems.

The effort has to be multi –disciplinary and multi-dimensional conducted by trained health and social workers, educated patients and families, communicators, community and opinion leaders, with the support of GCAE, bilateral and multilateral co-operation, international institutions and NGOs and pharmaceutical companies. Then this campaign can bring 'epilepsy, out of the shadows'[8].

It must be appreciated that more and more attention is now being paid to the problem of tribal health. The health problems of the tribals should be co-ordinated between medical doctors, social scientists, NGO's, etc. The need is to combine modern medicine with the traditional method of treatment. Many other field experiences emphasize also that working in close connection with traditional healers would give the primary health care worker a better opportunity to gain acceptance from the community and modify certain harmful practices.

## REFERENCES

1. S.C. Tiwari, (1994) *Socio-cultural and Genetico-environmental determinants of tribal health: measures for health development*—"Tribal Health in India": edited by Salil Basu; pp. 285-94.
2. Ishwar C Verma, (1994) *Medico-Genetic Problems of Tribal Communities—A challenge for Indian Scientist*—"Tribal Health in India": edited by Salil Basu; pp. 260-67.
3. Saraswati Swain, (1994) *Health Disease and Health Seeking behaviour of Tribal People of India*—"Tribal Health in India": edited by Salil Basu; pp. 13-25.
4. S.K. Das and K. Sanyal (1996) *Neuroepidemiology of Major neurological disorders in rural Bengal*—"Neurology India" 44; pp. 47-58.
5. Krishnamoorthy Srinivas, N. Subbulakshmy, (200) *History of Epilepsy- "Epilepsy in India"*—edited by B.S. Singhal & Devika Nag; pp. 2-6.
6. K.S. Mani, Geeta Rangan, (2000) *The Yelandur Model for Rural Epilepsy control in India*—"Epilepsy in India" pp. 16-31.
7. "Epilepsy out of the shadows". WHO, 2001.
8. Rajendra Kale-Bringing epilepsy out of the shadows. *BMJ* volume 315, 2-3.

# 2

# Mental Health Issues of Tribes

R.K. CHADDA

## Introduction

The word tribe refers to a group of people of the same race and sharing the same language, religion and customs, and often led by a chief (Oxford Advanced Learner's Dictionary). They have strong ethnocentric feelings but do not have social stratification and occupational specialization, and in social life have very strong kinship bondage. The tribal population forms a significant part of our country's population. Their social needs have often been neglected by the mainstream society. The health facilities are also often primitive in the tribal areas. The present paper focuses on the mental health aspects of the Indian tribals.

## Tribal Population in India

As per the 1991 census of India, there are 573 tribes in India with a population of 67.76 million (excluding the state of Jammu & Kashmir). They form 8.08 per cent of the total population of the country. The tribal areas of India can be broadly divided in six distinct regions: Central region, Western region, North-Eastern region, North-Western region, Southern region and the Island region. The largest concentration of the tribal population is in the middle of India (the states of Jharkhand and Chattisgarh specifically) and the north eastern states. Some of them are also living in the remotely located islands of Lakshadeep and Andaman & Nicobar. The Government of India has identified 74 primitive tribal communities in 15 states and union territories.

Most of the tribal groups in the country depend largely on agriculture and forests for their livelihood, speak a variety of languages and dialects, and have distinct socio-cultural characteristics. A number of them are landless labourers and marginal farmers. Most are economically weak, backward in education and are often not much concerned with sanitation and hygiene as per the general country standards, thus exposing them to a variety of health problems and not many resources to deal with them. However, the individual groups are mostly homogeneous, culturally firm, have strongly inbuilt magico-religious health care systems, and often like to survive and live in their own life-style. Many of them do not have reasonable access to the modern health facilities, and even where available these are not optimally utilized.

## Health Status of Tribes

General health status of the tribal is poor as compared to the modern society. They may suffer from some distinct health problems, not because they have some specific type of health, but because of specific placement in difficult areas and circumstances, in which they live. Because of the widely varying geo-climatic and ecological conditions, the different tribal societies depending on their uniqueness may have some specific health issues and problems of their own.

Widespread poverty, illiteracy, malnutrition, non-availability of safe drinking water and sanitary living conditions, poor maternal and child health services, ineffective coverage of national health programmes and consanguineous marriages have been found to affect the health status of the tribal adversely and also responsible for some of the specific illnesses including genetic disorders. Unfortunately, proper health services are not available in many of the tribal areas. Understandably, the common beliefs, customs and practices connected with health and disease influence their choice of treatment methods. The inadequate nature of facilities in many tribal areas, lack of respect in the staff manning these facilities for the indigenous culture and further inadequate attention towards these patients is often responsible for the non-acceptance and distrust of the tribal towards the modern medicine.

The gradual encroachment by the modern society on the natural resources of the tribal and depleting them of their habitat and exposing them to the apparently alien modern acculturation is a continuing stress, which could result in a variety of psychiatric problems.

## Tribal Perception of Etiology

The concept of health, disease, treatment, life and death among the tribes is as varied as their culture. The tribal society is often guided by the traditionally laid down customs, to which every member of the society is expected to conform. As per their beliefs, often the fate of the individual and the community depends on their relationship with the unseen forces, which intervene in human affairs. If someone offends them, the mystical powers punish the person and the society by causing sickness, death, or other natural calamities. There are gods for health, disease and calamities. They worship these deities to protect them from evil spirits, disease and epidemics (Sinha, 1996). Broadly speaking, the tribal believe in four types of spirits: (i) protective deities or spirits, believed to safeguard the welfare of the village and worshipped at community level, (ii) benevolent spirits, which are worshipped at the family and community level regularly, otherwise these might bring disease and other calamities, (iii) evil or malevolent spirits and deities controlling small pox, fever, abortion, etc., (iv) ancestral spirits, which are very benevolent spirits and protect the family members.

In the tribal society, disease is often perceived to be caused by breach of some taboo or rules of the society, or by the hostile spirits, the ghosts of the dead. There is a belief in both benevolent and malevolent spirits, the former playing a protective role, while the latter are considered to be responsible for causing disease and epidemics. Besides the belief in spirits, different tribe also believe in a number of other causes for various illnesses like imbalance of the three humours (*doshas*) of the body, lack of harmony with the supernatural world, activities of the ghosts, especially the unwanted and aggrieved ghosts, displeasure of deities, faulty diet, and immoderation or inappropriate behaviour in physical, social or economic matters.

The tribal are staunch believers in the natural history of diseases. As per the belief, the human life is governed by the sun, rain, wind and other elements, and when man falls out of harmony with nature, he becomes susceptible to disease and accidents. The treatment lies in correcting these influences by various magico-religious methods.

## Some Examples of Magico-Religious Practices

In the Santal tribe of Orissa, Bihar and West Bengal, one of the largest tribes in India, having an estimated population of more than 4.2 million, Thakurji is the supreme deity, which ultimately controls the entire universe. The weight of belief, however, falls on a court of spirits (*bonga*), who handle different aspects of the world and who must be placated with prayers and offerings in order to ward off evil influences. These spirits operate at the village, household, ancestor, and subclan level, along with evil spirits that cause disease, and can inhabit village boundaries, mountains, water, tigers, and the forest. A characteristic feature of the Santal village is a sacred grove on the edge of the settlement where many spirits live and where a series of annual festivals take place.

The most important spirit is Maran Buru (Great Mountain), who is invoked whenever offerings are made and who instructed the first Santals in sex and brewing of rice beer. Maran Buru's consort is the benevolent Jaher Era (Lady of the Grove).

A yearly round of rituals connected with the agricultural cycle, along with lifecycle rituals for birth, marriage and burial at death, involves petitions to the spirits and offerings that include the sacrifice of animals, usually birds. Religious leaders are male specialists in medical cures who practice divination and witchcraft. Similar beliefs are common among other tribes of north-east and central India such as the Kharia, Munda and Oraon.

## Mental Health Problems in Tribes

With a reasonably huge tribal population of about 68 million (should be quite more now), the Indian tribal religious concepts, terminologies, and practices are as varied as the hundreds of tribes. However, all of them are under constant pressure from the major organized religions, the outside missionaries working among tribal groups to gain converts, and from the process of integration into the national political and economic system that brings tribes into increasing contact with other groups and the various prestigious belief systems. In general, the tribes, which are geographically isolated in desert, hills, and forest regions or on islands, may be able to retain their traditional cultures and religions longer. In fact, those tribes, which apparently are in the process of the transition from hunting and gathering to sedentary agriculture, usually as low-status labourers, find their ancient religious forms in decay and their places filled by practices of Hinduism, Islam, Christianity, or Buddhism, and thus face constant psychosocial stress as a result of this changing identification.

The tribal are not immune to psychiatric illness, as once believed because of their being away from the stresses of the modern society. The mental illness can affect anyone, since the general stresses of the life would be faced by any society or culture. In case of the tribal, the additional continuing stress of being considered an odd or alien community in a rapidly changing modern society which is also encroaching upon one's habitat along with the general stresses of day-to-day life associated with various developmental, constitutional and genetic factors would make a tribal more prone to a psychiatric illness.

There has not been much investigation into the mental health problems of the Indian tribal. Carstairs (1958) was one of the earliest psychiatrists to have shown interest in psychiatric problems in his epidemiological studies in the rural areas of Rajasthan. Later, Carstairs and Kapur (1976), Nandi *et al.* (1977, 1980) have done some pioneering work on the area.

Nandi *et al.* (1980), in his extensive work, found a prevalence rate of 20 per 1000 of psychiatric disorders in two tribal communities (Munda and Lodha) in 28 villages scattered over two districts of the state of West Bengal. In this study, 2,363 subjects were assessed, who belonged to 506 families. Two more community groups, Brahmins and Scheduled Castes were also assessed in the study. The prevalence of psychiatric morbidity was higher in both the Brahmins (11%) and the Scheduled Castes (7%), as compared to the tribal population (2%). In the tribal, depression was the commonest psychiatric illness with a prevalence of 11.0 per 1000 followed by hysteria (3.0 per 1000), phobia (2.1 per 1000), schizophrenia (1.3 per 1000) and mania (0.4 per 1000). The study also found epilepsy and mental sub-normality in 2.5 and 4.7 per 1000 of the population respectively. Of the various tribal families, 11 per cent had one or more affected members. Depression was the commonest psychiatric illness in all the three community groups studied, and was twice more common in females than in males in tribal population and the Brahmins, the difference not significant in the Scheduled Castes.

Interestingly, anxiety states (generalised anxiety disorder and panic disorder) and obsessions were not seen in the tribal populations. Similarly, no cases of culture bound syndrome were found. In fact in one of the earlier studies on tribal population in Ghana, Field (1960) also did not find any cases of obsessions. Probably, the diseases of superego conflict (obsessions) are likely to be rare in the tribal culture (Wintrob & Wittkower, 1966). In the study by Nandi *et al.* (1980), obsessions were common in the Brahmin community, more so in women, a community which has a traditionally high moral and ethical standard, ingrained in the personality structure of its members. Though the total prevalence of psychiatric morbidity in the tribal community was lower than that in the Scheduled Castes and the Brahmins, prevalence of schizophrenia in the tribal was not much different from that in Scheduled Castes (1.3 and 1.7 per 1000 respectively). The figure was much higher at 7.2 per 1000 in the Brahmins.

As regards to the socio-economic status, the prevalence of psychiatric morbidity including psychotic disorders was higher in the upper socio-economic class. The socio-economic factors like better farm power, better housing and occupation were associated with higher mental morbidity.

The two tribes studied by Nandi *et al.* (1980), though quite distinct in their ethnicity, had many things in common in their cultural pattern. Social stratification and occupational specialization were yet to develop in them. The two tribes are known to have strong ethnocentric feeling and kinship bondage. Other commonalities included those in material and social heritage, general attitudes, values of life and group behaviour.

## Indigenous Health Practices among the Indian Tribal

The modern system of medicine has not made many roads in the Indian tribal population. Carstairs (1955) has pointed out that allopathic medicine does not fit in the social system of the villagers. The villagers expect to pay only after they are cured and feel that why a doctor immediately asks for fees are like a tradesman or shopkeeper. They do not understand why the doctor asks them so many questions as the traditional practitioners tell them what is wrong without asking any details.

Magico-religious practices are frequently resorted to for treatment of various diseases. There are also a number of indigenous practices, which incorporate considerable amount of practical know-how, derived over centuries of experience in the use of herbs and other substances to cure variety of illnesses. The tribal have hit upon some herbs in someway or other and come to know of its efficacy. Use of herbs is guided by this randomly or formally gained experience. The knowledge is often passed from one generation to the next. There was no documentation of such experience till recent past, but in recent years some herbs have been identified with treatment of specific illnesses. The choice of herbs and treatment depends according to availability of plants in the neighbouring surroundings. Some of these have also efficacy against psychiatric illnesses.

Some of the common herbs found to have efficacy against psychiatric symptoms and used by the tribal in different parts of the country include *Anatamul* (plant), *Aswagandha* (plant), *Sarpagandha* (plant), *Bigchanda* (plant), *Thankumi* (herb) (Narayan, 1986). The plant of *Anatamul* is used for treatment of nerve troubles, neuralgia, sciatica and paralysis. *Aswagandha* has efficacy against sexual weakness and is also an important component of many Ayurvedic drugs. *Sarpagandha* is another herb with established efficacy against psychosis as well as tension. It also reduces blood pressure. The plant of *Bigchanda* has also antipsychotic properties. *Thankumi* is another plant, which is used as a brain tonic and also having efficacy against dysentery, leprosy and skin diseases.

## Conclusion

The mental health issues in the Indian tribal have not been investigated much and only preliminary information is available about the prevalence of psychiatric morbidity in them. The nature of illnesses doesn't appear much different from the general population as per the available evidence. The tribal frequently resort to various magico—religious methods and some indigenous herbs for the psychiatric problems.

## REFERENCES

Carstairs, G.M. (1955): Medicine and faith in rural Rajasthan, In *Health, Culture and Community* (Eds. BD Paul). Russel Sage Foundation: New York, pp. 107-34.

——(1958): *Some problems of psychiatry in patients form alien cultures*. Lancet, i, 1217.

Carstairs, G.M. and Kapur, R.L. (1976): *The Great Universe of Kota—Stress, Change and Mental Disorders in an Indian Village*, London: The Hogarth Press.

Field, M.J. (1960): *Search for Security: An ethno-psychiatric Study of Rural Ghana*, Evansion: North Western University

Nandi, D.N., Mukherjee, S.P., Boral, G.C., Banerjee, G., Ghosh, A., Ajmany, S., Sarkar, S. and Biswas, D. (1977): Prevalence of psychiatric morbidity in two tribal communities in certain villages of West Bengal—A cross cultural study, *Indian Journal of Psychiatry*, 19, pp. 2-12.

Nandi, D.N., Mukherjee, S.P., Boral, G.C., Banerjee, G., Ghosh, A., Sarkar, S. and Ajmany, S. (1980): Socio-economic status and mental morbidity in certain tribes and castes in India—A cross cultural study, *British Journal of Psychiatry*, 136, pp. 73-75

Narayan, S. (1986): *Health, Forestry and Development. In Tribal Health-Sociocultural Dimensions* (ed) Inter-India Publications: New Delhi.

Sinha, U.P. (1996): Traditional tribal medicine and modern health care system. In *Tribal Health in India* (Eds), pp. 151-62.

Wintrob, R., and Wittkower, E.D. (1966): Magic and witchcraft in Liberia: Their psychiatric implications. *Transcultural Psychiatric Research Review*. 3, p. 149.

# 3

# Tribal Health in India: Perspectives in Medical Anthropology

GAUTAM KUMAR KSHATRIYA

## Introduction

The tribal populations of India are the indigenous groups. They form about 8.08 per cent of the total population. About 67.5 million persons have been enumerated in the country as being members of Scheduled Tribes. There are about 162 major tribes and 270 minor tribal communities. The tribal populations of India inhabit widely varying ecological and geo-climatic conditions (hilly, forest, desert, coastal regions) in different concentration with different socio-economic background. Tribal groups are homogeneous, culturally firm having developed strong magico-religious health care system of their own and they live and survive in their own style. Due to remoteness and isolation many tribal population are out-reach groups.

Scheduled Tribes constitute an overwhelming majority in Mizoram (94.75%), Lakshadweep (93.15%), Nagaland (87.70%), and Meghalaya (85.53%). Even though the tribal populations constitute a majority in these states/Union Territories, their contribution to the total tribal population is fragmentary. The states of Madhya Pradesh, Maharasthra, Gujarat, Rajasthan, Orissa, Bihar, West Bengal and Andhra Pradesh, however, account for by 83 per cent of the total tribal population of India, despite the fact that the numerical strength of non-tribal population in these states exceeds tribal population. The Census of India (1991) enumerates 573 notified Scheduled Tribes in India. Out of these 573 tribal groups, Government of India has identified 74 primitive tribal communities for taking up special development programmes. Criteria adopted for identification of primitive tribal groups are (a) pre-agricultural level of technology and economy largely based on hunting and food gathering (b) extremely low literacy, (c) small, stagnant and diminishing population. Incidentally both Andhra Pradesh and Orissa possess maximum number (12 each) of primitive tribal groups.

Among all the states and Union Territories both Andhra Pradesh (12) and Orissa (12) are found to posses of maximum number of tribal groups, followed by Bihar (9), Madhya Pradesh (7), Tamil Nadu (6), Gujarat (5), Kerala (5), Andaman and Nicobar Islands (5), Maharasthra (3), West Bengal (3), Karnataka (2), Uttar Pradesh (2), Rajasthan (1), Manipur (1) and Tripura (1). The figures in parenthesis represent number of primitive tribal groups (Working Group Report of Ministry of Welfare of ST, 1989).

## Sub-division of Indian Tribes

Depending upon the geographical location, Indian region can be sub-divided into seven distinct regions where the tribal population is largely concentrated. These are: (a) North Eastern Region comprising Arunachal Pradesh, Assam, Manipur, Meghalaya, Mizoram, Nagaland, Sikkim and Tripura, (b) Eastern region comprising West Bengal, Bihar and Orissa, (c) Northern region comprising Jammu and Kashmir, Himachal Pradesh, Uttar Pradesh and Rajasthan, (d) Central Region comprising Madhya Pradesh, (e) Western Region comprising Gujarat, Maharashtra, Dadar and Nagar Haveli, Goa, Daman and Diu, (f) Southern Region comprising Karnataka, Kerala, Tamil Nadu and Andhra Pradesh, and (g) Island Region comprising Andaman and Nicobar Islands and Lakshadweep.

## Ethno-demographic Characteristics

The tribal communities of India differ considerably from one another in race, language, culture and beliefs, in their myths and customs, and present a spectacle of striking diversity. There is bewildering variation in population size of the individual Scheduled Tribes, ranging from 31 Jarwas of Andaman and Nicobar islands to more than 7 million Bhils of Rajasthan, Madhya Pradesh, Maharasthra, and Gujarat (1981 census). Notwithstanding so much diversity, there are certain broad similarities between the mutually divergent tribal groups. Striking similarities are noticed in their mode of living. Each tribe lives in a definite area, has common dialect, cultural homogeneity and unifying social organization. It is worthwhile to look at various demographic indicators among Indian tribes, which are presented in Table 3.1.

**Sex Ratio**

It has been found to vary from tribe to tribe and from region to region. It varies from a low of 744 females per thousand male in Sherpas of Sikkim to a high of 1098 females per thousand males in Dudh Kharias of Orissa. Sex ratio may reflect favourable and unfavourable social and cultural condition against women. Most of the tribal population groups reveal a sex ratio much below the sex ratio of Indian National Population of 933.

***Crude Birth Rate (CBR) and Crude Death Rate (CDR)***

It is evident from Table 2.1 that CBR shows considerable heterogeneity among different tribal groups. CBR varies from a minimum of 22 in Bhutias of Sikkim to a maximum of 75 in Soliga of Karnata. CBR is invariably above 30 in most of the tribal groups in India.

Data on CDR on individual tribe is far from satisfactory. Only few studies have been reported and it can be seen from Table 2.1, that CDR varies from a minimum of 9 in Hill Korwas to a maximum of 25 in Oraons of Bihar. Data reflect a large range in CDR. This could be due to investigations being carried out in different years and in different geo-climatic tribal habitat and also due to inadequate systematic, well designed study. Nevertheless, a very low rate of rural tribal female literacy could be one of the major attributable factors for a high CBR and CDR in all the tribal populations besides other social, cultural, economical and technological factors.

**Total Fertility Rate (TFR) and General Fertility Rate (GFR)**

It is heartening to state that not many tribal population groups are investigated for basic demographic indicators like TFR and GFR.

Fertility rates give a variable picture among the Indian tribes. TFR varies from 3.14 among Mirdhas of Orissa to 6.16 among Soligas of Karnataka. TFR among various tribal groups is quite high in comparison to 3.8 for Indian National Population. Similarly, GFR varies from a minimum of 125 among Jaunsaris to a maximum of 188 among Soligas of Karnataka. In other words, tribal population of India, in general, reveal high fertility.

## Infant Mortality Rate (IMR)

It is unfortunate that IMRs for individual tribes are not readily available. It is a very sensitive indicator of overall health culture and health behaviour of a tribe. There are many factors that determine IMR like low birth weight, women's literacy, poor hygiene, poor sanitation, poverty, crowding due to high fertility, available and utilization of health services, the status of women in the society and many more.

Data on IMR were not comparable because these studies were conducted in different years. It is also seen that tribal populations living in the same habitat show tremendous variability in IMR, *e.g.* in Bastar it varies from 85 in Madias to 148 in Bhattras.

By and large IMR among Indian tribes varies from a minimum of 65/1000 live births among Sherpas to a maximum of 239/1000 live births among Gadabas of Andhra Pradesh. Mean IMR among Indian tribes was estimated to be 120.3 which is alarmingly higher than 65 for Indian National Population at this time. Although infections diseases account for the bulk of IMR, but the role of genetic and genetico-environmental disorders becomes equally important because their frequency is quite high in Indian tribal groups.

Available data do not allow any conclusion regarding the contribution of genetic and environmental factors in IMR among the Indian tribal groups. It is, therefore, necessary in view of a great inter-tribal difference in IMR, to conduct well designed systematic studies at micro level among different tribal groups so as to understand the magnitude of the IMR in proper perspective.

## Reproductive Wastage

Invariably, data on abortion and stillbirth are under-reported. One of the reasons could be their inability to share such sensitive information with the field workers who often stay there for a short period. Since most of the field workers are non-clinicians, it becomes difficult to persuade the tribal people regarding the rationale of seeking such information. It takes time before people are convinced about the purpose

**Table 3.1:** Demographic indicators among different tribal groups of India

| *Sl. No.* | *Particulars* | *Crude Birth Rate (CBR)* | *Crude Death Rate (CDR)* | *Sex Ratio* | *Total Fertility Rate (TFR)* | *General Fertility Rate (GFR)* | *Infant Mortality Rate (IMR)* | *Authors* |
|---|---|---|---|---|---|---|---|---|
| **1.** | **North India** | | | | | | | |
| | *Jammu and Kashmir* (Western Himalayas) | | | | | | | |
| | 1. Bodhs | 24.46 | 14.32 | 956 | 2.79 | 95.79 | 97.56 | Bhasin & Nag (1990) |
| | 2. Baltis | 23.57 | 16.84 | 961 | 3.12 | 98.59 | 163.26 | Bhasin & Nag (1990). |
| | 3. Brokpas | 27.17 | 21.74 | 947 | 3.09 | 119.05 | 200 | Bhasin & Nag (1990) |
| | *Himachal Pradesh* (Western Himalayas) | | | | | | | |
| | 4. Bods (High Altitude) | – | – | – | 4.11 | – | – | Prakash & Malik (1990) |
| | 5. Bods (Low Altitude) | – | – | – | 3.63 | – | – | Prakash & Malik (1990) |
| | 6. Gaddis (Middle Altitude) | 28.4 | 14 | 870 | 3.47 | 110.5 | 170.1 | Bhasin & Bhasin (1993) |
| | 7. Kinnauras | 21.06 | 10.0 | 1006 | 2.91 | 162 | 74.1 | Kshatriya (2004) |
| | *Uttar Pradesh* (Central Himalayas) | | | | | | | |
| | 8. Bhoksa | – | – | – | 6.45 | – | – | Garg *et al.* (1980) |
| | 9. Jaunsari | 32 | 11.8 | 889 | 3.84 | 125 | 81 | Kashtriya *et al.* (1997) |
| | 10. Buksa | – | – | – | 5.7 | – | – | Saxena (1990) |
| | *Rajastham* | | | | | | | |
| | 11. Bhils | – | 16.61 | – | – | – | – | Parsuram & Rajan (1990) |

(*Contd.*)

Table 3.1 (*Contd.*)

| Sl. No. | Particulars | Crude Birth Rate (CBR) | Crude Death Rate (CDR) | Sex Ratio | Total Fertility Rate (TFR) | General Fertility Rate (GFR) | Infant Mortality Rate (IMR) | Authors |
|---|---|---|---|---|---|---|---|---|
| **2.** | **West India** | | | | | | | |
| | *Maharashtra* | | | | | | | |
| | 12. Gonds | 44 | 22.97 | – | – | – | – | Parsuram & Rajan (1990) |
| | 13. Bhils | – | 20.09 | – | – | – | – | Parsuram & Rajan (1990) |
| | *Gujarat* | | | | | | | |
| | 14. Bhils | – | 23.09 | – | – | – | – | Parsuram & Rajan (1990) |
| | 15. Dhodia | 24.5 | 7.8 | 962 | 3.89 | 123 | 72 | Kshatriya (2004) |
| | *Rajasthan* | | | | | | | |
| | 16. Bhils | 34.05 | 9.22 | 904 | 5.7 | 193 | 93.9 | Kshatriya (2004) |
| **3.** | **East India** | | | | | | | |
| | *Sikkim* (Easter Himalayas) | | | | | | | |
| | 17. Bhutias | 22.22 | – | 996 | 3.15 | 93.22 | – | Bhasin & Bhasin (1995) |
| | 18. Lepchas | 20.87 | – | 849 | 3.07 | 92.19 | – | Bhasin & Bhasin (1995) |
| | 19. Sherpas | 19.61 | – | 744 | 3.01 | 90.91 | – | Bhasin & Bhasin (1995) |
| | 20. Bhutia (Lachen) | – | – | – | 4.6 | – | 76.3 | Das *et al.* (1982) |
| | 21. Bhutia (Lachen) | – | – | – | 3.79 | – | 220.34 | Das *et al.* (1982) |

(*Contd.*)

Table 3.1 (*Contd*)

| *Sl. No.* | *Particulars* | *Crude Birth Rate (CBR)* | *Crude Death Rate (CDR)* | *Sex Ratio* | *Total Fertility Rate (TFR)* | *General Fertility Rate (GFR)* | *Infant Mortality Rate (IMR)* | *Authors* |
|---|---|---|---|---|---|---|---|---|
| | *West Bengal* | | | | | | | |
| 22. | Santal | 37.2 | 10.9 | 913 | 5.5 | 168 | 94.8 | Sumana (1999) |
| 23. | Lodha | 31.2 | 11.8 | 902 | 3.3 | 133.3 | 99.2 | Sumana (1999) |
| 24. | Santal | 3.3 | 1.8 | 847 | 4.8 | – | 117 | Kshatriya (1999) |
| 25. | Sherpa | – | – | – | 4.53 | – | 65.8 | Gupta (1980)* |
| 26. | Sherpa | – | – | – | 7.44 | – | 72.1 | Gupta (1980)* |
| 27. | Kora | 41.81 | – | – | 4.2 | – | – | Datta (1990) |
| 28. | Oraon | – | – | 968.5 | | | | |
| 29. | Pahira | – | – | – | 4.97 | – | – | Basu (1967) |
| 30. | Toto | – | – | – | 7.63 | – | – | Dabnath & Sen (1983) |
| 31. | Lepcha | – | – | – | 7 | – | – | Mukhopadhyay (1982) |
| | *Meghalaya* (Eastern Himalayas) | | | | | | | |
| 32. | Pnar | – | – | – | – | – | 119.2 | Khongsdier (1992) |
| 33. | Hajong | – | – | – | – | – | 182 | Barua (1982) |
| 34. | Jaintias | – | – | – | – | – | 126.3 | Deka (1978)* |
| | *Nagaland* (Eastern Himalayas) | | | | | | | |
| 35. | Zemi | – | – | – | – | – | 86.1 | Bhomick *et al.* (1971)* |
| | *Orissa* | | | | | | | |
| 36. | Santal | 3.6 | 13 | 1019 | 4.6 | – | 127 | Kshatriya (1999) |
| 37. | Konds | – | – | – | 3.6 | – | 105.5 | Sharma (1979) |

(*Contd.*)

Table 3.1 (*Contd.*)

| Sl. No. | Particulars | Crude Birth Rate (CBR) | Crude Death Rate (CDR) | Sex Ratio | Total Fertility Rate (TFR) | General Fertility Rate (GFR) | Infant Mortality Rate (IMR) | Authors |
|---|---|---|---|---|---|---|---|---|
| 38. | Kutia Konds | – | – | – | 5.03 | – | 179.7 | Chetlapalli et al. (1991) |
| 39. | Dudh Kharia | 38.5 | 11.8 | 1098 | 5.39 | 164 | 102.4 | Kshatriya & Basu (1987) |
| 40. | Desia Kondh | – | – | – | 3.89 | – | 151.28 | Chetlapalli et al. (1993) |
| 41. | Dongaria Kondh | – | – | – | 3.87 | – | 153.11 | Khan (1993) |
| 42. | Mirdha | – | – | – | 3.14 | – | 116 | Choudhary et al. (1994) |
| | *Assam* | | | | | | | |
| 43. | Garo | – | – | – | 3.7 | – | – | Majumder (Paul), 2003 |
| | *Bihar* | | | | | | | |
| 44. | Santhal (S.T.) | | | 1074.7 | | | | Singh et al., (1999) |
| 45. | Surias (S.T) | | | 1054.1 | | | | Singh et al., (1999) |
| 46. | Mals (S.T.) | | | 1015.7 | | | | Singh et al., (1999) |
| 47. | Kumarbhags (S.T.) | | | 1092.1 | | | | Singh et al., (1999) |
| **4.** | **Central India** | | | | | | | |
| | *Madhya Pradesh* | | | | | | | |
| 49. | Bhils | – | 15.53 | – | – | – | – | Parsuram & Rajan (1990) |
| 50. | Khairwar | – | – | – | 4.85 | – | – | Sharma & Khan (1990) |
| 51. | Hill Korwas | – | 9 | 954.4 | – | – | – | Pandey & Tiwari (1993) |
| 52. | Madia | – | – | – | 5.6 | – | – | Skhatirya et al. (1993) |
| 53. | Muria | – | – | – | 5.64 | – | 123.5 | Basu & Kshatirya (1989) |
| 54. | Madia | – | – | – | 6.00 | – | 85.4 | Basu & Kshatirya (1989) |
| 55. | Bhatira | – | – | – | 5.95 | – | 148.5 | Basu & Kshatirya (1989) |

(*Contd.*)

Table 3.1 (*Contd*)

| *Sl. No.* | *Particulars* | *Crude Birth Rate (CBR)* | *Crude Death Rate (CDR)* | *Sex Ratio* | *Total Fertility Rate (TFR)* | *General Fertility Rate (GFR)* | *Infant Mortality Rate (IMR)* | *Authors* |
|---|---|---|---|---|---|---|---|---|
| | 56. Halba | – | – | – | 5.89 | – | 92.7 | Basu & Kshatirya (1989) |
| | 57. Gonds | 43 | 23.19 | – | – | – | – | Parsuram & Rajan (1990) |
| | 59. Oraon | – | 25.88 | – | – | – | – | Parsuram & Rajan (1990) |
| | 60. Muria Gond | – | – | – | 5.1 | – | – | Saha (1981) |
| | 61. Bhil | 43.5 | – | – | – | – | – | Chaudhary & Kumar (1976) |
| **5.** | **South India** | | | | | | | |
| | *Tamil Nadu* | | | | | | | |
| | 62. Kota | – | – | – | 3.73 | – | – | Ghosh (1970) |
| | 63. Irula | – | – | – | 5.03 | – | – | Reddy (1985) |
| | *Karnataka* | | | | | | | |
| | 64. Soliga | 75 | – | – | 6.16 | 188 | – | Murthy (1987) |
| | *Andhra Pradesh* | | | | | | | |
| | 65. Yanadi | – | – | – | 4.1 | – | – | Gurumurthy (1986) |
| | 66. Pradhan | – | – | – | 6.18 | – | – | Murthy & Ramesh (1978) |
| | 67. Gond | – | – | – | 4.52 | – | – | Murthy & Ramesh (1978) |
| | 68. Savra | – | – | – | – | – | 213.23 | TRI Hyd. (1980)* |
| | 69. Jatapu | – | – | – | – | – | 102.04 | TRI Hyd. (1980)* |
| | 70. Gadaba | – | – | – | – | – | 239.43 | TRI Hyd. (1980)* |
| | 71. Mooka Dora | – | – | – | – | – | 88.88 | TRI Hyd. (1980)* |
| | 72. Konda Dora | – | – | – | – | – | 102.56 | TRI Hyd. (1980)* |
| | 73. Hill Kolams | – | – | – | 5.8 | – | 70.59 | Murthy & Ramesh (1978) |
| | 74. Manue Kolam | – | – | – | 5.51 | – | 68.00 | Murthy & Ramesh (1978) |
| | 75. Chenchu | – | – | – | 5.7 | – | – | Sirrajuddin & Basu (1984) |
| | **Scheduled Tribes** | – | – | – | 3.06 | – | 84.2 | NFHS–2, 1998–99 |

of such information. This is just one of the several observation about the practical difficulties in obtaining information on such vital issues.

Table 3.2 presents the available data regarding reproductive wastage among different tribal population. It is apparent that such data are available for few populations only. It can be seen that incidence of stillbirths varies from Zero to 16.76 per cent in Kulhaiya of Bihar.

**Table 3.2:** Reproductive Wastage Among the Tribal Populations (K.C. Malhotra, 1994)

| *Tribe* | *State* | *Still births* ('A') | *Abortion.* *f* ('A) | *Reference* |
|---|---|---|---|---|
| Savra | Andhra Pradesh | 0.67 | 1.96 | TRl, Hyd., 1980 |
| Jatapu | Andhra Pradesh | 0 | 0 | TRI, Hyd., 1980 |
| Gadaba | Andhra Pradesh | 2.04 | 0.95 | TRI, Hyd., 1980 |
| M.Dora | Andhra Pradesh | 1.18 | 0 | TRI, Hyd., 1980 |
| Konda Dora | Andhra Pradesh | 0 | 0 | TRI, Hyd., 1980 |
| Hill Kalam | Andhra Pradesh | 3.00 | 1.40 | Murty & Ramesh, 1985 |
| M. Kolam | Andhra Pradesh | 1.70 | 2.20 | Murty & Ramesh, 1985 |
| Mishings | Assam | 7.40 | 4.88 | ? |
| Zemi | Nagaland | 4.35 | 7.50 | Choudhuri *et al.* 1971 |
| Jaintias | Meghalaya | 0.44 | | Deka, 1978 |
| Hajong | Meghalaya | – | 3.1 | Barna, 1982 |
| Konds | Orissa | 2.17 | – | Sharma, 1979 |
| Bhils | Rajasthan | 0..39 | 1.30 | Sarkar, 1978 |
| Garasia | Rajasthan | 029 | 2.04 | Sarkar, 1978 |
| Kota | Tamil Nadu | 0.09 | 0.21 | Basu, 1972 |
| Muria | Madhya Pradesh | – | 2.5 | Basu and Kshatriya, 1989 |
| Bhattra | Madhya Pradesh | – | 0.2 | Basu and Kshatriya, 1989 |
| Muria | Madhya Pradesh | 0.05 | 0.05 | Saha, 1981 |
| Kisan | Bihar | 12.35 | 6.10 | Pandey *et al.*, 2000 |
| Kulhaiya | Bihar | 16.76 | 9.25 | Pandey *et al.*, 2000 |
| Oraon | Bihar | 14.95 | 7.33 | Pandey *et al.*, 2000 |

The frequency of abortion varies from Zero in few populations to 9.25 per cent in Kulhaiya of Bihar. There is considerable heterogeneity between tribal populations with respect to reproductive wastage (Malhotra, 1994).

## Life Expectancy

A general indicator of the health of girls and women is their life expectancy. The expectation of life is the average number of years remaining to be lived by those surviving to that age. The expectation of life at birth is the life table function most frequently used as an index of the level of mortality. It also represents a summarization of the whole series of mortality rates for all ages combined as weighted by the life table stationary population. In those countries where mortality is higher, and where infant and child mortality is particularly high, the maximum of the expectation of life comes at a more advanced age (4 or sometimes 5 years) and the child of 10 years of age has an expectation of life often close to that of the newborn infant (Rolland Pressat, 1973). The expectation of life is the index most often used when one wishes to summarize the risk of mortality in a country.

Basu and Kshatriya (1989) estimated life expectancy at birth for Bastar tribal groups which was found to be less than 45 years for Muria, Madia and Bhattara and Halbars. A similar trend was obtained by Chattllapali *et al.* (1991) for Kutia Kondhs of Phulbani and by Datta (1990) for Kora of Midnapore. Life expectancy of less than 58 years were obtained by Basu and Kshatirya (1993), Kshatriya *et al.* (1993 and 1997) for Dudh Kharias of Sundergarh, Madias of Dantewara and Jaunsaris of Jaunsar Bawar.

Recently, Kshatriya (2004) has given estimate of life expectancy of birth for Dhodias of Gujarat as 62 years, for Bhils of Rajasthan as 54 and Kinnauras of Himachal Pradesh as 59 years. So, there is a steady improvement in life expectancy at birth over the years among the tribal groups as well as among other demographic indicators.

### *Ethnic Affinities*

On the basis of racial features, Guha (1935) considers that the tribal populations of India belong to the three races, namely (a) The Proto-Australoids—dark skin colour, sunken nose and lower forehead. These feature's are found among the Gond (Madhya Pradesh), the Munda (Chotanagpur), the Ho (Bihar) etc. (b) the Mongoloids-light skin colour, head and face are broad, the nose bridge is very low and their eyes are slanting with a fold on the upper eyelid. These features are found among the Bhotiya (Central Himalayas), the Wanchu (Arunachal Pradesh), the Naga (Nagaland), The Khasi (Meghalaya) etc. (c) the Negrito-dark skin colour, round head, broad nose and frizzly hair. These features are found among the Kadar (Kerala), the Onge (Little Andaman), the Jarwa (Andaman islands) etc.

Nevertheless, many tribal population of North West and Western region also show Mediterranean affinities as well (Bhilmina, Mina, Patelia, Kolis, Rathwas etc).

### *Linguistic Affinities*

The tribal populations of India have been found to speak 105 different languages and 25 subsidiary languages indicating a great deal of variety (IGNOU, 1990). Indian tribal group in general speak languages belonging to four major families of languages, namely Austro-Asiatic, Tibeto-Chinese, Dravidian and Indo-European family (Vidhyarthi, 1983).

### Economic Conditions

The economic life of tribal populations is specific in nature and vary significantly. Many tribal populations of Eastern, Southern and Central India (Chola Naicken, Juang, Birhor, Kadar, Chenchu, Hill Khadia, Makadia) and the Andaman Islands are efficient food gatherers and hunters. There are many tribal populations of North Eastern, Central and Eastern region (Khasi, Naga, Kutia Kondha, Korwa, Saora, Hill Muria, etc.) who still practice shifting cultivation. There are settled agriculturists (Bhil, Mina, Santal, Munda, Oraon, Gond etc.) at par with other peasant communities in many parts of Madhya Pradesh, Gujarat, Rajasthan, Maharashtra, Bihar, West Bengal and Orissa. And, there are urban industrial workers as well (Behura, 1995). The differences between the tribal groups are alarming. On the one hand there are Jarwas with virtually no contact with the outside world, on the other hand there are tribal industrial workers in Ranchi, Jamshedpur, Bacheli (Baster), Raurkela, Bhilai, etc.

### Literacy

Tribal populations are predominantly rural (92.6%) and they maintain their distinct cultural identity despite living in isolation. However, they differ greatly in the present level of development. Despite increase in literacy rate in post independence period, they have a literacy rate of only 23.6 per cent as against 65 per cent for General Population. Ironically, the rural tribal females have the lowest literacy rate of 12.7 per cent of all the social groups in India.

There are about 78 tribal groups with zero level of literacy. Several large tribes like Bhil, Meena, Rathwa, Santal, Khond have less than 5 per cent rural female literacy rate. On the other hand, a few tribal groups, mainly Christian converts, have higher female literacy rate (Singh, 1997).

**Concept of Health and Perception of Disease**

Although the concept of well-being and the notion of the disease varies between different tribal groups, yet in tribal habitat, a person is usually considered to be afflicted with some diseases if he/she is incapable of doing the routine work which is usually being expected to be carried out by that individual in the society, i.e. incapacitation from work is the universal index of poor health. Thus the concept of ill health becomes a functional one and not clinical. This is precisely the reason that among many tribal groups, *e.g.* Kutia Kondha, Muria, Madia, Bhattra, Halba, Jaunsari, Santal, Lodha, Kharia, Bhil, Rathwa, Mina, Jatapu, Saora, Pando, Khairwar, Oraon, Munda, Kinnauras, Dhodias and among many others; symptoms such as pains and ache, weakness, scabies, prolonged cough, mild fever, wounds, etc. are not taken seriously as symptoms of disease.

A tribal in general, hardly makes a distinction in the magnitude of fever. However, within the limits of their own respective worldview, most of the tribal societies have definite means for identifying and classifying various kinds of ailments and diseases. It may be worth while to state that at least one component of health is universally seen among the tribal societies, and that is, committing or omitting certain acts, in other words a breach of trust is thought to bring upon some kind of affliction on the individual or a family as a whole. Measles, tuberculosis, diarrhoea, cholera are some such diseases where individual's action may cause some concern to the family, clan or the village. Interestingly, the causation of such diseases is independent of the sanitary condition of the community/individuals. The fate of the individuals and the community depends on their relationship with unseen forces, which intervene in human affairs. If human beings offend them, the mystical power punish by causing sickness, death or other natural calamities. The tribal people believe in the presence of benevolent and malevolent spirits, the former playing a protective role, while the latter are considered being responsible for causing disease and epidemics.

It is a common observation across the tribal culture that the ancestral spirits play important role in the prosperity and protection of the family. And they have to be properly honoured for otherwise they will bring wrath on family members. These spirits are believed to bring a state of physical, mental and social well-being to the members of the family. There are many spirits who are feared because of their power to afflict people by bringing a number of diseases. The role of spirits, ghosts and deities in the tribal life in the causation and treatment of diseases is so important that the local tribal people have to seek the help of traditional diviners, medicine men, sorcerers (Sirha, Gunia, Bhua, Jani, Bhopa, Ojha, Pujari etc.) for appeasing, controlling or driving away the disease causing agents. The frequency of worshiping or getting in touch with malevolent spirits is more common because of their immediate effect on day-to-day life. The author's experience in Bastar, Phulbani, Mayurbhanj, Sundergarh, Panchmahals, Purulia, Dumka, Dehradun, Gadchiroli, Barmer, Valsad, Kinnaur, and Udaipur indicates that the practice of offering through sacrifice for the health related purpose is very common among the tribal people.

According to Jay (1970) there were at least 100 shamanistic performances and various correlated sacrifices per year in the tribal village of Central India taking into account only family related rituals. Sacrifices are very common for driving away the malevolent spirits and for worshipping the benevolent spirits.

Among the Santal, there exists a scientific theory of disease, which is in line with the modern theory of infections caused by bacteria. According to them, a disease can be caused by 'Tijio' germs, which can be large or microscopic (Gupta, 1986). The germs enter and are embedded in different parts of the body and can cause leprosy or hydrophobia. The germs are often believed to be collected by witches in order to spread diseases. The Santals also believe that evil men through their magical powers intrude the body with stones, wood, pebbles which causes unbearable pain, the 'Ojha' sucks these out from the body through rituals, and people believe that 'Ojhas' are responsible for curing their pain. Similar beliefs are shared by other tribal groups like Malpharia, Saoras of Bihar and Barias, Tadvi and Nayaka of Gujarat. Kondha of Orissa believe that men, animals, birds, reptiles and plants co-exits in symbiotic relationship. Any disturbance in this relationship can bring disastrous outcome. The Hill Bhuiyan and Saora of Orissa associated diarrhoea and dysentery in the rainy season to the substitution of cereal diet by jackfruits and seeds.

## Maternal and Child Health Care

Nutritional anaemia is a major problem for women in India and more so in the rural and tribal belt. In developing countries, it is estimated that at least half of the non-pregnant and two-thirds of the pregnant women are anaemic (U.N., 1984). This is particularly serious in view of the fact that both rural and tribal women have heavy workload and anaemia has a profound effect on psychological and physical health. Anaemia lowers resistance to fatigue, affects working capacity under conditions of stress and increases susceptibility to other diseases.

The nutritional status of pregnant women directly influences their reproductive performance and the birth weight of their children. It is observed that among most of the tribal population groups, staple diet is rice or minor millets except Mompas of Assam who consume wheat also (Basu *et al.*, 1985). Studies carried out at National Institute of Nutrition (1971) and Planning Commission of India (Sixth Five Year Plan, Government of India) reported a high protein calories malnutrition along the rice eating belts.

Surveys on the nutritional deficiencies (Gopalan, 1971) among the tribals show a high incidence of goitre, angular stomatitis among the Mompas of Assma and Vit. A deficiency among the Onges. A high incidence of malnutrition was observed (Ali, 1980; Basu *et al.*, 1990; Mahapatra and Das, 1990) in some primitive tribal groups in Phulbani, Koraput and Sundergarh districts of Orissa and also among Bhil, Garasia of Rajasthan, Padar, Rabari and Charan of Gujarat and Bonda of Orissa (Haque, 1990). Studies of tribal communities in Orissa conducted by Ali (1992) have found that an ecological inbalance caused by rapid deforestation which resulted not only in depleting food resources, but in prolonged droughts, adding to hunger and starvation. Studies carried out by NIHFW among the Gond (Muria and Madia), Bhatra and Halba tribal groups of Bastar district, Madhya Pradesh showed varying degree of malnutrition among them (Basu *et al.*, 1989).

Consumption of milk or milk products are tabooed in pre-school tribal children because milking of cow is a taboo among most of the tribal population groups. Pulses, milk and milk products and other animal foods which were the main sources of protein were lacking in the diets of tribal women of Trivandrum district, Kerala (Prema and Thomas, 1992). Average calorie consumption was found to be below the recommended level for normal, pregnant as well as lactating women. Consumption of calcium (in the form of tapioca and fish) was noticed to be the highest in normal women whereas it was poorest in the lactating women. Similar deficits of calcium in the diets of pregnant and lactating tribal women of Western and Central India was reported by Gopaldas (1987). The intake of iron and vitamin A were found to be low. Detailed clinical examination of the Kannikar tribal women showed that anaemia (90%), vitamin A deficiency (30%) and niacin deficiency (10%) were prevalent among them (Prema and Thomas, 1992).

In a survey conducted in Abujmarias of Bastar district by RMRC Jabalpur, a very high incidence of rickets induced genuvalgum (65%) was reported. Anaemia was found to be very common and 40 per cent had severe anaemia with hemoglobin levels of 7 gm/dl. ICMR bulletin (1996) documents high prevalence of goitre and intestinal parasites in Baigas of Baigachak area of Mandla district of Madhya Pradesh (MP). RMRC Jabalpur reported incidence of Goitre as 11.6 per cent among Bharias children below 5 years in Patal Kot valley in Chindwara district of MP. In 1995-96, RMRC Jabalpur carried out a study of fluoride osteopathy with genuvalgum syndrome in few villages of Mandla district. In Tilaipani village, 52 per cent children below 15 years of age had severe genuvalgum of grade IV and 73 per cent had marked dental fluorosis. Study among the Pauri Bhuniyas of Orissa showed (Ali, 1992) that 52 women as against 17 men in a sample of 268 persons suffered from diseases related to malnutrition. As a result of deforestation, additional distance and less fertile soil, the availability of food for the tribal family is reduced. This has implications particularly for the housewife who is responsible for the provision and distribution of food. In cases of shortage, she may even deprive herself of food in order to feed the others. Studies in this connection have shown that tribals in general are undernourished. For example, a study has shown that over 55 per cent of Kondhs consume less than 2000 calories per day (Patel, 1985) and most of them as little as 1700 calories (Sharma, 1979) compared to the ICMR stipulated requirement of 2400 calories.

In one of the study in Bastar district (Basu and Kshatriya, 1989), it was observed that maternal and childcare was largely neglected. Expectant mothers to a large extent are not inoculated against tetanus. From the inception of pregnancy to its termination, no specific nutritious diet is consumed by women. The consumption of iron, calcium and vitamins during pregnancy is poor. More than 90 per cent of deliveries are conducted at home attended by elderly ladies of the household. Maternal mortality directly related to pregnancy and childbirth has been found to be appreciably high among the tribal populations of Bastar district. In addition, a lot of females suffer from ill health due to pregnancy and childbirth in the absence of well-defined concept of health consciousness.

The chief causes of maternal mortality were found to be unhygienic and primitive practices for parturition. For example, it was observed that among Kutia Kondhs (Basu *et al.*, 1990), the delivery was conducted by the mother herself in a half squatting position holding a rope tied down from the roof of the hut. This helped her in applying pressure to deliver the child.

## Morbidity

Among the morbid conditions, yaws, leprosy, tuberculosis and malaria have been found to be quite prevalent in tribal areas. Yaws is caused by Treponema pertenue and cases has been reported from (Bastar) Madhya Pradesh, Tripura and Maharashtra (NICD, 1993). Incidence of tuberculosis has been found to be increasing in tribal areas as the tribals are coming more in contact with other non-tribals. Poor nutritional status is also one of the contributory factors. This was specially time for the tribal groups of Himachal, Bihar, Gujarat and West Bengal (Kinnaura, Gaddis, Rathwas, Bhils, Munda, Oraon and Santal).

Incidence of leprosy has been reported in Scheduled Tribes of Bihar, Madhya Pradesh, Orissa, Uttar Pradesh and Tripura. Incidence of malaria is widespread in almost all the tribal areas. Tribals who constitute 8 per cent of the total population contribute 25 per cent of the total malaria cases in the country. About 50 per cent of the *P. Falciparum* cases reported in India come from tribal population. Malaria is a major health problem in most of the tribal areas. Malaria control in tribal dominated forest areas is posing a difficult task due to technical and operational problems. Besides, a large number of cases of unspecified fever, URTI, UTI, accidental deaths, burn cases, diarrhoea, dysentery, skin diseases, diseases of oral cavities, etc. occur from time to time.

In certain tribal communities, STDs were found to be significantly high. In Jaunsaris of Chakrata Tehsil of Dehradun district, 17.12 per cent of polyandrous Jaunsaris were VDRL +ve. In Santhals of Mayurbhanjh district, Orissa, 8.90 per cent cases were VDRL +ve. In morbidity study of Kondha tribe in Phulbani district, Orissa, Swain (1990) reported 10 per cent syphilis in Desia Kondhs. In Toda tribal population of Nilgiri hills, high incidence of sexually transmitted disease has been reported. Health and nutrition surveys conducted by RMRC Port Blair among Andamanese in 1976 and 1989 reported that Anamanese suffer from syphilis, tuberculosis and anaemia. Married males and females of reproductive age group of Kairwar tribe of Kusmi block of Sidhi district were found to have a very high incidence of syphilis (57% in males and 70% in females). The study was conducted to find out the causes for high incidence of infertility among Khairwars (ICMR Bulletin, 1996).

Very little information is available about the prevalence of non-communicable diseases in tribal population. Studies carried out by NIN (Rao *et al.*, 1986) among the tribals of Sarguja, Jhabua and Bastar districts of Madhya Pradesh showed high incidence (53.9%) of Goitre (enlarged thyroid gland) in tribals of Sarguja district. Eye conditions like cataract, corneal opacity etc. were found to be in high frequencies (20.3%) in Bastar district. Cases of dental caries (5.1%) were noted in Jhabua. A few instances of cardiovascular diseases like hypertension, valvular heart disease were clinically found in Jhabua, Sarguja and Bastar.

## Genetic Disorders and Malaria

There are two genetic disorders, namely sickle cell anaemia and G-6-PD red cell enzyme deficiency which have been found to occur in rather high frequencies in Scheduled Tribes and Scheduled Caste populations. Both male and females are equally affected in case of sickling whereas males are more affected than females in G-6-PD deficiency cases. Both these genetic disorders have profound health implications in terms of morbidity for the affected persons.

Several human genetic makers have been found to provide an advantage against the malarial parasite, i.e. reducing susceptibility of the red cells to invasion by malarial parasite and none so far has been implicated for increase in susceptibility (Sharma, 1985, Ghosh, 1984). The most widely investigated markers is sickle cell trait (Allison, 1954). It has been reported that sickle cell hemoglobin (HbS) provides protection from Plasmodium falciparum infestation. Correlation between hemoglobin S (HbS) and malaria was noted by Neel (1956), Lehman and Hunstman (1966), etc. The first report about advantage of hemoglobin S (HbS) gene for malaria on India sample was published on Mahars of Aurangabad (Sharma, *et al.*, 1974).

Another such characteristic genetic trait is Glucose-6-Phosphate dehydrogenase (G-6-PD) red cell enzyme deficiency. It has been suggested that G-6-PD deficiency confers some resistance to falciparum malaria. Motulsky (1960) observed that there is a correlation between the high frequency of G-6-PD deficiency with malaria endemicity. Primaquine 8-aminaquinoline is known to produce hemolysis in G-6-PD deficient red blood cells. This drug is administered as gametocytocidal agent in Plasmodium falciparum infection. Its administration to all malaria cases may result in serious complications and may be fatal. Therefore, it is important to know the genetic background of populations/ethnic groups before recommending a dosage schedule (Sharma, 1995).

### *Sickle Cell Disease (HbSS)*

It is a haemolytic anaemia (shortened life span of red cell) leading to severe and often fatal anaemia. The disease is further characterized by enlarged spleen, painful crisis, organ damage, impaired mental functions, increased susceptibility to infection and ultimately early death under certain conditions. The patients tend to have shorter trunk with long legs, chronic leg ulcers and an overall asthenic (weak) built. The sickle cell disease has been found in 72 districts of Central, Western and Southern India. There are more than 35 tribal population groups showing a frequency of more than 19 per cent. It is estimated that approximately a staggering 50 lakh individuals are carriers (heterozygotes) among the tribals (DST Report, 1990). Prevalence rate upto 40 per cent of heterozygous form (sickle cell trait) has been reported in some tribes, i.e. Adiyan of Kerala, Irula, Paniyan, Mulukarumbha of Nilgiri Hills, Gonds of Raipur (Basu, 1994) and 32 per cent among Dhodias of Valsad, Gujarat, (Kshatriya, 2004).

### *Glucose-6-Phosphate Enzyme Deficiency (G-6-PD)*

It is an important enzyme of the red blood cell and its deficiency is inherited as an X-linked recessive trait. Males are strongly affected but expression in females varies greatly. This enzyme deficiency causes frequent haemolytic episodes by intake of commonly used drugs such as anti-malarias, antibiotics, analegesics etc. and also by the ingestion of broad bean "Vicia Fava". About 13 lakhs G-6-PD deficients are present in tribal population (DST, 1990). The prevalence is specially high among the tribes and scheduled castes of Madhya Pradesh, Maharashtra, Tamil Nadu, Orissa, Assam, (more than 15%) specially in hyperendemic malarial zones.

## Health Seeking Behaviour

It has been observed that there is great difficulty in persuading the tribal people to avail modern medical treatment because they have firm, rigid and well-developed system of primitive medicine. They hold firm belief that a disease is always caused by hostile spirits, ghosts or breach of some taboos. Henceforth, they seek remedies through magico-religious practices to propitiate the supernatural powers.

The cure or treatment of the disease is essentially sought through getting rid of the wrath of Gods, evil spirits and observance of punishment in case of breach of a taboo. "Sirha" and "Gunia" in Bastar, "Jani" in Mayurbhanj, "Bhagat-Bhua" in Valsad, "Vaid" in Gadchiroli, "Bhope" in Barmer, "Amchi/Lama" in Kinnaur, etc. are the first line of defence for tribal groups. Tribal groups also prefer herbal medicine, Ayurvedic medicine and modern medicine depending upon desirability, availability, accessibility, affordability and acceptability. More and more tribal groups are now coming into the fold of modern medical care.

Tribal groups of India have specific problems, some of these are in built problems of these communities and some are imposed upon them, which jeopardize their overall development and progress inclusive of their health. Therefore, the health care delivery system should be such designed for each specific group that it caters to their specific needs and problems by bringing their personal involvement. Research studies should be directed towards understanding their knowledge and concept of health, felt needs for promoting and ensuring greater acceptance of purposeful modern health care practices. A large nunber of recommendation obtained from different sources are given in Annexure 1.

It could be worthwhile to state here that besides progressive measures of economic and social development (including transport connectively) the role of health providers is the most important factor in improvising health status of the tribal groups in India. Amongst the health providers, the government health providers are the key players. I say so because my experience of over 20 years in tribal areas reveal that the role of primary health care providers is stupendous. They are catering to a large segment of the society remarkably well. The primary health care delivery model now functioning under Government of India is doing fairly well. It should be understood that it provides enough width for some amount of regional variability within certain limits. There is no need for any policy or programme shift at this juncture, because the model has not been exploited to its full potential. It is, therefore, recommended to strengthened the existing set up of the programme for better service out put, this can be achieved easily by

(a) Filling up the sanctioned vacant posts along with the strengthening of the health infrastructure at the district level
(b) Providing specific incentive and encouraging the primary health care providers for the services they are rendering to the tribal groups, and appreciating the constraints under which they functions.
(c) Generating primary health specific data for providers in order to meet the health needs of the community effectively.
(d) Strengthening economic and social development measure (ensuring at least 25 percent of primary women literates) together with sturdy and compact transportation system for accessibility.

## ANNEXURE 1

Basu (1993) provided following strategies in "Tribal Health Workshop"

- Socio-cultural and Environmental Awareness (six recommendations under this heading).
- Focus on Nutrition (four recommendations under this heading).
- Focus on MCH (three recommendations under this heading).
- Focus on Genetics Disorders (three recommendations under this heading).
- Focus on Health Education (four recommendations under this heading).
- Focus on Training (four recommendations under this heading).
- Focus on other measures (six recommendations under this heading). (It includes suggestion on mobile health unit, HAAT as a focus, cooperatives, and involvement of local leaders in decision making among others).

***World Bank Projects (1995, 1996)***

*Malaria*

- IEC component (six recommendations under this heading).
- Health services providers (twelve recommendations under this heading.
- Training (three recommendations under this heading).

*TB*

- IEC components (nine recommendations under this heading).
- Training of staff (three recommendations under this heading).
- Services component (eleven recommendations under this heading).

***Kshatriya (2000)***

- Formulation of realistic developmental plans based on needs of specific tribal group.
- Positive tribal culture/values, traditional skills should be encouraged and inducted into the main stream of life.
- Most of the tribal communities have a wealth of folklore related to health. Documentation of this folklore available in different socio-cultural system could provide the model for promoting appropriate health and sanitary practices in given eco-system.
- Encouraging the development of horticulture with emphasis on local fruits.
- Study of nutritional status and physical growth among tribal children in different ecological setting should be carried out for an effective strategy to plan nutrition intervention programmes.
- Hundred per cent immunizations for pregnant mothers and children below five years must be targeted.
- Attempts should be made to introduce oral rehydration therapy among different tribal population through their culturally accepted food habits.

- Simple kits should be provided at PHC level and staff to be trained for genetic disorder tests like sickling, G-6-PD enzyme deficiency, etc.
- Health education should be imparted by the local people (preferably women) with guidelines provided by health functionaries. It can also be imparted through distribution of leaflets and playing of audio and where possible video cassettes, preferably in local dialects at weekly markets, ghotuls, schools, etc. Health education through community participation.
- Organization of short-term orientation courses on tribal culture for health workers at district and sub-divisional headquarters.
- Training of tribal girls as nurses and midwives to generate better response.
- In a difficult tribal/hilly areas, Mobile Health Teams should be formed to provide more coverage. Tribal "HAATS" can be taken as the focal point of the activity.
- Awareness about STD and AIDS must be further enhanced.
- Local community leaders, clan chiefs must be involved in the decision making process, in which women must also be included.
- Efforts should be directed towards achieving a respectable literacy rate for women.

### *Health Care Delivery Model Proposed by NIHFW (2003-2004)*

Various aspects of existing health care delivery in Bastar district—the tribal district studied were with special focus on their implications for developing an alternative model. Based on these certain recommendations for better health care delivery for tribal population in the study district have been given below:

- Increase the number of health facilities and staff to fulfil the recommended norms.
- Health services are to be strengthened further to make them more efficient.
- Vacancies to be filled at the earliest through recruitment of appropriately trained staff.
- Revised personnel policy to attract more health personnel to

work in tribal areas though financial and academic incentives etc.

- Adequate, regular and appropriate training strategy for health personnel need to be evolved and monitored by higher authorities.
- Strengthening physical infrastructure.
- Develop linkages with the NGOs functioning in the district.
- *Dais* to be trained to enhance their skills and service capabilities and to be utilized efficiently.
- Local practitioners need to be identified and fully involved as true partners in health care delivery.
- Infrastructural strengthening at all levels from the village to the district headquarters for effective functioning of referral system.
- Mobile outreach units to provide health services.
- Mapping of the area indicating the levels of accessibility and resource facilities in the villages for the planning of activities and services for the people in the area.
- Ensuring timely availability of transport suitable to the situations.
- Involve panchayat in health matters.
- ISM&H to be made functional with required facilities and resources.
- Inter-sectoral involvement in the district needs to be promoted
- Component on water supply and sanitation to be strengthened.
- For adequate utilization of available services, local need based IEC efforts to be considered.
- Locally operating organized groups like mahila mandals, bhajan mandals etc. to be fully utilized.

## REFERENCES

Ali, A. (1980): Health and genetic problems of Kutia Kondhs of Burlubaru village Phulbani district, Orissa. *The Newsletter* (Govt. of India, Min. Home Affairs, Trib. Dev. Div., N. Delhi) 1: 103-114.

Ali, A. (1992) Nutrition: In: *State of India's Health.* A. Mukhopadhyay Ed. VHAI, New Delhi.

Alison, A.C. (1954): Protection afforded by sickle cell trait against malarial infection. *Brit. Med.* J., 1: 290.

Barua. S. (1982): Biodemographic factors associated with offspring mortality among the Hajongs of Meghalaya. *J. Ind. Antropol. Soc.*, 17: 143-146..

Basu, A. (1967): Selection intensity in the Pahiras. *Eugen. Quart.* 14: 241-242.

Basu, S.K. (1972), Jindal, A., and Kshatriya, G.K. (1990): Genetic and socio-cultural determinants of tribal health: A primitive Kutia Kondh tribal group of Phulbani district, Orissa.—*ICMR Final Report,* NIHFW.

Basu, S.K. (1972) c.f. Kshatirya, G.K.,: Ecology and health with Special Reference to Indian Tribes. *J. Hum. Ecol. Special issue*, 9:229-245 (1967)

Basu, S.K. and Kshatriya, G.K. (1989): Fertility and mortality in tribal populations of Bastar district, MP. *Biology and Society,* 6: 110-112.

Basu, S.K., Jindal, A. and Kshatriya, G.K. (1985): Genetico-environmental studies among the tribal populations of India: Consideration of approaches for promotion of health care. In: *Population Genetics and Health Care: Issues and Future Strategies.* S.K. Basu, A. Jindal (Eds.). *Techn. Report* 8, NIHFW, New Delhi.

Basu, Sumana (1998): *Health Need Assessment of Tribal Populations of District Midnapore, West Bengal.* Ph.D. Thesis. Unpublished Delhi University, Delhi.

Behura, N.K. (1995): Tribes in India: Planned development pp. 98-117: In: *Tribals in India: Development. Deprivation and Discontent.* A.K. Singh and M.K. Jabbi (Eds.). Har Anand, New Delhi.

Bhasin, M.K. and Bhasin, Veena (1995): *Sikkim Himalayas: Ecology and Resource Development:* Kamla-Raj Enterprises, Delhi.

Bhasin, M.K. and Nag, Shampa. (1998): Anthropo-demographic study among the population groups of Ladakh in Jammu and Kashmir, India. 3. Mortality differentials and determinants. *J. Hum. Ecol.*

Bhasin, M.K., Nag, Shampa (1999): Anthropo-demographic study among the population groups of Ladakh in Jammu and Kashmir, India: 2. Fertility differentials and determinants. *J. Hum. Ecol.*

Bhasin, V. and Bhasin, M.K. (1993): Ecology, population dynamics among Transhumani of Himalayan. A case study of Gaddis of Himachal Pradesh. *J. Hum. Ecol.*, 4:171.

Census of India (1981): Paper-I of 1992. *Final Population Totals.* Registrar General and Census Commissioner of India, Delhi.

Census of India (1991): Paper-I of 1992. *Final Population Totals.* Registrar General and Census Commissioner of India, Delhi.

Chetlapalli, S.K. (1993): A Study of Relationship Between Blood Group Polymorphism, Red Blood Cell Enzymes and Serum Proteins Interrelations Thereof and their Impact on Reproductive Performances among *Desia Kondhs of Phulbani District of Orissa.* Unpublished Ph.D. Thesis.

Chetlapalli, S.K., Khan, A.S., Kshatriya, G.K. and Basu, S. (1991): Estimates of fertility and mortality in Kuti Kondhs of Phulbani district, Orissa. *J. Hum. Ecol.*, 2: 177-180.

Choudhury, N.R. and Kumar, R. (1976): Demographic profile of Bhils. *Eastern Anthropologist,* 29: 273.

Choudhury, R.K., Naik, M. and Mohanty, M.K. (1994): Fertility and mortality among Mirdhas: A tribal community of Orissa. *J. Hum. Ecol.,* 5: 191.

Das, S.K. *et al.* (1982): Demography and demographical genetics of two isolated mountain villages of northern Sikkim. *J. Ind. Anthropol. Soc.,* 17: 155-162.

Datta, U. (1990): *Demographic Investigation Among the Koras of Midnapore District, West Bengal.* Unpublished Ph.D. Thesis. Ravi Shankar University, Raipur.

Debnath, S.K. and Sen, T. (1983): Selection intensity in the Toto of Jalpaiguri Hills, West Bengal. *J. Ind. Anthropol. Soc.,* 18: 79-81.

Deka (1978) *c.f.* Kshatirya, G.K.: Ecology and Health with Special Reference to Indian Tribes. *J. Hum. Ecol. Special issue,* 9:229-245 (2000).

DST Expert Committee (1990): Health, Drinking Water and Management of Genetic Disorders. *DST Technical Report Series,* DST, New Delhi.

Garg, S.K., Sankyan, A.R. and Tyagi, D. (1980): Selection intensity in the Bhoksa of Doon valley, Uttar Pradesh., India. *Bull. Anthropol. Soc. Ind.,* 28: 12-16.

Ghosh, A.K.: Selection intensity in the Kotas of Nilgiri Hills, Madras. *Soc. Biol.,* 17: 224-225.

Ghosh, T.N. (1984): Factors of human genits in malaria. Proc. Indo-UK Workshop on Malaria, New Delhi (Ed) V.P. Sharma, Malaria Research Centre, New Delhi.

Gopalan, C. (1971): *Nutritional atlas of India.* ICMR, New Delhi.

Gopaldas (1987) *c.f.* Basu (1994).

Guha, B.S. (1953): The racial affinities of people of India: Census of India 1993, Vol.1, Part III B Govt. Press, Shimla.

Gupta, R. (1980): Selection intensity in Sherpas. *Curr. Anthropol.,* 21: 136-137.

Gupta, S.P. (1986): Tribal concepts of health, disease and remedy. In: *Tribal Health: Socio-Cultural Dimensions.* B. Chaudhuri (Ed.). Inter-India Publications, New Delhi.

Gurumurthy, G. (1986): Culture and fertility among Yanadis. A tribal community in South India. *Eastern Anthropologist,* 39: 35-45.

ICMR Bulletin (1996): Highlights of tribal health research under ICMR. *ICMR Bulletin Vol.* 26 March-April.

Jay, E. (1970): *A Tribal Village of Middle India.* Anthropological Survey of India, Calcutta.

Khan, A.S. (1993): *Genetic Structure of Dongaria Kondh of Koraput district of Orissa with special reference to its impact on mortality and morbidity.* Unpublished Ph.D. Thesis.

Khongsdier (1992) *c.f.* Basu, Sumana (1998).

Kshatriya, G.K., Singh, P. and Basu, S. (1993): Fertility and mortality in Bison

Horn Madias of Dantewara tehsil of Bastar district of MP. *J Hum. Ecol.*, 4: 93.

Kshatriya, G.K., Singh, P. and Basu, S. (1997): Anthropo-demographic features and health care practices among the Jaunsaris of Jaunsar-Bawar, Dehradun, UP. *J Hum. Ecol.*, 8: 347.

Kshatriya, G.K. (1999): Estimates of fertility and mortality among the Santals of Mayurbhanj district, Orissa. Under preparation.

Kshatriya, G.K. (1999): Dimension of tribal health: Few considerations. Paper presented at National Seminar on Tribal Health. Feb. 16 through Feb. 18, 1999 organized by the Department of Anthropology, Doctor Harisingh Gaur University, Sagar.

Kshatriya, G.K. (2004): "Determinents of genetic and socio-cultural aspects of health vis-à-vis the role of health providers among the tribes costal, Desert and Himalayan regions. ICMR Final Report. (Unpublished).

Kshatriya, G.K. and Basu, S. (1992-93): Fertility and mortality trends in Dudh Kharia tribal population of Sundergarh district, Orissa. Paper presented at the *International Symposium on Human Genetics and variation and XVIII Ann. Conf. Ind. Soc. Hum. Genet.*, Hyderbad. Jan. 1993.

Lehman, H. and Huntman, R. (1996): *Man's haemoglobins*. North Holland Publishing company, Amsterdam.

Mahapatra, D. and Das, J. (1990): Nutritional Ecosystems of Orissa tribals. In *Cultural and Environmental Dimension on Health*. B. Chaudhuri (Ed.). Inter-India Pub. New Delhi.

Majumdar, G. (Paul) (2003): The Oraons of Barasat: A study of some aspects of demography. *J. Hum. Ecol.*, 14(2): 133-136.

Malhotra, K.C. (1994): Genetico-environmental disorders and their impact on mortality and morbidity profile among the tribal populations. In: *Tribal Health in India*. S.K. Basu (Ed.). Manak Publications Pvt. Ltd., Delhi.

Mukhopadhyay, B. (1982): Selection intensity in the Lepchas of Kalimpong sub-division. *Curr. Anthropol.*, 23: 577-578.

Murthy, G.B. (1987): The Soligas of B.R. Hills: A demographic study. *The Journal of Family Welfare*, 34: 54-58.

Murthy, J.S. and Ramesh, A.(1978): Selection intensities among the tribal populations of Adilabad district, Andhra Pradesh., India. *Soc. Biol.*, 25: 302-305.

Motulsky, A.G. (1960): metabolic Polymorphism and the role of infections diseases in human evolution, *Hum. Biol.* 32: 28-63.

National Family Health Survey India (1998-99) (NHFS-2), International Institute for Population Sciences, Mumbai.

National Institute of Nutrition (1971): ICMR, Hyderabad, *Annual Report*.

Neel, J.V. (1956): The genetic of human haemoglobin differences, problems and perspectives, *Ann. Human. Genel.* 21. 1.

Pandey, G.D. and Tiwary, R.S. (1993): Socio-cultural characteristics and health seeking behaviour of the Hill Korwas. *The Journal of Family Welfare*, 39: 44,.

Pandey, B.N., Mishra, S.K., Yadav, S. and Das Sharma, P. (2000): Foetal Wastage and Infant mortality in Four Endogamous Population of Purnia, District (Bihar), *J. Hum. Ecol.*, 11(6): 477-481.

Parsuraman, S. and Rajan, S. (1990): On the estimation of vital rates among the Scheduled Tribes in Western India. In: *Demography of Tribal Development.* A. Bose, U.P. Sinha and R.P. Tyagi (Eds.).

Patel, S.: *Ecology, Ethnology, and Nutrition* (1985)*: A Study of Kondh Tribals and Tibetan Refugees.* Mittal Publ., Delhi.

Prakash, M. and Malik, S.L. (1990): Differences in fertility in highlanders and lowlander Bods of Himachal Pradesh. *J Hum. Ecol.,* 1: 175-180.

Prema, L. and Thomas, F. (1992): Nutrition and health problems faced by Kanikar women. In: *Dimensions of Scheduled Tribes Development in India.* P.D. Tiwari and R.S. Tripathi (Eds.). Uppal Publ. House, New Delhi.

Rao, D.H., Mathur, Y.N., Radhaiah, G., and Rao, P.N. (1986): *Health and Nutritional Status of Tribals in MP.* NIN, ICMR Report, Hyderabad.

Reddy, K.N. (1985): *Irulas of Nilgiris; A study of Anthropological Demography.* Research Report. Tamil University: Tamil Nadu, India. Unpublished.

*Report of Sixth Five Year Plan (1980-85)* (1980): Planning Commission, Government of India, New Delhi.

Ronald, P. (1973) Demographic analysis, Methods Results and applications. *c.f.* Basu (1994).

Saha, S.S. (1981): Selection intensity: Inter and intra group variation. *J. Ind. Anthropl. Soc.,* 16: 185-187.

Sarkar (1978) c.f. Kshatriya, G.K.: Ecology and Health with Special Reference to India Tribes. *J. Hum. Ecol.* Special Issue 9:229-245 (2000).

Saxena, D.N. (1990): Family building, fertility and family welfare among two tribal communities of UP. In: *Demography of Tribal Development.* A. Bose, U.P. Sinha and R.P. Tyagi (Eds.). pp. 249-69.

Singh, Murlidhar, Singh, R. K., and Sinha, S.P. (1999): Biology of the Paharia and the Santhal tribes of the Rajmahal Region of Bihar, *J.Hum. Ecol.*, 10 (3): 183-190.

Sharma, K. (1978): Fertility and mortality in Kondhs: A tribal community of Orissa. *Man in India,* 57: 77.

Sharma and Khan (1990) *c.f.* Kshatriya, G.K.: Ecology and Health with Special Reference to India Tribes. *J. Hum. Ecol*. Special Issue 9:229-245 (2000).

Sharma, V.P. (1985): Genetic Epidemiology of Malaria—An India Perspective Tech Report No. 11, NIHFW, New Delhi.

Sharma, K. (1979): *The Kondhs of Orissa, An Anthropometric Study.* Concept Publishing Company, New Delhi.

Sharma, K.D., Kshirsagar, V.H. and Deshmukh, V.V. (1974): Evaluation of deficiency of erythrocyte, Glucose-6 phosphate dehydrogenase and sickle cell trail with malarial endemicity in a Mahar Population of 1099 subjects. (In) *Human Population Genetics in India* (eds.) L.D., Sanghvi *et al.* Orient Longman Ltd. New Delhi.

UN Report (1984): Health status of women. Improving concepts and methods for statistics and indicators on the situation of women. *Studies in Methods-Series F. No.* 33.

W.H.O. (1971): Family Planning in Health Services. *WHO Technical Report. Series* 476. Geneva.

Working Group Report (1989-90): *Report of the working group on the Development and Welfare of Schedule Tribes During Eighth Five Year Plan (1990-95).* Government of India, Ministry of Welfare, New Delhi.

# 4

# Indian Tribes and their Urgent and Emerging Health Status: An Over View

SWETANSU SEKHAR RATH

## Introduction

India occupies a unique position in the tribal map of the world. The tribal population groups of India are known to be the autochthonous people of the land. Tribals are often referred to as *Adivasi, Vanyajati, Vanvasi, Pahari, Adimjati* and *Anusuchit Jan Jati*, the latter being the constitutional name. The concept of tribe emerged in India with the coming of the British. Gradually, the concept of reservation emerged and through that emerged the idea of scheduled tribe in independent India. In India, 427 groups have been recognised as scheduled tribes. They form approximately 8 per cent of the total Indian population. These tribal groups inhabit widely varying ecological and geo-climatic conditions (hilly, forest, desert, etc.) in different concentrations throughout the country with different cultural and socio-economic backgrounds. Due to their remote and isolated living, it is difficult to reach them. The tribal population in India are generally homogeneously distributed, who are culturally firm and have their own, strong magico-religious health care system. They always prefer to live with in their own style. Orissa, having the highest number of tribal (62) and primitive tribal (13) groups of the country (556 and 75, respectively) constitutes a significant proportion (22.3%) of the total state population. Though several tribal groups have put into one category, each one is different at levels of development, and is distinct socio-culturally. There are several Integrated Tribal Development Agencies and Micro-project

Development Agencies functioning for the overall development of tribal and primitive tribal groups, respectively.

Health is an important aspect of development and nutrition plays a central role in determination of health and well-being of individuals and affect growth and development through out the lifecycle. Nutritional status of tribals depends on the consumption of food in relation to the needs that influence the ecosystem in which they live (Mohapatra and Das, 1990). The health problems of tribals are profoundly influenced by interplay of prevailing socio-cultural and economic factors, which are quite distressing. Hence, it is necessary to understand the food habits of tribals in view of their subsistence economy, social isolation and food insecurity. Their natural habitat renders them vulnerable to a host of astringent unsanitary living conditions, widespread poverty, illiteracy, ignorance, absence of safe drinking water, lack of personal hygiene and health education, poor utilization of maternal and child health services and ineffective coverage of health services. A considerable proportions suffer from malnutrition such as protein-energy and deficiencies of iron, vitamin A and iodine (Rao *et al.*, 1989; Bulliyya *et al.*, 2002). Their common superstitious beliefs, customs, practice and taboos connected with health and disease intimately related to treatment of diseases that affect the morbidity and mortality. Maternal and childcare is largely neglected, which is reflected in terms of high infant and maternal mortality rates (Kumar *et al.*, 1991). Malaria, meningitis, unspecified fevers, diarrhoea, respiratory infections and neonatal tetanus take a heavy toll (Basu *et al.,* 1993). A large number suffer from various communicable diseases like leprosy, tuberculosis, and venereal diseases transmitted through contact with non-tribals (Swain, *et al.*, 1990). Worm infestations are high due to semi-starvation, inferior food and unhygienic food habits, which in turn affect nutritional status. The acute food insecurity feature is commonly characterized with malnourishment, vulnerability and poor socio-economic condition. It is reported that more than half of the tribal population is not consuming the recommended requirement (Patel, 1985). Their diets are grossly deficient in animal protein, fats and vital nutrients like calcium, iron, riboflavin and vitamin A. Besides scarcity of food, they have superstitions and misconceptions regarding food in spite of all sufferings and starvations. Further extremes of magico-religious beliefs and taboos tend to aggravate the nutritional problems. A high prevalence of malnutrition is reported in primitive tribal groups such as Lanjia Saura, Kutia Kondh, and Paudi Bhuiyan. Protein-energy-malnutrition and iron and vitamin deficiencies are widely prevalent among preschool children. High rate of micronutrient deficiency is documented for adolescent girls, pregnant women and lactating mothers (Rao *et al.*, 1989; Vijayaraghavan *et al.*, 1997). Owing to hard work along with poor quality of food, females suffer from different ailments since their early age and survival tasks, which result in inevitable neglect and adverse effect on health during infancy.

Recently a number of studies on the tribes, their culture and the impact of acculturation on the tribal society and health aspect have been undertaken. There are studies relating to tribal and their socio-cultural problems, their economic rights, their participation in management, their access to employment, food aspect, etc. But these issues have not been properly focused in relation to the tribal health matters. Thus in this present era of quality care, effective formulation of health strategy seems to be more important not only for programme formulation but also for effective plan implications with the social milieu in the indigenous tribal groups.

## Urgent Health Needs Components

From various tribal studies it has been pointed out that the strong magico-religious belief system of the tribal not only restrains them from the modern impact but also hold very important role in their individual health status. The alarming threat of high infant mortality rate (IMR), maternal mortality rate (MMR), etc. has not only influenced the health map of nation but also affecting the population size of their tribal groups in particular. It is generally accepted fact that a problem among tribals varies from population to population and from area to area. Some major problems are highlighted here are as follows:

### *Maternal Health*

It is little surprise to mention that major tribal women consumed no specific nutritious diet of any kind during the inception of pregnancy to its completion. Among the Dudh Kharias, Santals tribal of Orissa, pregnant women have practiced the reduction of food intake because of the fear of recurrent vomiting and also to ensure that the baby may remain small and the delivery may be easier. The consumption of iron, calcium and vitamins during pregnancy were poor among the tribal. The habit of taking alcohol during pregnancy was found to be common among the tribal women and almost all of them continued their regular activities including hard labour even during advanced pregnancy. More than 90 per cent of the deliveries were conducted at home attended by elderly ladies of the household. No specific precautions were observed at the time of conducting deliveries, which resulted in an increased susceptibility to various infections. Services of paramedical staff were required only in difficult labour cases. Maternal mortality directly related to pregnancy and childbirth was found to be appreciably high among the tribal population all over India. In addition, a lot of females suffered from ill health due to pregnancy and child-birth in the absence of a well defined concept of health consciousness. As far as child-care was concerned, both rural and tribal illiterate mothers were observed to breastfed their babies. But, most of them adopted harmful practices like discarding of colostrum. Giving prelacteal feeds delayed introduction of breast-feeding and delayed introduction of complementary feeds. Vaccination and immunization of infants and children were inadequate among tribal groups. Poor nutritional status with its concomitant problems of poor body weight, poor weight gain during pregnancy, low haemoglobin levels, was one of the primary underlying causes of maternal mortality among tribals in India. More maternal deaths occurred in India in one week than in all of Europe in one year. Malnutrition, nutritional anaemia, poor medical facilities and unfavourable social conditions, were the major underlying causes for high maternal mortality among the tribal in India.

### *Nutrition*

The nutritional problems of different tribal communities located at various stages of development were full of obscurities and very little scientific information on dietary habits and nutritional status were available due to lack of systematic and comprehensive research investigations. Malnutrition was common and greatly affected the ability to resist infection and this lead to chronic illness and in the post-weaning period to permanent brain impairment. Good nutrition was a requirement throughout life and was vital to women in terms of their health and work. Nutritional anaemia is a major problem for women in India and more so in the rural and tribal belt. In developing countries, it was estimated that at least half of the non-pregnant and two-thirds of the pregnant women were anaemic (U.N., 1984). Nutrition also affected lactation and breasts feeding which were key elements in the health of infants and young children and a contributory factor in birth spacing. Scanning through available data, it was observed that among most of the tribal groups, the staple diet was rice or minor millets except the Mompas of Assam who consumed wheat also (Basu *et al.* 1985). Problems of Iodine deficiency disorder (IDD) also presently emerging as the problems of tribals of western Orissa (ICMR study, 2001).

### *Sexually Transmitted Diseases (STDs)*

Infections of the female genital tract were numerous and widespread. They constituted a large part of grade morbidity among women, and contributing to a continuous and physically draining fatigue. These infections were closely related to inappropriate care or poor hygiene in connection with childbirth, abortion or menstruation. They include the sexually transmitted diseases, which were most prevalent disease forms in the tribal areas. These infections were often untreated, as they were difficult to diagnose and would even lead to infertility. VDRL, a very sensitive test to diagnose if a person was suffering from syphilis or, not was found to be positive in 17.12 per cent cases (relative in dilution of 1.8 or more) of polyandrous Jaunsaris of Chakrata, Dehradun. Out of 17 per cent, 9.92 per cent was found among the Santals of Mayurbhanj district, Orissa, 8.90 per cent cases (relatively in dilution of 1.8 or more) of VDRL were observed, out of which 4.99 per cent were females and 3.91 per cent were males. (Basu *et al.*, 1993).

### *Genetic Disorders*

There are two genetic disorders, namely sickle cell anaemia and G-6-PD deficiency found to occur in high frequencies in Scheduled Tribe populations in Indian subcontinent. Both male and female were equally affected in the case of sickle cell anaemia whereas males were more affected than females in G-6-PD deficiency cases. Sickle cell disease (HbSS) valued a shortened life span of the red cell leading to severe and often fatal anaemia among the tribal group in India. The disease was further characterized by enlarged spleen, painful crisis, organ damage, impaired mental functions, and increased susceptibility to infection and untimely death. The sickle cell disease was found in 72 district of Central, Western and Southern India. There were more than 35 tribal population groups showing a frequency of more than 19 per cent.

### *Malaria*

Malaria is a major public health problem among tribes in India because of their inhabiting place and, the unawareness of disease. This disease is pandemic among infants and pregnant mothers among tribes resulting in high rate of infant and maternal death. Rapid ecological changes in the tribal area such as construction of irrigation projects, deforestation, increase in paddy cultivation, urbanization, industrialization and aggregation of different developmental activities lead to malariogenic conditions. Besides these, malaria being a local and focal disease has many facets and ecotypes. Malaria control especially in tribal area requires local community to understand the problem in the right perspective on the first hand.

### *Problems Associated with Family Welfare Programme*

While evaluating the impact of the family welfare programme on tribal women through a study of 300 tribal women of Tamian development block of Chindwara district of Madhya Pradesh, it was observed by Tekhre, (1989) that tribal women gave more attention to child welfare and child development programmes rather than mother care or family planning programmes. This may be because of their inherent maternal instinct and protectiveness towards their children. They contacted doctors more for antenatal care than postnatal care because of their concern with the welfare of the foetus in the womb and preparing for a safe labour. More than 90 per cent of the eligible couples of Jaunsaris and Santals were found to be aware of family planning methods whereas only 16 per cent Dudh Kharia couples were aware of family planning methods.

## Emerging Health Problem Components

### *Status of Tribal Women*

The status of women in a society is a significant reflection of the level of social health in terms of the level of social justice in that society. Women's status is often described in terms of their level of income, employment, education, health and child bearing capacity as well as the roles they play within the family, community and society. A tribal woman occupies an important place in the socio-economic as well as health structure of her own family as well as society. The Dhebar Commission Report (1961) mentions that the tribal women is not drudge or a beast of burden, she is found to be exercising a relatively free and firm hand in all aspects related to her social life unlike in non-tribal societies. The status of tribal women in matrilineal societies has been observed to be somewhat better that of women in a patrilineal society, e.g., their legal status is much higher than that of their counterparts in patrilineal societies and they have a significant role in the tribal health status. However, after a comparative analysis of the various indicators (political organization, religion, ritual practices etc.) among the different tribes of India, it has been observed that the status of tribal women is comparatively lower than that of tribal men. Moreover, the status of tribal women has gone from bad to worse as a result of the impact of social change which has affected the social structure of tribal society (Chauhan, 1990).

### *Sex Ratio*

Sex ratio (females per thousand males) measures the balance between males and females in human population. Large imbalances in this aspect affect the social, economic and community life in many ways. In a population closed to migration, the sex ratio is an indicator of the sex differential in mortality. A higher or lower sex ratio reflects the status of the socio-cultural, maternal and child health care programmes existing in the population. The sex composition of the population in India is found to be favourable to males. Female disadvantage in mortality attributed as the cause for the low sex ratio [F/M over the last 30 year, i.e. 941 (1961), 930 (1971), 935 (1981), 927 (1991) respectively]. As compared to the general population, there appears to be a more even distribution of males and females among the Scheduled Tribes, i.e. 987 (1961), 982 (1971), 983 (1981), 972 (1991). These suggest that the females in the tribal society are not neglected; the social and cultural values protected their interest. However, it may be pointed out that their sex ratio (972) in 1991 census shows a definite decline when compared to the 1981 census figure of 983.

It is observed from the data that the sex ratio of the Scheduled Tribes varied within the country, i.e. among the States it was highest in Orissa (1002) and lowest in Uttar Pradesh/Sikkim (914); among the Union Territories, it was highest in Dadra and Nagar Haveli (1022) and lowest in Daman and Diu (931). The sex ratio of the Scheduled Tribes in India was found to be near even in Arunachal Pradesh (998), Meghalaya (997), and Kerala (996). While conducting health related studies among the individual tribal population groups, the sex-ratio was found to exhibit a variable picture. Kutia Kondhs, a primitive tribal group of Kondhamal district, Orissa, had a low sex ratio of 920 females per thousand males as compared to the Scheduled Tribes of India (972) (Basu, 1990). This indicated a preponderance of female deaths among the Kutia Kondhs. One of the ascribed social reasons for this sex difference was the utter neglect and apathy towards proper rearing of the female and apathy towards proper rearing of the female children among them. A still lower sex ratio, i.e. 903 females per thousand males, was observed (Basu *et al.*, 1993) among the Jaunsaries, Chakrata tehsil, Dehradun district, Uttar Pradesh. It seemed quite logical, as the Jaunsaries were known to be a polyandrous tribal group. Higher sex ratio indicating a comparatively better health status among the tribal women of Dhudh Kharias of Sundergarh district, Orissa (1098 females/1000 males) and Santals of Mayurbhanj district, Orissa (1019 females per 1000 males) were found during investigations. (Basu, *et al.*, 1993). These sex ratio were much higher compared to the India's general population (927/1000) and the Scheduled Tribes (972/1000) in 1991. Datta (1990) while conducting demographic investigations among the Kora tribe found the sex ratio to be 882 females per 1000 males which was quite low compared to the all India Scheduled Tribal figure of 972.

**Table 4.1:** Sex Ratio in India and Tribal

| *Year* | *Sex Ratio—India* | *Tribal* |
|---|---|---|
| 1961 | 941 | 987 |
| 1971 | 930 | 982 |
| 1981 | 935 | 983 |
| 1991 | 927 | 972 |
| 2001 | 933 | n.a |

**Table 4.2:** Sex Ratio in Some Selected Tribes

| *Name of the Tribe* | *Sex Ratio* | *Reason* |
|---|---|---|
| Kutia Kondha | 920 | Female infanticides still exist; people are not liking girl child (1991) |
| Jaunsaries | 903 | Polyandrous tribal group |
| Dudh Kharias | 1098 | Better health status of the tribes in comparison to others (Basu, 1993) |
| Santal | 1019 | Better health status |
| Kora | 882 | High son preference |

## Literacy

Literacy is universally recognized as a powerful instrument of social change. The level of literacy is undoubtedly one of the most important indicators of social, cultural and health development among the tribal communities. Literacy is important for the young girl; it had correlations with the survival of her children. Infant mortality is found to decrease significantly when the mother is educated upto the primary level and above. The Indian tribes have been exposed to literacy only recently (Moonis Raza, *et al.*, 1990). By and large, their response to programmes of literacy and of formal education varied significantly between tribes and from regions. These responses depended on their socio-cultural, economic and demographic characteristics and on the magnitude and direction of the forces of modernization, such as urbanization and industrialization (Bose, 1970). The influence of Christianity in some tribal areas had also played a significant role (Madan, 1951). The census recognised an individual as literate if one could both read and write with understanding in any of the languages. According to thc 1991 census data, excluding Assam, Jammu and Kashmir, the literacy rate among the general population aged 7 years and above was found to be 52.19 (64.20 for males and 39.19 for females). Literacy among the tribals was found to be very low, i.e. 25.9 per cent and especially so among the tribal females (14.5%) (NSSO, 1991). Most of the literates among the Scheduled Tribes were literate only up to the primary level. Within the country, the level of literacy among the tribals varies widely. At one end were tribal communities like the Malapandaram, Suhang etc. in the South with hardly any literates among them, whereas on the other end, there were communities like Lushai in North-East Himalaya with more than 40 per cent literacy (Vidyarthi, 1983). The lowest level of literacy among the tribes was recorded in Andhra Pradesh (14.5%) and the highest in Mizoram (80.0%). The lowest level of literacy among the females was found in Rajasthan (4.1%). Among the territories, the highest literacy among tribals was observed in Lakshadweep (79.1%). Studies on some individual tribes revealed the following trends of literacy:

Low litracy rate (3.3%) was observed among the primitive Abhujmaria tribe of Bastar district, Madhya Pradesh (RMRC, 1992). The educational status among the Santal tribe of Mayurbhanj district, Orissa showed marked sexual differentials. 51.6 per cent males were found to be literate against 19.4 per cent females. A similar literacy trend was observed among the polyandrous Jaunsaris of Jaunsar Bawar, Dehradun, i.e. 45.79 per cent literate among the males and 15.26 per cent literate among females. Kora females of Midnapur district, West Bengal had a very low literacy level (2.66%) (Datta, 1990). The female literacy rate among the Dudh Kharia tribal group of Sundargarh district, Orissa was found to be much higher, i.e. 41 per cent as compared to that of the Scheduled Tribe females (14.5%) (Basu, *et al.*, 1993). Literacy among the tribals of the North Eastern region could be due to the influence of Christianity. Literacy among tribals in general had improved slightly over time. Marked improvement over 1981 was noticed in some of the states of North-Eastern, Western and island regions. In other, specially in the Eastern and Central regions and in some of the states of other regions, improvement in literacy level was still lagging behind (Sinha, 1990).

## Marriage Pattern and Age at Marriage

The cultural norms that particularly affect women's health are attitudes towards marriage, marriage practices, age at marriage, values attached to fertility and sex of the child, pattern of family organisation, her status in the society, decision making capability and ideal role demanded of women by social and cultural conventions (Kshatriya, 1992). All these determine her place in the family, her access to medical care, education, nutrition and other health resources.

**Table 4.3:** Literacy among Tribes in States

| *Major States* | *% Literacy Among Tribal* | | |
|---|---|---|---|
| | *Male* | *Female* | *Total* |
| Andhra Pradesh | 2.18 | 0.69 | 1.45 |
| Bihar | 3.93 | 1.26 | 2.62 |
| Gujarat | 4.34 | 1.86 | 3.11 |
| Madhaya Pradesh | 2.58 | 0.92 | 1.78 |
| Maharastra | 3.91 | 1.51 | 2.72 |
| Orissa | 3.21 | 0.94 | 2.06 |
| Rajasthan | 3.54 | 0.41 | 2.02 |
| West Bengal | 3.50 | 1.09 | 2.31 |
| Assam | 6.45 | 3.76 | 5.22 |
| Karnataka | 5.89 | 3.29 | 4.74 |
| Kerala | 5.98 | 5.15 | 5.59 |
| Tamil Nadu | 3.20 | 1.41 | 2.35 |
| Arunanchal Pradesh | 3.99 | 2.60 | 3.31 |
| Uttar Pradesh | 4.77 | 1.13 | 3.03 |
| Tripura | 4.98 | 2.33 | 3.75 |
| All India | 3.68 | 1.45 | 2.59 |

*Source*: NSSO Report (1991)

**Table 4.3(a):** Literacy among Some Selected Tribes

| *Name of the Tribe* | *Literacy* |
|---|---|
| Malapandaram, Suhang (Southern state tribes) | Very low literacy/ Very negligible |
| Lushai (North-easten Himalaya) | 40.00% |
| Abhujmaria (Madhaya Pradesh) | 3.30 |
| Kora (West Bengle) | 2.66 |

## *Marriage Practices*

India is characterized by the presence of a large number of endogamous castes, tribes and religious communities with different types of marriage practices. The pattern of marriages in India is largely government by three important regulations, namely (a) Endogamy (marrying within the group of birth) (b) Exogamy (marrying out) and (c) Consanguineous marriage. There is a greater incidence of consanguineous marriages specially among the population of the southern states, Muslim groups, Parsees and various tribal communities (Basu, 1985). In many tribal communities, cross-cousin marriages were preferred and practiced. The system of cross cousin marriage had proved to be beneficial to the females in terms of care and treatment at husband's place. It also avoided high bride price/dowry and maintained the property of the household. Consanguineous marriages may, however, result in an increased probability of abortions, miscarriage, stillbirths, neo-natal deaths, infant and juvenile deaths, physical and mental defects, susceptibility to infections diseases, etc. In Himalayan region, some of the tribes like Naga, Lusia, etc. practiced polygamy, which was for economic reasons to protect the property/land and get help in agricultural activities. On the other hand, some of the tribes in India practised polyandry because of less number of women available for marriage, e.g. Jaunsaris of Jaunsar-Bawar, Chakrata tehsil, Dehradun, Todas of Nilgiri hills. Formerly the Todas practised female infanticide, which resulted in less number of girls available for marriage.

### *Age at Marriage*

The age at which the girl was given in marriage depends on social values and norms. Among the tribals, virginity was not very much valued. Many of the tribal societies were lax towards pre-marital sex relation, which were considered as training in the art of love and sex life and often culminates in marriage (Vidyarthi and Rai, 1977). Girls in tribal societies were given in marriage generally after puberty. According to 1971 census at the national level, the age at marriage for tribal women was higher (16.39) than that of the rural women in general (15.39). The mean age at marriage of the tribal females in Assam, Gujarat, Himachal Pradesh, Kerala, Manipur, Meghalaya, Nagaland, Andaman and Nicobar Islands and Arunachal Pradesh was more than 18 years, the highest being in Nagaland (21.33). On the other hand, it was less than 15 years in Rajasthan and Uttar Pradesh, the lowest being in Uttar Pradesh (14.50). There were a few micro-level studies which dealt with the age at marriage of individual tribes, e.g. female age at marriage—Ao Naga (16-20 yrs.), Bhil (16 yrs.), Chenchu after puberty, Khasi (13-18 yrs.), Koli (12-16 yrs.), Bodh (19 yrs.), Gond (18 yrs.), Munda (18 yrs.), Oraon (16 yrs.) (Sinha, 1990). Mean age at marriage of Jaunsars was 12.2 yrs., Dudh Kharias 21.41 yrs., and Santals 17.87 yrs. (Basu, *et al.,* 1993).

**Table 4.4:** Age at Marriages in Selected Tribes

| *Name of the Tribe* | *Age at Marriage* |
|---|---|
| Ao Naga | 16-20 Year |
| Bhil | 16 Year |
| Chenchu | Soon after Puberty |
| Khasi | 13-18 Year |
| Koli | 12-16 Year |
| Bodh | 19 Year |
| Gond | 18 Year |
| Munda | 18 Year |
| Oraon | 16 Year |
| Jaunsari | 12 Year |
| Dudh Kharias | 21 Year |
| Soligas | 14.2 Year |
| Santhal | 17 Year |

Jaunsaris of Jaunsar-Bawar, Dehradun were a polyandrous tribe and they followed the custom of child marriage as a part of their cultural behaviour, which was still prevalent among them (Basu, 1993). Investigation showed that 33.83 per cent of the Jaunsari females got married before or at 8 yrs, 29.70 per cent in the age group 9-15 yrs, 30.33 per cent in the age group 15-20 years and the remaining 5.6 per cent got married above the age of 20 yrs. In the Northeastern region, the age at marriage was found to be relatively high whereas it was relatively low in the central region because of the influence of Hindu culture (Sinha, 1986). It was further observed from research investigations that the frequency of abortions, miscarriages, and stillbirths were found to be much higher in younger mothers below the age of 19 years. The major life threatening complications for very young mothers were pregnancy induced high blood pressure, anaemia and difficulty in delivery due to disproportion between the pelvic-size and the head of the baby.

## Fertility and Mortality

Studies on fertility and mortality trends among the tribal population of India have been found to be fragmented and isolated. Limited studies are available on infant mortality and hardly any study is available on maternal mortality among the tribal population. However, a brief review of the available studies is discussed zonewise.

**Table 4.5:** Fertility and Infant Martality in Tribes

| *Tribes* | *Fertility* | *Infant Mortality ('000)* |
|---|---|---|
| *North-Eastern Zone* | | |
| Lachen | 4.66 | 125 |
| Lachung | 3.79 | 135 |
| Hajong | 3.25 | 182 |
| *Northern Zone* | | |
| High Altitudes Bods | 4.11 | 125 |
| Low Altitude Bods | 3.63 | 97 |
| Tharu | High (6+) | 189 |
| Jaunsari | 4.26 | 79 |
| *Central Zone* | | |
| Koras | 4.18 | 206 |
| Toto | 6.9 | 211 |
| Kutia Kondha | 5.09 | 180 |
| Dudh Kharia | 5.39 | 102 |
| Desia Kondh | 3.89 | 151 |
| Dongria Kondh | 4.07 | 153 |
| Kharwar | 4.85 | 197 |
| Bhattars | 5.95 | 148 |
| Murias | 5.64 | 123 |
| Marias | 6.00 | 85 |
| Halbas | 5.95 | 92 |
| *Western Zone* | | |
| Mahadeo Koli | 4.45 | 90 |
| Thakar | 3.85 | 75 |
| *Southern Zone and Island Zone* | | |
| Chenchu | 5.06 | 275 |
| Irula | 6.05 | 245 |
| Onge | 6.55 | Very High |
| Andamanese | 6.04 | Very high |

## North-East Zone (Arunachal Pradesh, Assam, Meghalaya, Manipur, Mizoram, Nagaland, Sikkim and Tripura)

A few studies on fertility and mortality of individual tribes, besides two studies on tribes, in general were available from North-East zone. On the basis of the census data, Gogoi (1990) found that during 1961-71, the rate of growth of tribal population in North-East India was lower than that of the general population. This was mainly because of a very low natural growth rate of the tribal population in the region. Pandey (1990) observed high fertility and mortality in Mishmi tribal groups and attributed it to the low level of education and income, lack of knowledge of family planning method and importance of small family size, poor medical facilities, lack of proper sanitation and drinking water. Barua (1982) studied 196 pregnant women belonging to the Hajong tribe of West Garo hill district of Meghalaya. High infant mortality (18.2%) and prenatal mortality (3.1%) were reported among them. Das *et at.* (1982) studied two Lepcha village of northern Sikkim namely Lachen and Lachung and found the total fertility rate for Lachung and Lachen to be 4.66 and 3.79, respectively. The results on total fertility rate were more or less similar to the Indian national population. Differences between the two were possibly due to the socio-cultural factors. The number of surviving children per women in Lachung and Lachen were found to be 3.70 and 2.65, respectively. The net reproductive index was observed to be 3.6 in Lachung and 1.80 in Lachan.

## Northern Zone (Himalayan belt of Himachal Pradesh, Uttar Pradesh and Darjeeling district of West Bengal)

This zone has been better investigated and about 10 studies on individual tribes were available. Prakas and Maulik (1990) showed that high altitude Bodhs had higher fertility than the low altitude Bodhs. They also had higher mean number of children (4.11 per mother) as compared to the low altitude Bods (3.63 per mother). The altitudinal differences in fertility have been explained in terms of socio-cultural factors such as education, awareness, urban contact, and advancement in medical facilities, which were higher at low altitude. The differences have also been accorded to a stronger feeling in the altitude population that children were economic assets. Kumar and Mitra (1975) observed high infant mortality and fertility among 199 Tharu tribal women of Nainital. Despite the availability of modern facilities of treatment, Tharus had their own beliefs and concepts of diseases. Saxena (1990) in his study conducted among the Tharu and Buksa tribes of Uttar Pradesh reported that the Tharu and Buksa couples displayed a high level of fertility which was well reflected in the tendency to achieve higher order births even at younger ages. Basu, *et al.* (1993) while conducting research investigation on 481 households among the Jaunsaris of Jaunsar Bawar, Dehradun found a crude birth rate of 42.67 per thousand population and infant mortality rate of 79.64 per thousand live births. Polyandry and polygamy were found to co-exist in the study sample. Basu (1990) found that Lepchas ate fish and a type of tuber, viz. Diascoria, while Sherpas did not eat them. It was observed that diascoria had a fecundity-inhibiting function resulting in lower fertility among Lepchas as against Sherpas though both shared a similar physical environment.

## Central Zone (West-Bengal except Darjeeling district, Bihar, Madhya Pradesh, Eastern Maharashtra, Orissa and some parts of Andhra Pradesh)

Various scholars have investigated this zone quite in depth on fertility and mortality of reproductive health aspect from time to time. In this way, Datta (1990) reported from her study that Koras, a Scheduled Tribe of Midnapur, West Bengal had a mean of 3.30 surviving children in their completed age of fertility. She found the crude birth rate and total fertility rate to be 41.81 per 1000 population and 4.42 per 1000 Kora women, respectively. These values were relatively higher than the national figures for these measures. However, these values were in agreement with most of the tribal groups in India. Study among the Toto tribes of West Bengal conducted by the Demographic Research Unit of the Indian Statistical Institute, Calcutta revealed the average number of children born to women married for 20 years and over to be 6.9. Ray & Rath (1991) studied the fertility pattern of Juangs of Orissa. It was observed that the marital age specific fertility rate was highest (3.36%) among mothers in the 20-24 year age group whereas it was lowest (0.44%) among the 45-49 year age group. The total marital age-specific fertility rate was 1.157 among the Juang mothers. It was also observed that the Index of over all Fertility and the Index of Marital Fertility among the Juangs were 0.49 and 0.50 respectively. Basu and Jindal (1990) made an indepth study of a primitive tribal group, i.e. Kutia Kondhs of Tumdibandha block of Kondhmal district, Orissa. The average age at menarche among Kutia was found to be 14.5 years. It was observed that the average number of pregnancies per mother was 5.09 and 3.89 respectively among mothers of completed and incomplete reproductive life cycles. Infant mortality was found to be very high, i.e. 179.75/1000. The fertility record of Kutia Kondh mothers in various age groups indicated a total fertility of 5.0 estimated from the average fertility of the women in the group 45-49. Basu and Kshatriya (1992) studied the fertility and mortality trends among the Dudh Kharia of Sundergarh district Orissa. They reported that the estimated total fertility, crude birth rate, crude death rate and infant mortality rate were 5.39, 38.5, 11.80 and 102.4 respectively. All these demographic figures showed higher values than the Indian national population level according to the 1981 census. Satish Kumar (1993) reported that the average pregnancies per mother and infant mortality rate among the Desia Kondhs of Orissa were 3.89 and 151.28 respectively. Khan (1993) while investigating the Dongria Kondhs of Orissa found average pregnancies per mother and the infant mortality rate as 4.07 and 153.11, respectively. Choudhary and Kumar (1976) estimated the birth rate as 43.5/1000 among the Bhils of Jhabua district of Madhya Pradesh, Sharma & Khan (1990) observed that the average fertility rate among Kharwars of Sarguja district (M.P.) was 4.85. The highest reproductive wastage (9.67%) was observed in the age group of 40-44 years and the pre-reproductive mortality was highest (6.84%) among mothers in age group 35-39 years. Basu and Kshatriya (1988, 1989) reported the fertility and mortality estimates on the basis of demographic analysis of genealogical data collected from 792 households of the four tribal populations, namely Muria, Maria, Bhattras and Halba from Bastar district of Madhya Pradesh. The results of the study indicated that total fertility rates of 5.64, 6.00, 5.95 and 5.89 respectively for the four groups which were higher than the Madhya Pradesh rural non-tribal population and Indian national averages and was in accordance with high fertility levels among the tribal. The study groups showed higher mortality among males than females. A very high rate of infant mortality was observed among Bhattras (148.56) followed by Murias (123.25) whereas Marias (85.44) and Halbas (92.78) from the same area displayed lower IMR.

### Western Zone (Western Maharashtra, Gujarat, Rajasthan, Dadra, Nagar & Haveli, Goa, Daman & Diu)

Very few tribal studies on fertility and mortality aspects were available in this zone. Most studies showed the general trend of fertility and mortality among the tribes.

Parsuraman and Rajan (1990) discussed the estimation of vital rates among the Scheduled Tribes in Western India. A very high proportion of 0-14 population to the total population indicated a higher level of fertility and not so high mortality. Parsuraman and Rajan reported that there were significant differences in death rates among the tribal population in different states. It was high in Maharashtra followed by Gujarat. Sinha (1990) reviewed the fertility of tribal groups of Gujarat, M.P., Maharashtra and Rajasthan and found the general marital fertility rate to be 169.4 births/1000 females against 152.9 births/1000 females.

## Southern Zone (Andhra Pradesh, Kerala, Karnataka, Tamil Nadu)

The study of demographic and health determinants and infant deaths by Gurumurthy *et al.* (1990) among the Sugali tribal group in the Kalyanadurgam and Beluguppa blocks of Ananthapur district of Andhra Pradesh pointed out that out of 348 infant deaths 45.4 per cent were neonatal and 54.6 per cent were post neonatal. About 25 per cent infant deaths occurred due to dysentery/diarrhoea and 20 per cent due to maternal factors such as prematurity, birth injury, multiple birth, low birth weight, birth asphyxia and so on. The study of Sirajuddin *et al.* (1984) among the Chenchu tribal group of Achampet taluk of Andhra Pradesh found that the average number of surviving offsprings per married women and mortality in relation to live births were 3.67, 2.96 and 27.5 respectively.

Murty and Ramesh (1978) also found a high fertility and mortality among the Pardhans of Adilabad district. Basu (1967) conducted a demographic research work among the Irula of Tamil Nadu and reported the net reproductive index which was also an indication of their fertility as 1.31. It was also reported that mortality according to the age of the child was highest in the first year. Ghosh (1970) while studying the Kota tribe of Nilgiri hills, Madras found the average number of live births per women aged 40 years or more to be 3.73. Also the frequency or mortality before reproductive age, i.e., 15 year was 30.8 per cent. This also revealed a high mortality and fertility among the Kota tribe. Murty (1987) investigated the Soliga tribe in Karnataka in order to find out their fertility behaviour. The Crude Birth Rate (CBR), General Fertility Rate (GFR) and Total Fertility Rate (TFR) among the Soligas were found to be always higher in comparison to the general population of Karnataka. The unusual high fertility rate among the Soligas was influenced by their age at marriage, which was ultimately influenced by the age at menarche. The mean age of menarche among the Soligas was 13.2 years and the age of marriage was 14.2 years, which was very early. Early age of marriage, and low levels of family planning acceptance seemed to be responsible for the high fertility among the Soligas. The completed family size among the Soligas was 5.64.

**Island Region (Andaman and Nicobar Islands)**

Aggarwal (1967) found that among 45 ever married Onge women of the Andaman Islands, the mean number of children was 1.64 and the mean number of children per women was 1.13. Infant mortality was very high as revealed from the reproductive index, which was 0.51.

**Life Expectancy at Birth**

A general indicator of the health of girl and women is their life expectancy. The expectation of life is the average number of years remaining to be lived by those surviving to that age. The expectation of life at birth is the life table function most frequently used as an index of the level. It also represents a summarization of the whole series of mortality rates for all ages combined as weighted by the life table of stationary population. In those countries where mortality was higher, and where infant and child mortality in particular were high, the maximum expectation of life was at a more advanced age (4 or sometimes 5 years) and a child of 10 years of age had an expectation of life often close to that of the new born infant (Roland Pressat, 1973). Expectation of life was the index most often used when one wished to summarize the risk of mortality in a country. Basu and Kshatriya (1989) while studying the Bastar tribal groups of Madhya Pradesh estimated the average life expectancy at birth based on q5 values for Muria (Males 37.56 yrs. and females 40.07), Maria (Males 40.26 yrs. and females 45.30 yrs.) and Halba (Males 38.6 yrs. and females 41.46 yrs.) tribes and 41.1 years for all the four tribal group combined. Although these figures were comparable to the rural non-tribal population of Madhya Pradesh, they were far below the average life expectancy at birth of 58.6 yrs. For the Indian population, sex specific mortality differentials were observed with males experiencing highest mortality than females. The differences could only be attributed to the prevailing socio-economic, cultural and health care practices of the four tribal groups.

Chettlapalli *et al.* (1991) studied in depth a primitive tribal group, i.e. Kutiya Kondhs of Tumdibandha block of Phulbani district, Orissa and found the average life expectancy at birth based on q5 values for Kuttiya males to be 46.49 years and for Kutia females to be 41.93 years. Unlike the Bastar tribal group, Kuttia female life expectancy was found to be lower than males. Datta (1990) while conducting demographic investigation among the Kora tribal the expectation of life at birth to be 33.87 years and 29.70 years for males and females, respectively. The expectation of life when computed at age 10 for Kora males and females, however, was found to be 38.52 years and 35.13 years, respectively. Social scientists ascribed physiological stress while others viewed biological factors as the main cause of the difference in the mortality levels between the two sexes. Basu and Kshatriya (1993) studied demographic features and health care practices in Dudh Kharia tribal population of Sundergarh district Orissa. Using q5 values to estimate the average life expectancy, it was observed that the Kharia females showed a higher life expectancy (52.95 yrs) as compared to the males (51.02 yrs). Sex retio of Dudh Kharias (1101/1000) lent further support to the above observation. The general life style of Dudh Kharias was found to be relatively better than most of the surrounding tribal groups.

## Conclusion

In the tribal set-up health matters are diverse and some of these were built-in problems where as some others were imposed upon them, which ultimately jeopardized their overall development and progress towards a better quality health environment. It is therefore time to explore the health status of the tribal from different angles. The existing tribal health programmes are not only forcefully imposing plans but also do not explain/target the problem minutely, especially among the tribal folks. The tribal population in India can be summarized as, suffering from: deficiency of essential components in diet leading to malnutrition, protein calorie malnutrition and micronutrient deficiencies (vit. A, iron and iodine). Goiter of various grades is also endemic in some of the tribal areas. Water borne and communicable diseases: gastrointestinal disorders, particularly dysentery and parasitic infections are very common, leading to marked morbidity and malnutrition. To improve this, the habit of drinking safe portable water has to be emphasized along with advocating a change in defecation behaviour. Malaria and tuberculosis still remain as problem in many tribal areas, while the spectrum of viral and venereal (sexual) diseases have not been studied in-depth, due to the stigma attached to the topic. High prevalence of genetic disorders mostly involving red blood cells, genetically transmitted disorders like sickle cell anaemia, glucose-6 phosphate dehydrogenate deficiency and different forms of thalassaemia are also common. All these defects lead to the early destruction of red blood cells and add to the overall anaemia. Inbreeding practices, among the tribals are also common. Excess consumption of alcohol: The brewing of alcohol from Mahua flower and fruits has been practiced traditionally. However, the switch over to commercially available liquor is likely to be a major threat. Superstitions particularly related to health problems are major hindrances and over all extreme poverty is the root of all problems among tribals. Thus a better understanding of the health components along with community based health care delivery system may be the real solution to cater to the specific needs and problems associate with in the tribal community.

## REFERENCES

Basu, A. (1990): Anthropological approach to tribal health (In) *Tribal demography and development in North-East India*, (ed. Ashish Bose, Tiplut Nagbri & Nikhlesh Kumar).131-142. B.R. Publishing Corporation, Delhi.

Basu, S. and G. Kshatriya (1989): Fertility and mortality in tribal populations of Bastar district, Madhya Pradesh, India. *Biology and Society, 6:* 100-112.

Basu, S.K. (1992): Health and culture among the underprivileged groups in India (In) *State of India'a Health* (ed. Alok Mukhopadhyay). Voluntary Health Association of India, pp. 175-186.

Basu, S.K. and A. Jindal (1990): Genetic and socio-cultural Determinants of tribal Health: A primitive Kuttiya Kondhs tribal group of Phulbani district. Orissa. *ICMR final report*, NIHFW.

Basu, S.K. *et al.* (1993): Socio-cultural dimensions, demographic features, maternal and child health care practices and sexually transmitted diseases in Santals of Mayurbhanj district, Orissa.

Basu, S.K. *et al.* (1993): Study of socio-cultural, demographic characteristics, maternal and child health and sexually transmitted diseases among the polyandrous Jaunsaris of Jaunsar-Bawar, Dehradun.

Bose, A.B. (1970): Problems of education development of Scheduled Tribes, *Man in India*, Vol. L (1) pp. 26-51.

Brandon, R.R. & Dixit, B.N. (1988): Sericulture for tribal women in J.P. Singh, N.N. Vyas & R.S. Mann (Eds.) (1988): *Tribal women and development*. Udaipur: MLV Tribal Research and Training Institute, Tribal Area Development Dept. Rajasthan.

Census of India (1971): *Female age at marriage,* Series 1, paper 4.

Census of India (1991): *Paper-1 of 1992: Final Population totals.* Registrar General and Census Commissioner of India. New Delhi.

Chaudhuri, Buddhadeb (1990): Social and environmental dimensions of tribal health (In) *Cultural and environmental dimensions of health* (ed.) by B. Chaudhuri. Inter-India Publications.

Chaudhuri, B. (eds.), *Dimension on Health,* Inter-India Pubilcation, New Delhi. pp. 192-206.

Chauhan, Abha (1990): *Tribal women and social change in India.* A.C. Brothers, Etawah.

Chetlapalli *et al.* (1991): Estimates of fertility and mortality in Kutia Kondhs of Phulbani district. *Orissa J. Hum. Ecology,* 2 (1): 117-120.

Choudhury, N.R. and R. Kumar (1976). Demographic profiles of the Bhils. *Eastern Anthropologist,* V-29:3:273-280.

D'Souza, V.S. (1990): *Development planning and structural inequalities: The response of the underprivileged.* New Delhi: Sage.

Dalton, E.T. (1872): *Descriptive Ethnography of Bengal,* Calcutta.

Dhebar, U.N. (1961): *Report of Scheduled Areas and Scheduled Tribes Commission,* New Delhi.

Durning, A.T.(1992): *Guardians of the Land: Indigenous Peoples and the Health of the Earth.* World watch Paper 112.

Durning, A.T.(1993): *Supporting indigenous peoples in Worldwatch Institute's State of the World, 1993.* New York: Noston & Co.

Fernandes, W. (1991): "Power and powerlessness. Development projects and displacement of tribals,"*Social Action,* 41 (3).pp. 243-70.

Fernandes, W. (1993). Indian tribals and search for an indigenous identity. *Social Changes.* 23 (2&3).

Firth, R. (1946): *Human Types.* London: Nelson.

Furer-Haimendorf, Von. C. (1943): *The Chenchus: Jungle folk of Deccan,* London: Macmillan and Company.

Ghosh, A.K. (1970): Selection Intensity in the Kota of Nilgiri Hills. Madras. *Social Biology,* 17:224-225.

Gogoi, J.K. (1990): Tribal demography in North-East India. Some preliminary observation. In: *Tribal demography and development in North-East India* (ed. Ashish Bose, Tiplut Nangbri & Nikhlesh Kumar). 85-94. B.R. Publishing Corporation, Delhi.

Gopalan, C. (1971): *Nutritional Atlas of India.* ICMR, New Delhi.

Grigson, W.V. (1938): *The Maria Gonds of Bastar.* Oxford: Oxford University Press.

Hunter, W.W. (1973): *Orissa.* London: Smith Elder.

Hutton, J.H. (1921): *The Sema Naga.* London: Macmillan.

Kar, P.C. (1982): *The Garos in Transition.* Cosmo Publications, New Delhi.

Kumar, N & A.K. Mitra (1975): Reproductive performance of Tharu women East. *Anthrop.* 28 pp. 349-57.

Madan, T.N. (1951): Education of tribal India. Eastern *Anthropologist* Vol. V (4) pp. 179-82.

Mahapatra, D.K., J.Das (1990): Nuritional Ecosystems of Orissa tribal in *Cultural and Environmental Dimension on Health* (ed. Buddhadeb Chaudhuri).

Majumdar, D.N. (1973): *A Glimpse of Garo Politics in North Eastern Affairs.* London: Longman.

Mann, K. (1987): *Tribal Women in a Chaging Society.* Mittal Publications, Delhi.

Menon, Geeta (1987): Tribal Women. Victims of the development process. *Social Action*, Vol. 37.

Menon, Geeta (1991): Ecological transitions and the changing context of women's work in tribal India. *Purusartha,* 14, pp. 291-314.

Murthy Venka, G.B. (1987): The Soligas of B.R. Hills: A demographic study. *Journal of family welfare,* Vol. XXXIV, No. 154-58.

Murty, J.S. and A. Ramesh (1978): Selection Intensities among the tribal population of Adilabad district. Andhra Pradesh. *Social biology*, 25: 302-305.

National Institute of Nutrition (1971): Indian Council of Medical Research, Hyderabad: *Annual Report.*

National Sample Survey organization, Government of India (1991): *A report on living conditions of Tribals and Non-tribal Areas*, No. 380.

Parsuraman, S. and S. Rajan (1990): On the estimation of vital rates among the Scheduled Tribes in Western India. In: *Demography of tribal development* (eds. A. Bose, U.P. Sinha and R.P. Tyagi).

Patel, Shirsha (1985): *Ecology, Ethnology and Nutrition: A study of Khondh Tribals and Tibetan Refugees.* Mittal Publication, Delhi.

Post-gradute Department of Psychology, Ranchi University, Ranchi.

Prakash, M. and S.L. Malik (1990): Differences in fertility in High landers and lowlanders Bods of Himachal Pradesh. *Journal of Human Ecology* 1 (2): 175-180.

Prema, L and Thomas, F. (1992): Nutrition and health problems faced by Kanikkar women (In) *Dimensions of Scheduled Tribes development in India* (eds P.D. tiwari and R.S. Tripathi). Uppa; Publishing House, New Delhi.

Pressat, Roland (1973): *Demographic Analysis, Methods, Results, Applications.*

Ray, A. and A. Rath (1991): Indian tribals fertility patterns from Orissa. *Man in India 1991* (special) 71(1): 235-239.

Raza, Moonis, Ahmad Aijazuddin and Nuna Sheel Chand (1990). Special pattern of tribal literacy in India. In *Demography of tribal development* (eds. Bose, Sinha and Tyagi). B.R. Publishing Corporation, Delhi.

Rivers, H.H.(1973): *The Todas.* London: Macmillan.

Roy Burman, B.K. (1988): Challenges of development and tribal women of India, in J.P. Singh, N.N. Vyas & R.S. Mann (Eds.). *Tribal women and development*. Udaipur: MLV Tribal Research and Training Institute, Tribal Area Development Department, Rajasthan.

Sachchidananda (1978): Social structure, status and Mobility patterns the case of tribal women, *Man in India*, Vol., 58 No. 1.

Satyanarayana, R. & Behera, D.K. (1986): Socio-economic responsibility of tribal women: A micro-study of the Kissan of Western Orissa. *Tribal Women and Development*. Agenda Papers, Theme I, P.15.

Saxena, D.N. (1990): Family building, fertility and family welfare among two tribal community of UP In *Demography of tribal development*. (eds. A.Bose, U.P. Sinha and R.P. Tyagi). pp. 249-269.

Sen, D.K. (1956): Some notes on the fertility of Jaunsari women. *Eastern Anthropologist* V. 10, No. 1 60-67.

Sharma, B.D. (1991): Report of the Commissioner for Scheduled Castes and Scheduled Tribes. *Twenty-ninth Report*. New Delhi: GOI.

Sharma, K.K.N. and A.S. Khan (1990). Fertility and mortality trends of the Khairawar tribal women of Madhya Pradesh. *Man in India* 70 (4): 446-453.

Sharma, Krishan (1979): *The Kondhs of Orissa: An Anthropometric Study*. Concept Publishing Company, New Delhi.

Shashi, S.S. (1978): *The Tribal Women of India*. Delhi: Sandeep Prakashan.

Shiva, Mira (1992): Women and Health. In *State of India's Health* (ed. Alok Mukhopadhyay), Voluntary Health Association of India. pp. 265-301.

Singh, A.K. (1993): *Tribes and Tribal Life*. Vol.3. Approaches to development in tribal context. New Delhi: Sarup & Sons.

Singh, A.K. Jayaswal, M. & Hans. A. (1991): Understanding the health of the tribals. *Social Change*. 21(1), 3-22.

Singh, A.K., Sinha, S.K., Singh, S.N., Jayaswal, M. & Jabbi, M.K. (1987): The myth of the healthy tribal. *Social Change*, 17(1), 3-23. Refer also: *The myth of the healthy tribal*. Report of ICMR Task Force on Health Modernity Education Project.

Singh, B. (1993): *An outline of work to be taken up on tribal women*. Working Papers: NCW.

Singh, J.P., Vyas N.N. and Mann, R.S. (1988): *Tribal Women and Development*. Rawat Publications, Jaipur.

Singh, K.S. (1988): Tribal women: An Anthropological perspective. In *Tribal Women and Development* (eds. Singh, Vyas and Mann). Rawat Publications, Jaipur.

Singh, K.S. (1988): Tribal women: An anthropological perspective, in J.P. Singh, N.N. Vyas & R.S. Mann (Eds.) *Tribal Women and Development*. Udaipur: MLV Tribal Research and Training Institute, Tribal Area Development Department, Rajasthan.

Singh, K.S. (1993a): Tribal Perspectives—1969-1990 in Miri M.(Ed.). *Continuity and change in tribal society*. Shimla Indian Institute of Advanced Study. pp. 5-10.

Singh, K.S. (1993b): *Status of Scheduled Tribes. Some reflections on the debate.*

Sinha, U.P. (1990): Demographic profile of tribal population in India. In *Demography of Tribal Development* (eds. Bose *et al.*) B.R. Publishing Corporation. Delhi.

Sirajuddin and Arabinda Basu (1984): Population structure, consanguinity and its effect on fertility and mortality among Chenchu of Andhra Pradesh. *Hum.Sci. 33.:* 179-200.

Swain, S., S.C. Jena and P. Singh (1990): Morbidity status of the Kondha tribes of Phulbani (Orissa). In *Cultural and Environmental Dimensions on Health* (ed. Buddhadeb Chaudhuri). Inter-India Publications, New Delhi.

U.N. Report (1984): V. Health Status of Women. Improving concepts and methods for statistics and indicators on the situation of women. *Studies in Methods—series F.No. 33.*

Vidyarthi, L.P. (1983): Tribes of India. In *Peoples of India: Some Genetical Aspects.* XV International Congress of Genetics, Dec. 12-21, ICMR, New Delhi.

Vidyarthi, L.P. and Rai, B.K. (1977): *The Tribal Culture of India*, Concept Publishing Company, Delhi.

# 5

# Nutrition and Health among the Tribes of India

P. DASH SHARMA

## Introduction

Good health is difficult to define, but it is certainly more than just the absence of disease. It reflects a state of mental, social and physical fitness and well-being of the individual and is strongly influenced by his or her lifestyle. Health and nutrition are very intimately related aspects of an individual's biological status. Both are under the influence of hereditary and environmental factors.

Human beings need a wide range of nutrients to lead a healthy and active life and these are being derived through the diet which man consumes daily. Food contains various substances that are required for growth, development and maintenance of the body. These substances are called nutrients which are proteins, carbohydrates, fats, vitamins, and minerals. The amount of each nutrient that is required by man depends upon his age and physiological status. Adults need nutrients for maintaining constant body weight and ensuring proper body functions. Infants and young children who are growing rapidly require nutrients not only for maintenance of body functions but also for growth. Infants and young children require relatively more nutrients (2-3 times) per kg body weight than the adults. In special physiological conditions like pregnancy and lactation, adult women need additional nutrients to meet the extra demand for foetal growth and maternal tissue expansion in pregnancy and milk secretion during lactation. These extra intake of nutrients are essential for the normal growth of an infant in uterus and during the early postnatal life.

Health is a multifaceted aspect and has been defined by WHO as "a state of complete physical, mental and social well-being and is not merely the absence of disease or infirmity". Health and the related problems are very much interlinked with the socio-economic conditions of the community, particularly the tribes who are living in remote and inaccessible areas where health care and development services of the government are not available. So there is an urgent need to understand the concept of health among the tribes and their traditional knowledge and health seeking behaviour. The health seeking behaviour of the tribal groups is associated with their beliefs, customs and practices. Health status of different communities particularly the tribal group is influenced by their way of life including their social and economic conditions, nutrition and living conditions, dietary habits, housing, education, child rearing practices, socio-religious beliefs, taboos and superstitions, etc.

In the present study I will confine my discussion on the health and nutritional status of some of the tribes of India. The tribal groups in India inhabit widely varying ecological and geo-climatic conditions (hills, forests, deserts, etc.) and are at different stages of social, cultural and economic development process. The scheduled tribes differ considerably from one another in their biological characteristics, language, cultural practices and beliefs, and in their socio-economic characteristics. The health of these tribal groups is a function of the interaction between socio-cultural practices, genetic characteristics and the environmental conditions (Basu, 1996). The overall health status of the tribal community is dependent upon the effects of environment in which they live, genetic characteristics, cultural patterns and the lifestyles of the tribal groups, health care delivery service in tribal areas, and their detached attitude largely in accepting the modern health care services at the initial stages of the disease. Basu (1996) suggested that there is an urgent need for initiating area specific, group specific, health need specific action research studies among the tribal communities in India so that the health oriented action research studies ultimately help the authorities in formulating effective need based health care strategies among the various tribal groups in India.

The wide spread poverty, illiteracy, malnutrition, non-availability of safe drinking water and unhygienic living conditions and poor maternal and child health services, have been reported in several studies as the possible contributing factors for dismal health conditions prevailing among the tribal communities in India. It has been found that certain areas like Madhya Pradesh, Orissa, Rajasthan, Gujarat, Assam and in some other areas, certain diseases like goitre, yaws, malaria and guinea-worm are endemic (Government of India, 1989). Primitive tribal groups of India have special health problems because of their ignorance, unhygienic conditions, lack of health education and non-availability of health care facilities in their habitation areas.

There is a general agreement that the health status of the tribal population in India is very poor and many scholars have tried to establish this with the help of morbidity, mortality and health statistics (Basu 1986, 1993, 1996; Bardhan *et al.*, 1989; Rizvi, 1986; Roy Burman, 1986; Swain *et al.*, 1990; and many others). The low health status of the tribal community in general is closely linked with factors such as their poverty, illiteracy, lack of infrastructure facilities for medical care in the area where they inhabit.

A significant percentage of 8.08 per cent of the Indian population (excluding Jammu & Kashmir) have been enumerated as a member of the scheduled tribes as per 1991 Census of India. The Census of India enumerates 573 notified scheduled tribes in India. Out of these 573 tribal groups, only 74 tribal communities have been identified as 'Primitive Tribal Groups' in India. The tribal communities in India inhabit widely varying ecological and geo-climatic conditions in different concentrations throughout the country and are having distinct biological, cultural and socio-economic characteristics.

## Measure of Health Status

Malnutrition has been defined (Jelliffe, 1966: 8) as a pathological state resulting from a relative or absolute deficiency or excess of one or more essential nutrients, this state being clinically manifested or detected only by biochemical, anthropometric or physiological tests.

Clinical examination of individuals is an important practical method for assessing the nutritional status of an individual and a community. The method is based on examination for changes, believed to be related to inadequate nutrition, that can be seen or felt in superficial epithelial tissues, specially the skin, eyes, hair and buccal mucosa, or in organs near the surface of the body, such as the parotids and the thyroid glands. Occasionally this may be supplemented in the field by certain physical tests with or without instrumental aids, such as the testing of the ankle jerk. This method has the advantage as it is relatively inexpensive as neither elaborate field equipment nor a costly laboratory is required. Though the method is simple but it has its own limitations (Jelliffe, 1966: 10-11). (For descriptive list of selected clinical signs for malnutrition one may refer to Jelliffe, 1966:16-95.)

Age and body weight largely determine the nutrient requirements of an individual. Body weight and heights of children reflect their status of health and growth rate, while adult weight and height represent what can be attained by an individual with normal growth. Height unlike weight, once gained cannot be lost as weight is not affected by chronic malnutrition. The nutritional goal of any country would be to provide adequate nutrition and health support to its population so that they attain their full genetic potential in growth and development.

Anthropometric measurements (Vijayaraghavan, Singh and Swaminathan, 1971) of Indian children up to 14 years belonging to well-to-do groups have shown that they grow at rates similar to those of the children in the developed countries.

Available earlier data on well-to-do Indian children (Vijayaraghavan, Singh and Swaminathan, 1971; Hanumantha Rao, Satyanarayana and Sastry, 1976) indicate that their height and weights correspond to National Centre for Health Statistics (NCHS), up to the age of 14 years in the case of boys and 12 years in the case of girls. The heights and weights according to NCHS standards are given in Table 5.1.

Malnutrition in children in the tropics is important not only because it is common but also because it highlights important relationships between infection, immunity and nutrition which are of universal application.

All malnourished children show reduced growth and muscle protein deficiency. Two 'polar' types of protein energy malnutrition (PEM) are recognised, they are Marasmus and Kwashiorkor, but many children have a mixed clinical picture (Cowen and Heap, 1993:259).

Marusmus occurs in infants aged under 1 year when maternal milk supply is interrupted by death or illness, and in older children in time of famine. The child has clearly lost muscle and subcutaneous fat. The skin is dry and wrinkled and there is no peripheral oedema. The hair is thin and dry. Body temperature is low. The child looks anxious but moves less than normal and may be hungry, but vomit any foods offered. Such children are susceptible to diarrhoeal and respiratory infections, trachoma and vitamin A deficiency.

**Table 5.1:** Reference body weight and heights of children and adolescents according to NCHS

| *Age (in years)* | *National Centre for Health Statistics* | | | |
|---|---|---|---|---|
| | *Boys* | | *Girls* | |
| | *Height (cm)* | *Weight (kg)* | *Height (cm)* | *Weight (kg)* |
| 0 | 50.5 | 3.3 | 49.9 | 3.2 |
| 1/4 (3 m) | 61.1 | 6 | 60.2 | 5.4 |
| 1/2 (6 m) | 67.8 | 7.8 | 66.6 | 5.4 |
| 3/4 (9 m) | 72.3 | 9.2 | 71.1 | 8.6 |
| 1 | 76.1 | 10.2 | 75 | 9.5 |
| 1.5 | 82.4 | 11.5 | 80.9 | 10.8 |
| 2 | 85.6 | 12.3 | 84.5 | 11.8 |
| 3 | 94.9 | 14.6 | 93.9 | 14.1 |
| 4 | 102.9 | 16.7 | 101.6 | 16 |
| 5 | 109.9 | 18.7 | 108.4 | 17.7 |
| 6 | 116.1 | 20.7 | 114.6 | 19.5 |
| 7 | 121.7 | 22.9 | 120.6 | 21.8 |
| 8 | 127 | 25.3 | 126.4 | 24.8 |
| 9 | 132.2 | 28.1 | 132.2 | 28.5 |
| 10 | 137.5 | 31.4 | 138.3 | 32.5 |
| 11+ | 140 | 32.2 | 142 | 33.7 |
| 12+ | 147 | 37 | 148 | 38.7 |
| 13+ | 153 | 40.9 | 155 | 44 |
| 14+ | 160 | 47 | 159 | 48 |
| 15+ | 166 | 52.6 | 161 | 51.4 |
| 16+ | 171 | 58 | 162 | 53 |
| 17+ | 175 | 62.7 | 163 | 54 |
| 18+ | 177 | 65 | 164 | 54.4 |

Children with Kwashiorkor are usually aged 18 months to 4 years and have been weaned from the mother's breast. Muscle loss occurs but subcutaneous fat is preserved, and there is obvious peripheral oedema. The hair is dry, straight and depigmented. The skin is scaly and glistening, peeling and hyperpigmented, especially on the legs. The abdomen is distended and the liver enlarged. The child is fractious and irritable and often has diarrhoea. Clinical Vitamin A defiency may be present.

Children with mixed 'marasmic kwashiorkor' have a varied picture with muscle loss, oedema and damaged skin (Cowen and Heap, 1993:259). The diagnosis of the malnutrition syndrome is primarily clinical. Anthropometric documentation is essential for the individual child and for the study of the community. Body weight on a centile chart is a measure of current nutritional status, allowing for the presence of oedema; body length or height indicates previous progress in growth. Children with kwashiorkor have low serum albumin, potassium, zinc, magnesium and calcium levels and low blood sugar, and may be anaemic with defective blood clotting.

The treatment of marasmus requires the provision of adequate nutrients appropriate to the age of the child, with powder or cow's milk as the basis, involving the mother if possible at all stages.

The management of kwashiorkor is more complicated. Clinical dehydration at present should be treated with oral rehydration solution. Adequate intake of protein and calories require frequent feeds of a mixture of skimmed milk, vegetable oil and sugar (sucrose or glucose), followed by cereals, pulses, rice, eggs and meat or fish according to availability. Supplement of potassium and magnesium and vitamin A are important in early treatment, and should be followed with additional iron, folic acid and B vitamins. Children with kwashiorkor may also have tuberculosis and malaria may also complicate convalescence (Cowen and Heap, 1993:261).

Prevention of childhood malnutrition in a community depends on:

1. Adequate community food supplies;
2. Education of mothers in the use of nutritious foods which are cheap and available in their community;
3. Primary health care programmes including monitoring of child development, treatment of or immunization against common infections, provision of vitamin A supplements.

In India, prevention of childhood malnutrition is not possible at the present situation because of the extremely inadequate infrastructure facilities for health care in rural India, where the people are poor and there are no adequate food supplies in interior villages, parents are illiterate, and primary health centres are almost non-existent in the villages.

Report of the facts and figures about the existing health care infrastructure in the State of Jharkhand shows an 'unhealthy figures'. According to the Government of India guidelines, there should be 7260 health sub-centres in rural areas but there are only 4462. The situation is more pathetic in areas where a large number of sub-centres are non-existent. It makes for painful reading of the annual report published by the undivided Bihar that from 1990 to 2000 not a single new sub-centre was set-up anywhere in the entire state. The 'unhealthy figures' reported in *Hindustan Times*, HT Ranchi Live (Saturday, October 11, 2003) are as follows:

| *Health Centres* | *Should Be* | *IS* | *Gap* |
|---|---|---|---|
| Health Sub-Centre | 7260 | 4462 | 2798 |
| Primary Health Centre | 561 | 193 | 368 |
| Community Centres | 211 | 37 | 174 |
| Sub-Division Hospitals | 35 | 16 | 19 |
| Hospital Posts | 1740 | 0 | 0 |

The Chief Minister and Health Minister of Jharkhand have assured to revamp the health sector in rural areas of Jharkhand by the year 2007. This is the situation prevailing in a highly concentrated tribal population of the State of Jharkhand. We can presume that the situation is not better in other rural areas of the various states of India where there is large concentration of tribal groups.

An overview of the population, health and social development scenario of Jharkhand was presented by UNFPA adviser Dr. Almas Ali and Dr. B.P. Thiagarajan of Population Foundation of India. The report says that the root cause of overall poor health status of Jharkhand is poverty — both income and human related, social deprivation, low literacy rate, specially among females, and structural inequalities in terms of class, caste and sex. The report gives the nutritional status of Jharkhand as follows (Reference: State-Level Advocacy Conference on Population Stabilization, Health and Social Development, held at Ranchi on 18 November 2003):

- 1 in 9 children dies in the first year of life.
- Girls are more likely to be stunted and boys wasted.
- 54 per cent children under 3 years are underweight, 49 per cent stunted and 25 per cent wasted.
- Just 26 per cent children aged 6-9 months receive breast milk and mushy food.
- Only 6.5 per cent children are fully vaccinated.
- 32 per cent children were never vaccinated.
- 2 out of 5 women are undernourished.
- Anaemia in young children is 70 per cent.

- Anaemia in women is as high as 72.5 per cent.
- 40 per cent women have chronic energy deficiency.

This shocking presentation had other bad news: All the 31 Scheduled Tribes including the nine primitive tribes, are severely disadvantaged. In comparison to other states, the situation is very poor in terms of infrastructure for personal hygiene, sanitation, water supply, education—especially among the females and the number of girls schools, employment, health consciousness and also availability, affordability and accessibility of the health services.

Malnutrition is the single most important risk factor for spread of diseases in Jharkhand. About 54 per cent of children up to 3 years of age are underweight, 49 per cent are with stunted growth, while 25 per cent are wasted and 70 per cent suffer from anaemia. The ratio of children suffering from malnutrition is higher in rural areas and among the disadvantaged groups particularly Scheduled Tribes. Based on body mass index, 41 per cent women are undernourished and 73 per cent have some degree of anaemia. Only 56 per cent of households in the state use iodised salt at recommended levels. This was the report by CARE (a prominent NGO in Jharkhand) and the report specified that malnutrition among Scheduled Castes and Scheduled Tribes in the State is highest in the country. Almost in all the health and nutrition indictors right from immunisation to check up of pregnant women, Jharkhand is far below the national average. The report further observed "Reason for existing plight is multi-dimensional. People in the State are largely rural based and are even oblivious of the fact and even lack awareness about health behaviour. The concept of immunising the children against deadly diseases is yet to catch up. The lack of knowledge and adherence to traditional practices of healing hinder their belief to accept modern medicines." (Report by CARE; *Hindustan Times*, Ranchi Live, February 3, 2004).

So this is the situation in a tribal concentrated region like Jharkhand. It may be assumed that the situation is not very different in other areas particularly in States of Madhya Pradesh, Chattisgarh, Orissa, where there is large concentration of the tribal groups.

It would be appropriate to discuss the methodology of assessing the health and nutritional status of a community before we discuss specific tribal communities where health and nutritional studies have been carried out by earlier researchers.

**Assessment of Nutritional Status**

Anthropometry is the most important parameter in the assessment of protein energy malnutrition (PEM). Anthropometric methods commonly in use are: Weight for age; Height for age; Weight for height; Weight/Height ratio; Weight (kg)/Height $(cm)^2$ (which is known as Body Mass Index); Head circumference, Chest circumference, Calf circumference, Skin-fold thickness (triceps, calf), and Bangle test. Most of the parameters stated are not useful although some may be very simple. They only indicate that the child is malnourished but do not give information about the nature of malnutrition, i.e. Acute (short duration), Chronic (long duration) or consequence of past malnutrition. Also these do not differentiate wasting or stunting or a combination of wasting or stunting (Bhattacharyya, 1995). For the correct assessment of malnutrition in a child, the measurements of weight and height and knowing the age are sufficient. Weight for age is low in acute, chronic and past malnutrition and hence does not differentiate these types. Height for age is normal in acute malnutrition but low in chronic and past malnutrition. Weight for height is low in acute and chronic malnutrition but normal in past malnutrition. A combination of height for age and weight for height differentiate acutes, chronic and past malnutrition. The malnutrition can be graded arbitrarily into mild, moderate and severe degrees using either SD or percentage of NCHS (National Centre for Health Statistics, USA) median. However, NCHS data should be used as a 'reference' and not as 'standard', as regional and national standards are of limited use (Bhattacharyya, 1995). Classification of protein energy malnutrition is either clinical or anthropometric or a combination of both. Commonly used classifications are of Gomez (anthropometric), Waterlow (anthropometric), Bhattacharya (clinical), Composite (Wellcome Trust), and of Indian Academy of Pediatrics.

Anthropometric measurements and composite indices for the assessment of nutritional status of infants, preschool children, adolescents and adults was elaborated by Jelliffe (1966:50-79; Visweswara Rao and Singh, 1970; and others). "Nutritional anthropometry is concerned with the measurement of the variations of the physical dimensions and the gross composition of the human body at different age levels and degree of nutrition" (Jelliffe, 1966:50). Visweswara Rao (1995) elaborately discussed anthropometry for the assessment of various forms of malnutrition which is concisely presented here and will be helpfull for our later discussion. Bhattacharyya (1995) delivered a lecture at Anthropological Survey of India on 31 March, 1995 discussing 'anthropology in the assessment of malnutrition in children'.

It was found that weight for age is the measurement by which all forms of malnutrition should be assessed and indeed this has advantage as a working approximation in community surveys. Acute malnutrition obviously results in early weight loss, mainly due to depletion of subcutaneous fat and muscle or at least in failure to put on weight (Jelliffe, 1966). This leads to anthropometric disproportion, especially between weight and height that is low weight for height (Jelliffe, 1966; *cf.* Visweswara Rao, 1995:196). Diets chronically inadequate in calories and proteins lead to nutritional dwarfs or 'bonsai babies' who are apparently well proportioned and whose malnutrition is not evident unless exact ages are known (Jelliffe, 1966).

Weight for age gives a good indication of size at different stages of life. Height gives an indication of linear growth over a period. Precise birth date or calendar age is usually unobtainable in developing countries like India, particularly in rural communities. When calendar year of child is not known it appears to us of limited value in assessing the grades of malnutrition.

## The Methods and Classification of Malnutrition

The methods of diagnosis and classification of marginal or moderate forms of protein calorie malnutrition (PCM: the usual signs of protein calorie malnutrition in adults and school children are; diminished subcutaneous fat and muscle wasting) are the following:

*Gomez Classification*: This has been widely used. It was originally introduced as a prognostic tool for hospitalised cases of protein calorie malnutrition (PCM). A serious problem associated with this classification is that it does not distinguish between deficit in weight for height or deficit in height for age and all the deficit in height or weight for height produce deficit in weight for age. Grades of malnutrition by Gomez classification are likely to be combinations of current and chronic malnutrition (Jelliffe, 1966; Visweswara Rao, 1955). Gomez classification grades as are as follows (cited from Bhattacharyya, 1995): (see Gomez *et al.*, *J.Trop. Pediat.*, 1956. 2: 77-83).

| *Grades* | *Percentage of 50th Percentile of Boston value* |
|---|---|
| I | 90-75 |
| II | 75-61 |
| III | less than 60 |

*Waterlow's Classification*: This method of nutrition assessment consists of classification of children into four groups (Visweswara Rao, 1955):

(a) Present malnutrition (with low weight for height),
(b) Past malnutrition (with low height for age, and in the extreme cases, nutritional dwarfs),
(c) Present + past malnutrition (with low weight for height and low height for age), and
(d) Normals (with normal weight for height and normal height for age).

**Waterlow's Classification**

| | | *Weight for Height (%)* | |
|---|---|---|---|
| | | *Low (L)* | *Normal (N)* |
| *Height for age* | Low (L) | LL | LN |
| | Normal (N) | NL | NN |

where,

LL = low height for age and low weight for height (i.e. stunted and wasting).
LN = low height for age only (or short for age/stunted or dwarf).
NL = normal height for age and low weight for height (wasting only).
NN = normal height and normal weight for height.

Critical limit of height for age (%) = below 100 – 2SD of height for age (%)
Critical limit of weight for height (%) = below 100 – 2SD of weight for height (%).

On the basis of investigation carried out at the National Institute of Nutrition, Hyderabad, the following two approaches will be of use for prevention and diagnosis of protein-calorie malnutrition (Visweswara Rao, 1979, 1980, 1995; Visweswara Rao *et al.*, 1981, 1986).

Height for age and Weight/Height$^2$ and
Modified Waterlow's classification

*Waterlow's Classification:* If modified on the following lines (Visweswara Rao *et al.*, 1979; Visweswara Rao, 1980) will be of use for better estimation of mild or severe forms of malnutrition. The classification is as follows:

| | | Weight for Height (%) | |
|---|---|---|---|
| | *Less than 80%* | *80-90%* | *90% or above* |
| Less than 3rd percentile (or below 90% of standard) | LL* | LM | LM |
| *Height for age* | | | |
| 3rd percentile or above (or above 90% of standard) | NL | NM | NN |

*Note*: *Abbreviations as earlier given.

The children having weight for height in between 80 per cent and 90 per cent of the standard can be taken as with moderate forms of malnutrition.

Waterlow's classification as presented by Bhattacharyya, 1995 (see Waterlow, 1973. Lancet, 2:87-89).

| *Height for Age* | *Stunting* |
|---|---|
| 90-94% | Mild |
| 85-89% | Moderate |
| Less than 85% | Severe |
| Weight for height | Wasting |
| 80-89% | Mild |
| 70-79% | Moderate |
| Less than 70% | Severe |

Height for age and Weight/Height$^2$

The index weight/height$^2$ which is known as Body Mass Index (BMI) was found independent of age and sex (Visweswara Rao, 1995). Longitudinal studies showed that children with weight/height$^2$ value more than 1.5 to have food growth status with no incidence of protein calorie malnutrition (Visweswara Rao, 1980, 1995). The classification is as follows:

**BMI (Weight/Height²) Value**

| Height for age | Less than 1.35 | 1.35-1.50 | Less than 1.50 |
|---|---|---|---|
| Less than 3rd percentile (or below 90% of standard) | LL | LM | LN |
| Greater than 3rd percentile (or above 90% of standard) | NL | NM | NN |

*Note*:

BMI: Weight in grams/height in centimetres squared.
LL : Chronic and current severe form of malnutrition;
LM : Chronic and current moderate form of malnutrition;
LN : Chronic malnutrition only (short for age, stunted or dwarf);
NL : Current severe form of malnutrition (normal height and low BMI/weight or height);
NM : Current moderate form of malnutrition;
NN : Normal height for age and normal BMI/weight for height.

Bhattacharyya (1995) presented two more classifications for the assessment of malnutrition which are as follows:

**Wellcome Trust Working Party Classification**

| *Weight for Age % of Harvard* | *Oedema* | |
|---|---|---|
| | *Present* | *Absent* |
| 80-60 | Kwashiorkor | Under nutrition |
| < 60 | Marasmic- Kawashiorkor | Marusmus |

*Source*: *Lancet*, 1970, 2:302-307.

**Indian Academy of Pediatrics Classification**

| *Grades* | *Clinical Syndrome* | *Oedema* | *Weight for Age % of Standard* |
|---|---|---|---|
| I | Underweight | – | 71-80 |
| II | Underweight | – | 61-70 |
| III | Marusmus | – | 51-60 |
| IV | Marusmus | – | less than 50 |
| IK | Kwashiorkor | + | 71-80 |
| IIK | Kwashiorkor | + | 61-70 |
| IIIK | Marasmic kwashiorkor | + | 51-60 |
| IVK | Marasmic kwashiorkor | + | less than 50 |

*Source*: *Indian Pediatrics*, 1972, 9: 360. (Cited from Bhattacharyya, 1995)

Some of the other anthropometric indices which are commonly used for the assessment of nutritional status of a community are the following:

### *Pignet's Index*

Pignet's index includes stature, body weight and chest circumference for its calculation.

*Pignet Coefficient*: Stature in cm. (chest circumference in cm + weight in kg)

The formula itself indicates that the value of index increases with decline in the measurements of weight and/or chest circumference. The mean Pignet coefficient of 16 or so can said to be physically sturdy or good and that with a mean value of more than 30 or so can be taken to be physically weak or poor (Ivanovsky, 1932; referred by Keys *et al.*, 1950). The following quantitative gradations of Pignet's index is used for getting relative measure of body build of different individual and population as a whole.

| | | | |
|---|---|---|---|
| Below 10 | Very strong | 21-25 | Average |
| 10-15 | Strong | 26-30 | Weak |
| 16-20 | Good | Above 31 | Very weak |

### *Weight-Height Index*

The formula of Weight-Height index is:

$$\text{Weight (kg)} \times 100/\text{Height (cm)}$$

It gives an overview of the body build and thus suggest the nutritional status of the population. The assessment is done on the basis of the rated values as follows:

| | |
|---|---|
| 41.6-50.5 | Above normal |
| 40.6-41.5 | Normal |
| 31.6-40.5 | Threatened |
| 28.6-31.5 | Pre-cachetic |
| 20.6-28.5 | Cachetic |

### *Body Mass Index*

This index is also calculated from the measurements of weight and height. It is also known as a good indicator for measuring nutritional status of adult individual.

Weight (Kg)/height (M) (Johnston, 1987), considering the index value 18.5 or more as an indicator of normal nutritional status of an individual, the categories are given below:

| | |
|---|---|
| Normal | 18.5 |
| Mildly under-nourished | 17.0-18.4 |
| Moderately under-nourished | 16.0-16.9 |
| Severely under-nourished | 16.0 |

## Nutritional Status of Some Tribes of India

In the present paper I shall limit my discussion to some of the tribes of India with particular reference to the State of Jharkhand, West Bengal, Orissa and Madhya Pradesh, and the information have been culled down from published and unpublished reports of various authors. Though nutritional assessment have been made by many researchers through diet surveys among many tribes however I will limit my discussion only to those tribes where nutritional assessment have been made through anthropometric measurements.

### *Jharkhand*

In an extensive study Gupta on the tribes of Chotanagpur plateau (1974:81-83), had discussed the intake of food, nutrients, adequacy of diets and nutritional status of children. Gupta (1974) has also presented stature and weight measurements of four tribal groups (103 Asur, 22 Korwa, 103 Sauria Paharia and 26 Birhor) of Chotanagpur, which are primitive tribes in Chotanagour region. Table 5.2 gives the height and weight measurements of tribal children from 5 to 15 years as recorded by Gupta (1974) but he has not estimated the nutritional status of the children as based on the various indices as discussed earlier. However he mentions that calorie consumption is highest among the Saurias and lowest among the Birhors. The main source of calories of these tribes were rice and millets, roots and tubers as observed by Gupta during the field survey. Gupta has also presented a comparative growth curve of Birhor, Asur, Korwa and Sauria Paharia children for stature and weight. He found that the Asur and the Sauria Paharia children have better growth than the

Korwa and the Birhor children. He found that the Korwa and Birhor children subsists mainly on the forest economy. According to Mitra (1940) and Lal (1954), the Paharia children were smaller and lighter than the Santal (tribal) children. The rate of growth in height and weight of the Santal children reflected better intake of food, but deficiencies of calcium, vitamin A, and vitamin B2, were considerable. The authors noticed more nutritional defects in children due to deficiency of several nutrients (Gupta, 1974: 83).

**Table 5.2:** Average Stature and Weight of Asur, Korwa, Sauria Paharia and Birhor Children and their Comparative Growth from 5 to 15 years of Age

| *Age-group (in years)* | *Asur Children (103)* | | *Korwa Children (22)* | | *Sauria Children (103)* | | *Birhor Children (26)* | |
|---|---|---|---|---|---|---|---|---|
| | *Stature (cm)* | *Weight (lbs)* | *Stature (cm)* | *Weight (lbs)* | *Stature (cm)* | *Weight (lbs)* | *Stature (cm)* | *Weight (lbs)* |
| 5 | 102.1 | 31 | 100.5 | 29.0 | 94.2 | 31.0 | 90.5 | 26 |
| 6 | 108.9 | 36 | 105.2 | 32.5 | 112.9 | 38.6 | 99.6 | 34 |
| 7 | 115.4 | 37.8 | 112.1 | 36.5 | 117.2 | 42.7 | 104.5 | 35 |
| 8 | 118.3 | 42 | 112.7 | 37.5 | 120.4 | 46.0 | 113.4 | 39 |
| 9 | 123.7 | 48.4 | 119.1 | 44.0 | 125.5 | 49.7 | 118.7 | 46 |
| 10 | 126.8 | 50.1 | 123.6 | 46.5 | 126.8 | 53.0 | 123.9 | 48 |
| 11 | 130.8 | 56.4 | 126.5 | 47.5 | 136.6 | 65.8 | 125.2 | 53 |
| 12 | 138.9 | 64.1 | 130.3 | 52.5 | 137.9 | 67.4 | 132.7 | 54 |
| 13 | 141.6 | 69 | 130.3 | 52.5 | 146.4 | 81.7 | 143.2 | 77 |
| 14 | 148.6 | 88.2 | 143.5 | 79.0 | 150.9 | 91.2 | 148.9 | 78 |
| 15 | 156.4 | 104.2 | 156.1 | 90.5 | 156.2 | 102.8 | 153.7 | 89 |

*Note*: 1 lb = 0.4536 kg; (figures have been rounded to 1 decimal point by the present author).

Sengupta (1988) presented a study on the nutritional status of the Ho tribe of Singhbhum of southern part of Jharkhand. Nutritional survey was conducted by Dr. N.K. Sengupta and his team for 15 years (from 1970 to 1985) covering about 30 villages around the town of Chaibasa, covering the Ho and other tribes of Singhbhum as well as other non-tribal residing in the town of Chaibasa.

We shall only discuss the anthropometric measurements presented by Sengupta (1988) covering the Ho tribal children (a major tribe of Jharkhand).The analysed data presented by the author is as follows:

**Table 5.3:** Anthropometric measurements on Ho tribal children

| *Age (in years)* | *Number* | *Male* | | | *Female* | | |
|---|---|---|---|---|---|---|---|
| | | *Wt.(kg)* | *Ht.(cm)* | *Arm (cm)* | *Wt.(kg)* | *Ht.(cm)* | *Arm.(cm)* |
| 0 to 1 yr. | 2800 | 7.0 | 66.1 | 11.4 | 8.0 | 55.5 | 9.5 |
| 1 to 2 yr | 5000 | 8.0 | 76.0 | 12.0 | 7.0 | 74.2 | 12.0 |
| 2 to 3 yr. | 4900 | 10.5 | 86.0 | 12.8 | 10.0 | 81.6 | 12.7 |
| 3 to 4 yr. | 4700 | 12.0 | 96.0 | 13.5 | 11.5 | 93.0 | 13.0 |

**Table 5.4:** Mean ± SD Values of Heights and Weights of Children of Ho, Other Tribes, Urban Children of Chaibasa and Children of Well-to-do Indians

| | *Ho Tribe* | | *Other Tribes* | | *Urban* | | *Well-to-do Indians* | |
|---|---|---|---|---|---|---|---|---|
| | *Male n=170* | *Female n=180* | *Male n=180* | *Female n=150* | *Male n=90* | *Female n=60* | *Male n= ?* | *Female n=?* |
| *Measurements* | | | | | | | | |
| Height | 69.5 ± 4.73 | 69.0 ± 6.59 | 71.6 ± 5.96 | 70.0 ± 8.64 | 69.3 ± 4.24 | 71.0 ± 7.16 | 80.2 | 78.5 |
| Weight | 6.9 ± 1.07 | 7.4 ± 1.01 | 7.8 ± 1.89 | 7.4 ± 1.90 | 7.9 ± 1.90 | 8.8 ± 2.32 | 10.5 | 9.8 |

**Table 5.5:** Nutritional Status of Children as per Gomez Classification (Weight for age as percentage of standard)

| | *Ho tribals* | | | *Other tribes* | | | *Urban* | | |
|---|---|---|---|---|---|---|---|---|---|
| | *Male* | *Female* | *Pooled* | *Male* | *Female* | *Pooled* | *Male* | *Female* | *Pooled* |
| **Gomez Grades** | | | | | | | | | |
| 90% (Normal) | 1 | 1 | 2 | 5 | 4 | 9 | 1 | 3 | 4 |
| | 4.2 | 44.8 | 4.5 | 20 | 22.3 | 20.9 | 10 | 37.5 | 22.2 |
| 75-90% Grade I | 6 | 7 | 13 | 7 | 2 | 9 | 5 | 4 | 9 |
| (Mild malnutrition) | 25 | 33.3 | 28.9 | 28 | 11.1 | 20.9 | 50 | 50 | 50 |
| 60-75% Grade II | 9 | 11 | 20 | 9 | 6 | 15 | – | 1 | 1 |
| (Moderate malnutrition) | 37.5 | 52.4 | 44.4 | 36 | 33.3 | 34.9 | | 12.5 | 5.6 |

## *Orissa*

Anthropometric measurements from seven States according to age and sex. The body weight of preschool children as per cent of the NCHS standards for given age and sex were presented by Bulliyya (2003). In an extensive study on the nutritional status of young children in Orissa, Bulliyya (2003) presented the assessment of nutritional status. The children were classified into body weight deficit groups (PEM) based on Gomez classification. His findings are presented in Table 5.6, which will also help us to understand the comparative picture of the different states. It is evident from Table 5.6 that 92.5 per cent, 91.2 per cent and 96.7 per cent of rural children suffer from under weight as measured by 75 per cent weight-for-age by NCHS during the three periods of NNMB surveys during 1975-79, 1988-90 and 1996-97, respectively (NNMB, 1979; 1991 and 1999). There is only a slight decline in severe degree of underweight (< 60%) from 14.9 per cent in 1975-79, to 10.7 per cent in 1988-90 and 4.1 per cent in 1996-97 as evident from the Table. Data on tribal children show high rates of malnutrition when compared to the rural children in different periods. A similar state of decline was observed in nutritional status of tribal children of Orissa during the periods 1985-87 (93.2%) and 1988-99 (96.7%) (NNMB, 2000; cited from Bulliyya, 2003:61).

**Table 5.6:** Nutritional status of preschool children in Orissa and other States

| *India and its States* | *Gomez Malnutrition Grade* | | | *NNMB Surveys* | | |
|---|---|---|---|---|---|---|
| | *Rural* | | | *Tribal* | | |
| | 75-90 | 60-75 | < 60 | 75-90 | 60-75 | < 60 |
| India (8 States pooled) | 31.6 | 47.5 | 15.0 | 24.5 | 51.6 | 19.8 |
| | 37.6 | 43.8 | 8.7 | 34.4 | 51.5 | 8.6 |
| | 40.6 | 44.3 | 6.2 | – | – | – |
| Kerala | 35.7 | 46.5 | 10.3 | 23.0 | 56.1 | 15.7 |
| | 47.4 | 32.9 | 2.0 | 38.7 | 48.2 | 7.2 |
| | 50.7 | 25.1 | 2.0 | – | – | – |
| Tamil Nadu | 34.2 | 47.0 | 12.6 | 34.7 | 51.5 | 9.2 |
| | 42.0 | 45.8 | 4.2 | 33.1 | 55.0 | 7.6 |
| | 49.2 | 33.5 | 2.9 | – | – | – |
| Karnataka | 31.1 | 50 | 14.3 | 15.1 | 49.7 | 32.9 |
| | 38.1 | 48.8 | 8.3 | 46.2 | 43.1 | 2.4 |
| | 39.0 | 45.4 | 6.2 | – | – | – |
| Andhra Pradesh | 32.4 | 46.1 | 15.4 | 24.3 | 53.4 | 18.9 |
| | 39.5 | 44.3 | 7.5 | 36.8 | 46.8 | 10.1 |
| | 38.1 | 47.6 | 7.1 | – | – | – |
| Maharashtra | 25.4 | 49.5 | 21.9 | 23.6 | 59.0 | 15.2 |

*Source*: Bulliyya, 2003, p. 64.

The effect of maternal factor, such as mother's education, employment, nutritional status, nutritional knowledge and adherence to food taboos and beliefs related to child's nutrition, was studied by Acharya (2003) in relation to nutritional status of preschool children (1 to 5 years) of a slum area in Bhubaneswar. The study was conducted on 215 slum children of general population (non-tribal) following the techniques of nutritional anthropometry and interview. The study by Acharya indicate that nutritional status of the children deteriorates with mother's low nutritional status, poor nutritional knowledge, adherence to food taboos and beliefs. Further, mother's employment at home keeps the children in better nutritional health than her unemployment or employment away from home. The study being on a non-tribal population so details have not been discussed here. However, the results obtained by Acharya appears to be applicable to tribal children also.

### West Bengal and Orissa

In a study of the nutritional status of the Oraons of Sunderban, Bhattacharya (1995) reported on the weight/height index of different populations of West Bengal, Orissa and Bihar. Only the tribal populations reported by him is presented here.

**Table 5.7:** Weight/Height Index of Some Tribal Populations of West Bengal, Orissa and Bihar

| *Population Groups* | *Weight/Height Ratio* | *Authors* |
|---|---|---|
| Juang of Orissa | 28.20 | Roy and Roy, 1982 |
| Santals of West Bengal | 29.33 | Roy and Roy, 1982 |
| Kharwar of Bihar | 31.95 | Bhattacharya *et al.*, 1972 |
| Oraons of Sunderbans | 31.65 | Bhattacharya, 1995 |

In Indian context, with special reference to the tribal situation Roy and Roy (1982) opined that the index value below 28 may be considered as malnourished while the values beyond 28 and below 31 represent unsatisfactory state of nutrition.

The weight/height index upto 28 can be rated as gross undernutrition (Roy and Roy 1969) while values between 28.1 to 31.0 can be stated as mild undernutrition. Bhattacharya, Haque and Biswas (2004) in their study on the Toto and Bondo primitive tribes of eastern India found the distribution of weight/height index (in per cent) as follows (Table 5.8):

**Table 5.8:** Distribution of Weight/Height Index (in per cent) of the Two Groups

| Index | Values | Male | | Female | |
|---|---|---|---|---|---|
| | | *Toto n=86* | *Bondo n=68* | *Toto n=77* | *Bondo n=94* |
| – | 22 | 0 | 0 | 0 | 04.26 |
| 22.1 | 25 | 0 | 07.35 | 01.30 | 17.02 |
| 25.1 | 28 | 0 | 25.00 | 02.60 | 28.72 |
| 28.1 | 31 | 08.14 | 41.18 | 25.97 | 30.85 |
| 31.1 | 34 | 29.07 | 25.0 | 53.25 | 12.77 |
| 34.1 + | | 62.79 | 01.47 | 16.88 | 06.38 |
| Total | | 100 | 100 | 100 | 100 |

Body mass index is widely accepted as a singular physical status index *vis-à-vis* the index of obesity. A wide range of values between 18.5 and 24.99 have been taken as normal values (WHO 1995). Some authors suggested values between 18.5 to 20.0 as low weight normal. In any case, more than half of the male and about one-third of the female of the Bondo have this index values below the normal indicating poor physical status. In case of the Toto, less than four per cent of the male and a solitary female have the index value below 18.5. More than 94 per cent of the male Toto and about 99 per cent of the female Toto are normal in physical status as per WHO (1995). Two persons have been found to be obese also among the Toto (Table 5.9). Thus the nutritional status or the physical status of the Toto is comparable with the international standard as a whole (Bhattacharya *et al.*, 2004).

**Table 5.9:** Distribution of body mass index among the Toto and the Bondo

| Index Values | Male | | Female | |
|---|---|---|---|---|
| | *Toto n=86* | *Bondo n=68* | *Toto n=77* | *Bondo n=94* |
| < 16.0 | 0 | 4.41 | 1.3 | 8.51 |
| 16.0 – <17.0 | 0 | 11.77 | | 11.7 |
| 17.0 – <18.5 | 3.49 | 35.29 | 0 | 11.7 |
| 18.5 – <25.0 | 94.19 | 48.53 | 98.7 | 65.96 |
| 25.0 – <30.0 | 2.32 | 0 | 0 | 2.13 |
| 30.0 – <40.0 | 0 | 0 | 0 | 0 |
| Total | 100 | 100 | 100 | 100 |

Rao (1995), was of the opinion that 80 per cent and above weight for height can be inferred as normal state of nutrition. Below 80 is graded into different types of malnutrition. Over 120 per cent is stated to be obese. If we consider 80 per cent and above weight for height as normal, we will observe that only seven percent male and 1.3 per cent female of the Toto are in under nourished state, which can be considered as negligible. In case of the Bondo, as high as 65 per cent male and one fourth of the females are grossly undernourished. Almost half (48%) of the Bondo female are in marginal malnourished state, having weight for height, values between 80 to less than 90 per cent of the standard. Thus, three-fourth of the Bondo female are in unsatisfactory state of nutrition, while two-third male are grossly malnourished (Bhattacharyya, 2004; see Table 5.9).

Bhattacharya *et al.* (2004) concluded from their study that the Bondo tribal population of Orissa is in alarming stage of malnutrition while the Toto of West Bengal is better nutritionally as compared to many caste populations.

In an earlier study Sharma (1979) reported on the nutritional status of the Konds of Orissa. The study was conducted on the Konds (also spelled as Khonds) of three villages covering 51 households of Sagada range of Orissa of Kalahandi district. The study covered the morphological characteristics and body composition of the Konds with special reference to nutrition, fertility, mortality and morbidity studies. The nutritional study on Konds was based on diet survey, food and food habits. He concluded from his study that Kond diet is inadequate according to the accepted standards. Its deficiencies are both qualitative as well as quantitative. Such an inadequate diet is reflected in the wide prevalence of under-nutrition and or malnutrition in the Konds (Sharma, 1979:44-45).

Ghoshmaulik and Karmahapatra (1995) reported on the health situation of the Juangs of Keonjhar district of Orissa. The Juang is a primitive tribe of Orissa. The study reports on the nutritional intake, physique, haemoglobin concentration, arterial blood pressure and some observable diseases and sickness, and the socio-economic conditions of the Juangs. Their study present a dismal picture of nutritional intake by the Juangs. They observed that the nutritional intake has resulted in under nourishment of 50 per cent of the Juang children, and further 4 per cent of them are in Grade IV. Weight and height measurements of 361 Juangs (below 18 years = 79; and between 18 to 30 years = 282 individuals) have been taken to estimate the body mass index (BMI). Table 5.10 gives the values reported by Ghoshmaulik and Karmahapatra (1995) on the body mass index of the Juangs. Table 5.10

suggest that 65 per cent of the Juangs of the study area possess very lean physique devoid of any fat, only 3 per cent of them show sturdy body with tendency to get fatty. Thus the nutritional intake of the Juangs has made them undernourished.

**Table 5.10:** Body Mass Index (BMI) of the Juangs of Keonjhar

| *BMI* | *Sex* | *< 18 yrs.* | *> 18 yrs.* | *Total (Male + Female)* | |
|---|---|---|---|---|---|
| | | | | Abs. | (%) |
| 20 | Male | 43 | 81 | 235 | 65.1 |
| | Female | 27 | 84 | | |
| 20-24 (Normal) | Male | 3 | 64 | 115 | 31.8 |
| | Female | 46 | 42 | | |
| 25-29 | Male | 0 | 6 | 11 | 3.5 |
| | Female | 0 | 5 | | |
| Male + Female | | 79 | 282 | 361 | 99.9 |

## *Madhya Pradesh*

Abujhmaria is a primitive tribe of Chattisgarh inhabiting Abujhmarh region of Bastar division. The area is covered with dense forest and hilly terrain. Mitra and Sahu (2004) presented a report on the health and nutrition of Abujhmaria school children. They considered that preschool children constitute the most vulnerable segment of the population and their nutritional status is considered to be a sensitive indicator in community health and nutrition. The objective of the investigation by Mitra and Sahu was first to identify and describe the types and frequencies of malnutrition prevalent among Abujhmaria preschool children and the second objective was to analyze the impact of ICDS services, if any, on nutritional and health status of the Abujhmaria children.

Nutrition and health status of Abujhmaria preschool children residing in twenty villages of Abujhmarh were conducted during the year 2002 by the authors. The result of their investigations have been presented as follows. The authors have discussed and analysed the nutritional status of the Abujhmaria children based on the following indices suggested by Jelliffe (1966), Visweswara Rao and Singh (1970), Waterlow (1972), Ghosh and Tejaswini (1976) and Waterlow *et al.* (1977) for grading malnutrition. The NCHS growth standard was used as a reference to evaluate the nutritional status.

**Jelliffe's Index**

| | | | | | | |
|---|---|---|---|---|---|---|
| **1. (a) ICDS** | | | | | | |
| Normal | 54 | 32.34 | 62 | 34.07 | 116 | 33.24 |
| Grade–I | 45 | 26.95 | 56 | 30.77 | 101 | 28.94 |
| Grade–II | 38 | 22.75 | 36 | 19.78 | 74 | 21.20 |
| Grade–III | 30 | 17.96 | 28 | 15.38 | 58 | 16.62 |
| *Total* | 167 | 100.00 | 182 | 100.00 | 349 | 100.00 |
| **(b) Non–ICDS** | | | | | | |
| Normal | 42 | 21.97 | 51 | 29.31 | 93 | 25.41 |
| Grade–I | 58 | 30.21 | 53 | 30.46 | 111 | 30.33 |
| Grade–II | 45 | 23.44 | 49 | 28.16 | 94 | 25.68 |
| Grade–III | 47 | 24.48 | 21 | 12.07 | 68 | 18.58 |
| *Total* | 102 | 100 | 174 | 100 | 366 | 100.00 |
| ***Grand Total*** | | | | | | |
| Normal | 96 | 26.74 | 113 | 31.74 | 209 | 29.23 |
| Grade–I | 103 | 28.69 | 109 | 30.62 | 212 | 29.65 |
| Grade–II | 83 | 23.12 | 85 | 23.88 | 168 | 23.5 |
| Grade–III | 77 | 21.45 | 49 | 13.76 | 126 | 17.62 |
| *Total* | 359 | 100 | 356 | 100 | 715 | 100.00 |

**Waterlow's Index**

| | | | | | | |
|---|---|---|---|---|---|---|
| **2. (a) ICDS** | | | | | | |
| Normal | 74 | 44.31 | 68 | 37.36 | 142 | 40.69 |
| Grade – I | 32 | 19.16 | 57 | 31.32 | 89 | 25.50 |
| Grade – II | 39 | 23.35 | 38 | 20.88 | 77 | 22.06 |
| Grade – III | 22 | 13.18 | 19 | 10.44 | 41 | 11.75 |
| Total | 167 | 100.00 | 182 | 100.00 | 349 | 100.00 |
| **(b) Non–ICDS** | | | | | | |
| Normal | 69 | 35.94 | 61 | 35.06 | 130 | 35.52 |
| Grade – I | 52 | 27.08 | 63 | 36.21 | 115 | 31.42 |
| Grade – II | 41 | 21.35 | 26 | 14.94 | 67 | 18.31 |
| Grade – III | 30 | 15.63 | 24 | 13.79 | 54 | 14.75 |
| Total | 192 | 100.00 | 174 | 100.00 | 366 | 100.00 |

*Source*: Mitra and Sahu, 2004 (unpublished manuscript, in press)

Mitra and Sahu (2004) found that the most satisfactory method of nutritional grading is based on expressing observed weight of a child as a percentage of normal weight for his/her chronological age. Using weight deficit method of Jelliffe as a tool for nutritional grading it was observed that prevalence of protein calorie malnutrition (PCM) among Abujhmaria children is mostly of mild to moderate type. ICDS children had better nutritional status than non-ICDS children. Chi-square value show significant difference between the ICDS and non-ICDS children for various grades of malnutrition ($\chi^2 = 5.28$; d.f. = 1; $0.20 > p > 0.10$).

Gangopadhyay (2004) in her study on the Kamar of Raipur district of Chattisgarh (formerly Madhya Pradesh) found a grim picture of the nutritional status of the community. Their diet is deficient in all most all the nutrients excepting iron, the consumption of which is at nearly satisfactory level. The anthropometric data also supports the result of diet survey by representing poor body build through various indices. The value of Pignet's index and Weight-Height index of both males and females indicate poor physical status of the population. Mean body mass index also indicate that the population is mildly "undernourished". The nutritional status of the Kamar has been presented through Table 5.11(a) and 5.11(b).

**Table 5.11(a):** Nuritional indices among the Kamar male (n= 50) of Raipur

| *Characters* | *Mean* | ± | *S.E.* | *S.D.* |
|---|---|---|---|---|
| Body Mass Index | 7.9 | ± | 0.22 | 1.59 |
| Weight/Height Index | 28.6 | ± | 0.39 | 2.77 |
| Pignet's coefficient | 37.6 | ± | 0.91 | 6.41 |

**Table 5.11(b):** Nutritional indices among the Kamar female (n=50) of Raipur

| *Characters* | *Mean* | ± | *S.E.* | *S.D.* |
|---|---|---|---|---|
| Body Mass Index | 7.8 | ± | 0.25 | 1.74 |
| Weight/Height Index | 28.6 | ± | 0.39 | 2.77 |
| Pignet's coefficient | 26.4 | ± | 0.37 | 2.62 |

The Hill Korwa is one of the primitive tribes of Madhya Pradesh and Bihar (before bifurcation of the States on 15th November, 2000). Sharma and Mukherjee have reported on the nutritional status of the Hill Korwas of Surguja district of Madhya Pradesh (1995). The authors studied only the age independent parameters, i.e. weight/height$^2$ (Rao and Singh, 1970) and mid-arm/head circumference (Kanawati and Mclaren, 1970). Their observations are as follows:

**Table 5.12:** Nutritional Assessment of the Hill Korwa Children by Age Independent Ratios

| *Number of Children (1 to 10 years)* | *Weight/Height$^2$* | | *Mid-arm/Head circumference* | |
|---|---|---|---|---|
| | *< 0.0015* | *> 0.0015* | *< 0.310* | *> 0.310* |
| Male (n = 107) % | 75.70 | 24.30 | 65.40 | 34.60 |
| Abs. | 81 | 26 | 70 | 37 |
| Female (n = 77) % | 89.60 | 10.40 | 49.20 | 20.80 |
| Abs. | 69 | 8 | 71 | 16 |
| Total (n = 184) % | 81.50 | 18.50 | 71.20 | 28.80 |
| Abs. | 150 | 34 | 131 | 53 |

Reliability of such age independent parameters have been established by several studies for understanding the magnitude and dimension of malnutrition, especially among rural/tribal populations where it is difficult to estimate the correct age (Gupta *et al.*, 1979, 1981). The weight/height$^2$ ratio among the Hill Korwa suggest that 81.50 per cent children are malnourished whereas midarm circumference/head circumference ratio suggest 71.20 per cent of Hill Korwa children are malnourished.

## Conclusion

Extensive investigations have been done by anthropologists on diet surveys and nutritional anthropometry which have contributed significantly in the understanding of the nutritional status of the tribal populations of India who are living in different ecological set-up which in many ways differ from the general population of the country. The present paper reflects the nutritional status of some of the tribal groups with particular reference to the states of Jharkhand (part of Bihar), Orissa, Madhya Pradesh (including Chattisgarh of the present), and West Bengal. Most of the tribes mentioned in the paper, namely, Abujhmaria, Asur, Korwa, Sauria, Paharia, Birhor, Kamar, Hill Korwa, Bondo, Toto, Juangs and Kharwar are primitives tribes of India, excepting the Santhals (Santals), Ho, and the Oraons, who are settled agricultural tribal populations. In the present paper no comparative study has been done on the nutritional status of the tribes, as different authors have estimated the nutritional status of the tribes following different classificatory methods. However, one thing clearly transpires from this general review that there is an alarming state of malnutrition among the tribes of India in general, and particularly among the primitive tribes of India.

We have yet to see what the government thinks about this situation and what are the plans and the programmes of the authorities to mitigate the sufferings of the primitive tribal groups and to elevate their nutritional status so that they can live without hunger. Authorities must not think that they are still surviving, as they are breathing, and be happy about it.

## REFERENCES

Acharya, P.K. (2003): Maternal factors and nutritional status of preschool children. *Man in India*, 83 (1&2): 109-119.

Bardhan, A., S.K. Sinha, K. Gopinath and A.K. Brahmbhatt (1989): A diagnostic study of factors responsible for lesser or no utilisation of health facilities among the Bhills of Madhya Pradesh. PAC Report (Mimeographed). National Institute of Health and Family Welfare: New Delhi.

Basu, Salil (1986): Genetic, socio-cultural and health care among tribal groups of Jagdalpur and Konta tehsils of Bastar district (Madhya Pradesh). In: A.K. Kalla and K. S. Singh (eds.) *Anthropology, Development and Nation Building*, pp. 87-105. Concept Publishing Company: New Delhi.

Basu, Salil (1993): Health scenario and health problems of the tribal population in India. In: Mrinal Miri (ed.), *Continuity and Change in Tribal Society*. Indian Institute of Advance Study: Shimla

Basu, Salil (1996): Need for action research for health development among tribal communities in India. *South Asian Anthropologist*, 17(2): 73-80.

Bhattacharyya, A.K. (1995): Summary of a Lecture delivered before the Participants of the Referesher Course for Junior Level Scientific Officers of the Anthropological Survey of India, Eastern Regional Centre, Calcutta on 31 March, 1995. *(Lecture Topic, pp. 1-6, Memiographed).*

Bhattacharya, K.K. (1995): Nutritional status of Oraons of Sunderban, West Bengal. *South Asian Anthropologist*, 16: 99-104.

Bhattacharya, K.K., S.K. Biswas and J.K. Roy (1972): Studies on diet, body build and some aspects of infant nutrition: Kharwars of Palamau district in Bihar. *Bull. Anthropological Survey of India*, 21: 69-78.

Bhattacharya, K.K., M. Maque and T.K. Biswas (2004): Nutritional status of two primitive tribes of Eastern India. In: P.Dash Sharma (ed.), *Anthropology of Primitive Tribes of India*, Serials Publications: Delhi (in press).

Bulliyya, Gandham (2003): Secular deterioration in nutritional status of young children: An alarming menace for the state of Orissa. *Man in India*, 83(1&2):49-71.

Cowan, G.O. and B.J. Heap (1993): *Clinical Tropical Medicine*. (First edition). Chapman & Hall: London.

Gangopadhyay, Shampa (2004): Nutritional status of the Kamar of Madhya Pradesh. In: P.Dash Sharma (ed.), *Anthropology of Primitive Tribes of India*, Serials Publications: Delhi (in press).

Ghosh and T.Tejaswini (1976): Quick nutritional screening by mid-arm circumference or a bangle. *Ind. Pediatrics,* 12:15.

Ghoshmaulik, S.K. and R.K. Karmahapatra (1995): Health situation of the Juangs of Orissa. *South Asian Anthropologist,* 16:79-83.

Government of India (1989): Report of the Working Group on Development and Welfare of Scheduled Tribes during Eight Five Year Plan (1990-1995). Government of India, Ministry of Welfare (November 1989): New Delhi.

Gupta, Satya Prakash (1974): *Tribes of Chotanagpur Plateau: An Ethno-nutritional and Pharmacological Cross-section.* Bihar Tribal Welfare Research Institute (Government of Bihar, Welfare Department): Ranchi.

Gupta, S.K., S.K. Chaturvedi and R.C. Gupta (1979): Weight/height$^2$ ratio in assessment of protein calorie malnutrition. *Indian Journal of Paediatrics,* 46: 187-190.

Gupta, K., B.N.S. Walia and A. Narang (1981): An evidence of age independent anthropometric parameters for the assessment of protein calorie malnutrition. *Child Health,* 23: 5-10.

Jelliffe, Derrick B. (1966): *The Assessment of the Nutritional Status of the Community* (with special reference to field surveys in developing regions of the world). World Health Organization: Geneva.

Johnston, F.E. (1987): *Nutritional Anthropology*. Alan Liss Inc., New York, pp. 288. (*cf.* Gangopadhyay, 2004a)

Kanawati, A.R. and D.S. Mclaren (1970): Assessment of marginal malnutrition. *Nature*, 228:573.

Keys. A., J. Brozek, A. Henscheb, O. Michelsen and S.L. Taylor (1950): *The Biology of Human Starvation.* University of Minnesota Press: Minneapolis.

Lal, S.B. (1954): Changes in dietary habits and physique of aboriginals of Santal Parganas, a district of Bihar. *Ind. J. Med. Res.,* 42(2): 167-179.

Mitra, K. (1940): Investigations into the dietary and physique of aboriginals in Santal Parganas, a district of Bihar. *Ind. J. Med. Res.,* 28(1): 117-132.

Mitra, Mitashree and Narayan Sahu (2004): Nutritional status of Abhujmaria preschool children. In: P.Dash Sharma (ed.), *Anthropology of Primitive Tribes in India*. Serials Publications: New Delhi (in press).

NCHS (1976): National Center for Health Statistics Growth Curves for Children 0-18 Years. *United States, DHEW Publication No. (PHS) Series 11 (165) 78-1650, Rockville,* MD. 22-29.

NNMB (2000): National Nutrition Monitoring Bureau. Diet and Nutritional Status of Tribal Populations. Report on First Repeat Surveys, Hyderabad, pp. 1-24. National institute of Nutrition: Hysderabad.

Rizvi, S.N.H. (1986): Health practices of the Jaunsaries: A socio-cultural analysis. In: B.Chaudhuri (ed.), *Tribal Health: Socio-Cultural Dimensions*, pp. 223-246. Inter-India Publications: New Delhi.

Roy, B.C. and S.K. Roy (1982): *Hunger and Physique*. Memoir No. 55. Anthropological Survey of India: Calcutta.

Roy Burman, B.K. (1986): Morbidity and nutritional status of the scheduled tribes of India. In: B.Chaudhuri (ed.), *Tribal Health: Socio-Cultural Dimensions*, pp. 85-98. Inter-India Publications: New Delhi.

Sharma, K.K.N. and B.M. Mukherjee (1995): Nutritional status among the tribal Hill Korwa children of Madhya Pradesh. *South Asian Anthropologist*, 16: 95-98.

Sengupta, N.K. (1988): A note on the survey and investigation on some physical conditions and nutritional patterns in relation to the tribal people in Singhbhum. *Man in India*, 68(4): 473-476.

Sharma, Krishan (1979): *The Konds of Orissa: An Anthropometric Study*. Concept Publishing Company: New Delhi.

Swain, S.S.C. Jena and P. Singh (1990): Morbidity status of the Khond tribe of Phulbani (Orissa). In: B.Chaudhuri (ed.), *Cultural and Environmental Dimensions of Health*, pp. 177-191. Inter-India Publications: New Delhi.

Vijayaraghavan, K., Darshan Singh and M.C. Swaminathan (1971): Heights and weights of well-nourished Indian children. *Indian J. Med. Res.*, 59: 643.

Visweswara Rao, K. (1955): Anthropometry for the assessment of various forms of malnutrition— available approaches and their relative merits. *Man in India*, 75(2): 195-207.

Visweswara Rao, K. and D. Singh (1970): An evaluation of the relationship between nutritional status and anthropometric measurements. *American Journal of Clinical Nutrition*, 23:83-93.

Visweswara Rao, K. (1979): Validity of some clinical signs as early indicators of PCM in preschool children. *Indian Journal of Medical Research*. 67: 779-785.

Visweswara Rao, K. (1980): Efficiency of anthropometric indices for the diagnosis of malnutrition. *Courier*, 30: 113-121.

Visweswara Rao, K., G. Radhaiah, S.V.S. Raju, M.C. Swaminathan (1981): Relative importance of various anthropometric measurements and indices for an evaluation of nutritional status. *Indian Pediatrics*, 18: 223-231.

Visweswara Rao, K., N. Balakrishna and K. Adinarayana (1986): Critical limits of some anthropometric measurements and indices for the assessment of the nutritional status of preschool children. *Indian Journal of Nutrition and Dietetics*, 23:88-89.

# 6

# Anthropometric Measurement to Monitor Growth of Tribal School Going Children

SUMAN SINGH GUSAIN

## Introduction

Children are a critical resource whose growth and well-being will determine to a large extent the course of a country socio-economic and demographic future. Therefore appraisal of the progress of a country in the field of health can be made from time to time with the help of growth studies. The use of anthropometric measurement as a health indicators is becoming more important and practicable. To assess the growth and development pattern of local regions, a multi-country study was initiated by World Health Organisation (WHO, 1985).

A number of growth studies in India reveal that the height and weight of poor socio-economic group fall below the third percentile value of children (Gopalan, 1968). As a part of this initiate the growth and development of school going children was assessed in a tribal area of District Udham Singh Nagar.

Aykroyd and Rajgopal (1936), Wilson and Mitra (1938), Majumdar and Bahadur (1951), Majumdar (1958), Singh (1969, 1970), Mukerji and Kaul (1970), Nath (1972), Sikri (1972), Gupta *et al.* (1973, 1974), Bhandari *et al.* (1975), Malik and Singh (1978), ICMR (1989), Nath, Sachdeva and Chauhan (1991) and many others have stressed primarily on height weight studies including the socio-economic status and nutritional aspects in different part of the country.

The present study has been conducted on Tharu (boys and girls) in the age range of 5 to 14 years with a view to observe the growth pattern among tribal children as well as sexual diamorphism among them. Tharus are the second largest of the five Schedule Tribes of the newly state Uttaranchal. They are spread over a vast tract between Tanakpur and Kashipur. Though, Tharus are found in many state of India. They inhabit Udham Singh Nagar (Khatima and Sitarganj tehsil); Lakhimpur Khiri, Gonda, Bahraich and Gorakhpur in Uttar Pradesh; Champaran and Darbhanga districts of Bihar; their total population was 1,18,558 only (According to 1991 censes). Tharus are usually short statured, yellow complexioned, broad faced and plane nosed people showing lot of signs of mongoloid racial stock.

## Material and Methods

The present study is based on 400 school going children (200 boys and 200 girls) in the age range 5 to 14 years. All the subject belong to primary and high schools of Sidha, Balkhera, Piplia-Pistor and Sundar Nagar situated in tribal settlement area of Sitarganj Tehsil of District U.S. Nagar in a newly formed state of Uttaranchal. The subjects were measured for height and body weight in accordance with the standard measurement techniques recommended by Martin and Saller (1959) with modification suggested by Winner and Laurie (1969). Each subject's age was recorded from the subject and verified from the school records. While formulating age categories, age group five included all those subject who have completed 4 ½ year age and are up to 5 ½ (5 years 5 months 30 days). Thereby providing us average age as 5-0 years and so on up to 14 years.

## Result and Discussion

Variation in mean height and weight of the tribal school going children (boys and girls) have been presented in Tables 6.1 and 6.2. It is observed that the girls are taller than the boys at 5, 6 and 13 years while at remaining ages the boys are taller. In order to assess the sex differences, t-test has been applied which reveals that the apparent differences in the mean height differ significantly at 9 to 11 years while at remaining ages the sex differences are not significant (Table 6.1).

**Table 6.1:** Mean Height of School going Children in Tharu Tribe of U.S. Nagar

| *Age in Years* | *Nos.* | *Mean Height of School Going Children* | | | | | | *t-test* |
|---|---|---|---|---|---|---|---|---|
| | | *Boys* | | | *Girls* | | | |
| | | *Mean* | *S.D.* | *S.E.* | *Mean* | *S.D.* | *S. E.* | |
| 5 | 20 | 111.5 | 5.4 | 1.21 | 112.5 | 8.4 | 1.88 | 0.45 |
| 6 | 20 | 116.9 | 5.9 | 1.32 | 119.7 | 7.3 | 1.63 | 1.34 |
| 7 | 20 | 122.1 | 4.1 | 0.92 | 121.5 | 4.4 | 0.98 | 0.45 |
| 8 | 20 | 128.8 | 3.1 | 0.69 | 126.8 | 4.3 | 0.96 | 1.69 |
| 9 | 20 | 130.7 | 2.5 | 0.56 | 127.3 | 1.2 | 0.27 | 5.48* |
| 10 | 20 | 134.7 | 1.8 | 0.40 | 129.8 | 1.4 | 0.31 | 9.60* |
| 11 | 20 | 135.4 | 2.2 | 0.49 | 133.2 | 2.6 | 0.58 | 2.89* |
| 12 | 20 | 137.8 | 2.8 | 0.63 | 136.3 | 7.1 | 1.59 | 0.89 |
| 13 | 20 | 142.6 | 4.9 | 1.09 | 142.9 | 1.0 | 0.22 | 0.27 |
| 14 | 20 | 146.8 | 3.7 | 0.83 | 144.5 | 5.7 | 1.27 | 1.51 |

* Significant at 5 per cent level.

**Table 6.2:** Mean Weight of School going Children in Tharu Tribe of U.S. Nagar

| *Age in Years* | *Nos.* | *Mean Weight of School Going Children* | | | | | | *t-test* |
|---|---|---|---|---|---|---|---|---|
| | | *Boys* | | | *Girls* | | | |
| | | *Mean* | *S.D.* | *S.E.* | *Mean* | *S.D.* | *S.E.* | |
| 5 | 20 | 14.0 | 1.5 | 0.33 | 15.3 | 2.5 | 0.56 | 2.00* |
| 6 | 20 | 17.8 | 3.4 | 0.76 | 18.9 | 3.5 | 0.78 | 1.02 |
| 7 | 20 | 19.7 | 1.5 | 0.33 | 19.2 | 1.4 | 0.31 | 1.10 |
| 8 | 20 | 22.4 | 2.3 | 0.51 | 21.3 | 5.3 | 0.74 | 1.23 |
| 9 | 20 | 23.8 | 1.9 | 0.42 | 22.4 | 1.6 | 0.36 | 2.54* |
| 10 | 20 | 24.1 | 1.3 | 0.29 | 23.6 | 2.3 | 0.51 | 0.85 |
| 11 | 20 | 24.8 | 1.8 | 0.40 | 25.6 | 1.6 | 0.36 | 1.48 |
| 12 | 20 | 25.8 | 2.1 | 0.47 | 27.0 | 3.4 | 0.76 | 1.35 |
| 13 | 20 | 27.1 | 2.8 | 0.63 | 28.3 | 3.2 | 0.71 | 1.26 |
| 14 | 20 | 34.1 | 3.9 | 0.87 | 30.6 | 2.8 | 0.63 | 3.27* |

* Significant at 5 per cent level.

It is further observed that boys are heavier than the girls at 7 to 10 and 14 years, while at remaining age the girls are heavier. To assess the sex differences, t-test was applied which reveals that the apparent differences in the mean weight of boys and girls differ significantly at

5, 8 and 14 years while at remaining ages, the sex differences are non-significant.

## Summary

It may be concluded from the present study that the Tharu children (boys and girls) do not exhibit much variation in their height and weight during 5 to 14 years of age as the sex differences in both the body dimensions are by and large non significant at most of the age groups.

It is also observed that the apparent differences in height are more pronounced at ages 8 to 14 years except at 13 years where the girls outgrow the boys. While in case of body weight, a reverse trend is witnessed as the girls are by and large heavier that the boys from 11 to 13 years while at 14 the differences are highly pronounced.

These variations could be due to nutritional variation as the food intake between males and females of any population varies with females being more diet conscious than males.

## REFERENCES

Aykroyd, W.B and Rajgopal, K. (1936): The state of nutrition of school children in South Indian (part-1): *Ind. Jour. Med. Res.* 24: 419-37.

Bhandari, B., Jain, A.M. *et al.* (1975): Nutritional and health status of rural school boys of Udaypur District: *Ind. Jour. Pediatrices* 42:186.

Gopalan, C. (1968): Health problem in pre-school children: Worldwide experience special problem and preventive programmes–1, India. *J. Trop. Ped.*, 14. 228-232.

Gupta, V.M., Murthy, N.S. *et al.* (1974): Correlation study of weight height and mid-upper arm circumference in infant: Ind. *Jour. Med. Res.* 62: 1678-1681.

Gupta, M., Agrawal, K.N. and Manuwari, A.H. (1973): Nutritional status of preschool children, *Ind. Peds.* 19:81.

I.C.M.R. (1989): Growth and physical development of Indian infant and children. *I.C.M.R. Technical report series No. 18*, New Delhi.

Majumdar, D.N. and Bahadur, S. (1951): Anthropological study of growth among school children in Lucknow. *Eastern Anthropologist*: 1-26.

Majumdar, D.N. (1958): Differences between the morning and evening measurement of stature; *Sankhya*; 19, 296-298.

Malik, S.L., Singh, I.P. (1978): Growth trends among Bods of Ladakh—a high altitude population. *Amer. Jour. Physical Anthropo.* 48 (2) 171.

Mitra, D.D. (1939): A study of diet and nutrition in North Bengal, upper Assam and Calcutta: *Ind. Jour. of Med. Res.* 27: 441-450.

Mukherji, B. and Kaul, K.K. (1970): Anthropometrics observation on urban primary school children. *Ind. Jour. of Med. Res.* 58:1257-1271.

Nath, S. (1972): A study of age change of different biological variable in the Jat. Boys of Meerut, U.P. Ph.D. Thesis University of Delhi. Delhi (Unpublished).

Nath, S. Sachdeva, V. Chauhan (1991): progression of maturation sequence in stature and liner measures of extremities and sex differences among Lodhan of Bengal. *Ind. Jour. Phy. Anthro. and Hum. Gen.* 17:205-218.

Singh, R. (1970): A cross-sectional study of growth in five somatometric traits of Punjabi boys aged 11-18 years; *Ameri. Jour. Phys. Anthrop.* 32:129-138.

Vijayaraghavan, K. (1976): Growth and development of Indian children, *Indian J. Phisiol. and Pharma col.*, 20. 26p-276.

W.H.O. document (1985): MCH/MNH 86.1.

# 7

# Risk Factor of HIV/AIDS among Tribals in India

MRIDULA PALIWAL

## Introduction

India has the dubious distinction of being the country with the largest number of HIV infection (according to G.V., Satyawati Director of ICMR). The deadly HIV/AIDS disease is dangerously spreading among the tribal areas due to the lack of awareness. The people in the rural and tribal areas are unaware about the diseases and mode of its transmission. The most dangerous aspect of the problem is that people do not disclose their problems and thus a large number of HIV positive cases remain unreported. The role of the health department to help detect the exact number of HIV infected people is also faulty.

According to UNAIDS programme, HIV estimate among tribal is believed to be 0.1 per cent of the adult population, i.e. 70,000–80,000. At the national level, among the reported cases of HIV, the most common modes of transmission are heterosexual transmission, blood and blood products, homosexual transmission, infected drug use and MCT. The reality of HIV/AIDS among tribal in India is now raising its head.

The tribal population group form 8 per cent of the total population of India. These tribal groups inhabit widely varying ecological and geo-climatic conditions in different concentrations throughout the country and are distinct biological isolates with characteristic cultural and socio-economic background. Tribal groups are homogenous, culturally firm and have developed strong magico-religious health care system.

The highest number of tribes is represented by the State of Orissa (62) and the lowest of Sikkim (2). The largest tribal population around 15.4 million reside in M.P. 74 primitive tribal communities have been identified. The literacy among the Tribal is very low (25.9%) specially so among the tribal female (14.5) (NASSO) 1991. The lowest level of the literacy among females was found in Rajasthan.

**Dimensions of Tribal Health in India**

The culture of the community determines the health behaviour of the community in general and individual members in particular. The health behaviour of the individual is closely linked to the way he or she perceive various health problem alongwith access to various health care institution.

Primitive tribal group in India have special health problem and genetic abnormalities like sickle cell aneimia, G-6-PD red cell enzyme deficiency and STD. *Insanitary condition, ignorance, lack of personal hygiene and health education* are the main factors responsible for a majority of health problems.

Some of the problems indicated by investigations in tribal areas include:

(a) Endemic diseases like malaria, introduced from outside or otherwise like TB, influenza, dysentery, high infant mortality and malnutrition. These diseases also reflect that there can exist possibility of HIV infection as TB and STD are found in great number among the tribals.

(b) Venereal disease include abortion, inbreeding, addiction to opium, custom of eating tubers of DIOSCERA (may cause steritity as it contain substances used in oral contraception).

(c) Nutrition, anaemia is a major problem for women in India and more so in the rural and tribal belt. Anaemia lowers resistance to fatigue, affects working capacity under conditions of stress and increases susceptibility to other diseases. Tribal diets are generally grossly deficient in calcium, vitamin A, B, C riboflavin and animal protein.

Similarly *crude birth practices* were found to exist in some tribal groups like Kharias, Gonds, Santals, Kutia Khondhs of Orissa, Santals, Jaunsaries, and Kharias, etc. More than 90 per cent of deliveries are conducted at home attended by elderly ladies of the household. No specific precautions are observed at the time of conducting deliveries, which resulted in an increased susceptibility to various infections. These practices also increase the risk of mother to child Transmission of disease like HIV/AIDS.

Sexually transmitted diseases are most prevalent diseases in the tribal areas. VDRL was found to be positive in 17-12 per cent cases (reactive in dilution of 1.8 or more) of *polyandrous Jaunsaris* of Chakrata, Dehradun. Out of 17 per cent, 9.92 per cent was found among males and 7.19 per cent among females. Among Santals of Mayurbhanj Distt. Orissa 8.90 per cent cases of VDRL were observed, out of which 4.99 per cent were females and 3.91 per cent were males.

Malnutrition was common and greatly affected the ability to resist infection, leading to chronic illness and the post weaning period leading to permanent brain impairment. A high incidence of malnutrition was observed in some primitive tribal groups in Phulbani, Koraput and Sundergarh districts of Orissa and also among Bhils and Garasia of Rajasthan and Padars, Rabrig, and Charans of Gujarat and Bondas of Orissa.

## Health, Indigenous Knowledge System and Herbal Treatment of HIV/AIDS

Proper nutrition is the best frontline drug for AIDS and nutritional deficiency in part contribute to the more rapid onset of AIDS among HIV positive people in all the area. For to restricting the spread of epidemic among the already torned tribal groups, their nutritional level, hygienic condition and other health improving measures have to be undertaken besides reducing susceptibility of infection to Malaria, TB, STD which can further increase the risk of HIV among the tribal population.

In the various areas, herbal therapies is widely in use by HIV positive people. Among the tribal where modern medicine system is not in full-fledge, the people primarily take indigenous herbal medicine at the time of need. *Cadres of traditional health practitioners, spiritualists, birth attendants and herbalists* are found in every village, in poor urban neighbourhood, and in tribal areas.

The traditional health providers have a high degree of credibility and are usually the first source of help sought by individuals when they become ill. And the risk of infection on HIV/AIDS can be reduced by imparting awareness, knowledge and preventive measures through these traditional health practitioners, spiritualist, birth attendants, traditional midwives and herbalists as these are the integral part of the tribal's traditional culture.

Tribal health providers have herbal medicine for every common health problem. These herbal therapies may be effective in curing certain of the opportunistic infections that come with AIDS. Perhaps some of the herbal therapies have some of the anti-retroviral qualities for, e.g. Turmeric a naturally occurring spice has shown promise. Tribals also use Keezhanelli, a common weed in Tamil Nadu in South India, for centuries as a treatment of Hepatitis A (for this Dr. Sumit Solomon, Director of the Y.R.G. centre for AIDS research and education in Chennai took a sample of Keezhanelli to St. Michaels Hospital in London for chemical analysis). The chemical analysis result showed that Keezhanelli had some antiretroviral properties as a reverse transcriptase.

In the tribal areas, tradition healers are better positioned than medical doctors to care for the patients. As they can dispense herbal medicine to reduce opportunistic infections and to boost up the immune system of those who are HIV positive and can serve as caring counselors. The cost of consultation with a traditional healer and the price of herbal drugs are relatively low. Further traditional healers are perceived as being more approachable, informal, and community centered that are medical doctors as the doctor patient relationship is often hierarchical, depersonalized, and governed by bio chemical principles.

So far as the diagnosis of the disease is concerned, the tribal face great difficulty, particularly when they are confronted with any thing different from the common diseases of every day occurrence. Due to this, many opportunistic infection like STI and STD are not reported as sometime tribal relate them with supernatural power, or with any mystic figure.

## Cultural Practices and Risk of HIV

India is an ancient country with multi dimensional culture. In tribal societies, cultural values prescribed provide opportunities on social relation, through the institution of *marriage, youth dormitories,* etc. The youth dormitories play a very important role in relation to the health of the tribal, on the one hand it gives sex related behaviour education, on the other hand it also bring a platform for the risk of STD. But this institution can be used in a better way to control the spread of HIV. Given the close relation of religions and culture, HIV is challenging traditional sexual customs. With the lower literacy rate among most of the tribal, the risk of HIV has increased. Various marriage practices also increase the risk of HIV/AIDS and other opportunistic infections.

*Marriage Practices*—The pattern of marriage in India is largely governed by three important regulations, namely (a) endogamy, (b) exogamy, (c) consanguineous or *sapinda* marriage.

There is a greater incidence of *consanguineous marriages* specially among the population of the southern states, Muslim groups, Parsees and various tribal communities. Consanguineous marriages may, however, result in an increased probability of abortions, miscarriage, stillbirths, neonatal deaths, and increase susceptibility to infectious diseases, etc. In Himalayan region, some of the tribes like Naga, Lusia, etc. practiced polygamy. On the other hand, some of the tribes in India practice polyandary for example Jaunsaris of Jaunsar-Bawar, Chakrata tehsil, Dehradun and Todas of Nilgiri hills. These types of marriage practices like polyandry, polygamy, etc. set tribal population at the risk of HIV/AIDS and STD infections. Among tribal, age at which the girl was given in marriage depend on social values. Furthermore, virginity was not very much valued. Many of the tribal societies were lax towards pre marital sex relations, which were considered as training in the art of love and sex life and often ended in marriage. This sets them on the risk of opportunistic infections. Jaunsaris were a polyandrous tribe and they followed the customs of child marriage as a part of their cultural behaviour, which was still prevalent among them. These cultural practices contribute to a continuous and physically draining fatigue. The risk is closely related to inappropriate care or poor hygiene in connection with child birth, abortion, etc. The presence of *STD* was reported from Jaunsaris of Chakrata, Dehradun, Santals of Mayurbhanj district Orissa, polyandrous Toda tribal group of Nilgiri hills, Desia Kondhs, Andamanese, tribal group of Madhya Pradesh, Rajasthan, Mysore, Laccadive and Minicoy islands.

These practices will need to be reformed in the light of the reality of AIDS, but as evidenced from the rest of the world, it will take time and much education to change their behaviour, which has been normative for so long.

With these cultural practices there are some other major risk factors for the tribal concerning HIV. These are:

1. Lack of HIV/AIDS knowledge.
2. Lack of access to HIV barrier contraceptives in the remote locality.
3. Migration which take men and women away from their homes sometimes more than six months at a time putting them at higher risk for engaging in unsafe sexual practices.
4. Stress of immigration, where generally uncertainty over the future leads to employment limitations which in turn may lead to drug and alcohol use.
5. Social approval for the use of alcohol and few drugs as a part of tradition and some time related with strong religious practices.
6. Expense and prejudices associated with the preventive measure of HIV such as related with condom.

The great default in the estimation of the HIV/AIDS cases is that the method of collecting the cases is standardized not as it is unable to reflect the real scenario of HIV/AIDS in India. The number of reported cases which were taken by NACO through SACS are not reliable as the centres or the hospitals which records the HIV/AIDS cases are very few and touch only the fringe of the population instead of whole population. The situation becomes worse when we know that the hospital which provide regular care for the HIV/AIDS patients are very few, although on papers patients can get health care in any hospital. Various hospitals refuse to admit HIV/AIDS patients. For example, in UP the recorded cases are only 1,083 in 2003 whereas according to an N.G.O. AWARE, and few members of UPSACS who were working on HIV/AIDS, there is the possibility of three lakhs patients in UP, which also has a sizeable population of tribal. The devil of HIV/AIDS is on increase in the state of UP, and UP is not counted in the category of high risk states like Tamil Nadu, Maharashtra, etc., With this we can imagine the condition of HIV/AIDS among tribal in the high risk states.

Further help provided for the HIV/AIDS patients is not enough for the urban population and so it is not difficult to imagine the picture of the rural and tribal areas. Moreover, the worse situation is that there is no specific programme running for tribals and in the coming days it would cause a serious stroke on the health status of the tribal as well as of the nation.

In the present scenario of HIV/AIDS in India, if we really want to restrict its spread we have to spread the knowledge of HIV/AIDS in all the groups and areas, and not only among those who are infected or come in the risk groups but also among those whose condition is vulnerable and due to this they can be easily gripped by the infection at any moment. With specific reference to the tribals who are governed by their own tradition, it is not an easy job to teach them about HIV/AIDS. As we can come in front of various cultural restraints, we have to use their specific cultural patterns for this task. This need a very serious step and effort. We can save tribal group, as the HIV/AIDS infection rate is very low among them. With the help of target intervention we can restrict the spread of HIV/AIDS among any group.

**HIV Epidemic in Various States/UTs in Four Stages**

| | | |
|---|---|---|
| A | Generalized epidemic<br>HIV prevalence among antenatal women as more than 5 per cent | Nil |
| B | Concentrated Epidemic-1<br>HIV prevalence among antenatal women as more than 1 per cent and less than 5 per cent | Maharastra, Karnataka, Andhra Pradesh, Tamil Nadu and Manipur |
| C | Concentrated Epidemic-2<br>HIV prevalence among antenatal women as less than 1 per cent | Gujarat, West Bengal, and Nagaland. |
| D | Low level epidemic<br>HIV prevalence among STD clinic attendees as less than 5 per cent | Punjab, Haryana, Himachal Pradesh, Chandigarh, Uttar Pradesh, Rajasthan, Orissa, Assam, Kerala, Meghalaya, Sikkim, Arunanchal Pradesh. |

## REFERENCES

Basu, S.K. (1993): *Tribal Health in India*, Manak Publisher, New Delhi.

Basu, S.K. (1993): *Tribal Health (in) Rural Health*, Nutritional Institute of Health and Family Welfare, New Delhi.

Bosh, A.B. (1970): Problems of education development of scheduled tribes, *Man in India,* Vol. L (1).

National Family Health Survey (NFHS-2) India 1998-99 International Institute for Population Sciences, Mumbai, India.

Patton Cindy, (2002) *Globalizing AIDS*, Theory out of bonds, Volume 22. University of Minnesota Press, Minneaplis, London.

Roy, Debubrata (2001) *Community action on HIV for Indian NGOs*, Voluntary Health Association of India 2001, Published by VHAI press.

Singhal Arvind, Evert M. Rogers, (2003): *Combating AIDS communication strategy in Action*, Sage Publications, New Delhi,Thousand Oaks, London.

# PART II

# DEMOGRAPHIC AND ECOLOGICAL ASPECTS OF TRIBAL HEALTH

# 8

# Ecology, Diet and Health Status among Tribes: A Study in Pasuvulabanda Village of Visakha Agency Area, Andhra Pradesh

V. SUBRAMANYAM

## Introduction

Recent surveys of Third World food needs, carried out by Food and Agriculture Organization (FAO) shows that hunger and malnutrition continue to be urgent problems throughout the underdeveloped countries including India. The main shortages are in protective foods—proteins, vitamins and minerals. Lot of debate is going on this issue especially in the third world countries. Studies on food science and technology are much felt need of the hour. Food technology is the bridge between economic activity of food production and nutrition. In the field of nutrition, efforts to define the nature, extent and consequences of malnutrition in various parts of the world are achieving some success in persuading government to plan their agricultural production in relation to nutritional needs.

Geographical and ecological conditions determine the availability of foods. Differences exist in climate, soil and relative abundance of food materials (meat or vegetables). Dietary habits are closely associated with ecological and cultural behaviour of a human group. Cultural influences on food preferences, beliefs about the properties of food and taboos and the social role of food in the family and community can all have important effects on food needs and provision (S.J. Atkinson, 1992). The influence of technology on food habits is also very strong. For instance presence or absence of efficient means for obtaining, transporting, processing, storing and preparing food has a significant effect upon nutrient content and consequently upon nutritional and health status. The nutritional problems can be derived from inborn errors of metabolism.

The tribal population in our country is mostly distributed in the forest zones of *eastern ghats*, western *ghats,* central, north eastern and *himalayan* mountains. The forest dwelling population in India is estimated around 48 million. Through ages, they have established symbiotic relationship with forests and adapted to such ecosystems. Some of the earlier studies on the problem revealed that the incidence of malnutrition is very high among the tribal population (Tiwari and Sharma, 1989). Nutritional deficiency diseases like kwashiorkar, endemic goiter, anaemia, pellagra and beriberi were prevalent among them. Other *manifestations* were pot bellied school children, small body sizes, underweight adolescents and short life spans. Another set of nutritional problems develop from unsanitary food supplies and water contamination, less calories of food in take, which have much reflections on the health status of tribes. The tropical disease malaria is still rampant in the tribal areas of India. Long sufferance from malnutrition added with chromic diseases definitely reduces working capacity among the tribals. Ultimately they may not able to contribute for the societal or national development.

The present research paper forms the part of UGC minor research project report entitled "Ecology of malnutrition in the agency area of Visakhapatnam; food resources, habits and deficiencies". This study was carried out in a tribal habitat called Pasuvulabanda of *Chintapalle Mandal*, selected purely on the basis of purposive sampling. Conventional anthropological methods were used to collect the empirical data and also secondary source of data were collected from ICDS unit *Chintapalle* and ITDA *Paderu.* The data was analysed manually with electronic calculator. The paper provides ecological and cultural back ground of tribes, population structure, tribal composition in the village, dietary habits, nutritional deficiencies and health disorders. It also explains the role of government established Nutritional Rehabilitation Centre (*Anganwadi school*) in elevating the nutritional and health status among tribals, and suggests the ways and means for the effective functioning of nutritional and health programmes in specific to the study villages and other tribal areas in general.

## About the Field Village

*Pasuvulabanda* is one of the revenue villages of *Chintapalle Mandal* of Visakhapatnam district. It is situated in the north-western side of Chintapalle. The distance between the village and the *Mandal* headquarters is about 5 kilometres, a *katcha* road connects the village from *Chintapalle.* This village consists of another seven hamlets, namely China *Kothuru*, *Valmikicolony*, *Veedhulabailu*, Samara *Veedhi*, *Gurugudem*, *Goyyalametta* and *Gadedalametta*. All these hamlets are scattered with in the radius of three kilometres. Each hamlet is surrounded by agricultural fields and forest. Except *Valmikicolony*, the other hamlets are situated on the foot hills of eastern ghats. Fruit bearing trees like Jack, Mango and Tamarind are commonly found in each hamlet. Each hamlet is considered as a habitat for single or several tribal groups.

## Tribal Composition in Pasuvulabanda

The entire revenue village consists of eight habitats including Pasuvulabanda. The main village inhabited by the tribes like *Bagata, Gadaba, Konda Kammara, Valmiki and Madiga* (Scheduled Caste). It is a multi-tribal settlement, where as the other hamlets are single tribe habitats. *Valmiki* colony is the settlement of *Valmiki* tribe, *Chinakotturu* is a *Khond* settlement, *Veedhulabailu* is inhabited by *Nooka Dora* tribe, *Goyyala Metta* is the *Bagata* settlement, *Samaraveedhi, Gurugudem,* and *Gadedala Metta* are the habitats of *Gadaba* tribe. A hamlet is very small in size, not exceeds more than 28 households.

## Population Structure

The entire revenue village consists of 158 households with total population of 775. Out of total population 390 (50.32%) are males and 385 (49.68%) are females. Table 8.1 shows the tribewise population in all eight settlements of Pasuvulabanda. From the table it is noted that males population is slightly higher than that of female population. In regard to population size in accordance to tribe/caste wise, *Gadaba* is numerically dominant, followed by *Nooka Dora, Bagata, Valmiki, Khond, Kondakammara* and *Madiga.*

Table 8.2 shows the age and sexwise population of the study village. Out of the total population, 25.29 per cent of them (both males

**Table 8.1:** Tribewise Distribution of Population in Pasuvulabanda Revenue Village

| SNo | Name of the Village/Hamlet | Name of the Tribe Caste | No.of House-holds | % to Total Households | Males | % to Total Population | Females | % to Total Population | Total Males and Females | % to Total Population |
|---|---|---|---|---|---|---|---|---|---|---|
| 1. | Pasuvulabanda (main village) | Bagata | 14 | 8.86 | 42 | 5.42 | 32 | 4.13 | 74 | 9.55 |
| | | Gadaba | 4 | 2.53 | 9 | 1.16 | 6 | 0.77 | 15 | 1.93 |
| | | Konda-kammara | 4 | 2.53 | 9 | 1.16 | 9 | 1.16 | 18 | 2.32 |
| | | Valmiki | 2 | 1.27 | 4 | 0.52 | 6 | 0.77 | 10 | 1.29 |
| | | Madiga | 4 | 2.53 | 9 | 1.16 | 8 | 1.03 | 17 | 2.14 |
| 2. | Valmiki colony | Valmiki | 22 | 13.93 | 44 | 5.68 | 43 | 5.55 | 87 | 11.23 |
| 3. | China Kotturu | Khond | 16 | 10.13 | 50 | 6.45 | 46 | 5.94 | 96 | 12.37 |
| 4. | Veedlula Bailu | Nooka Dora | 25 | 15.82 | 58 | 7.48 | 66. | 8.52 | 124 | 16.00 |
| 5. | Samara Veedhi | Gadaba | 26 | 16.46 | 60 | 7.74 | 62 | 8.00 | 122 | 15.74 |
| 6. | Gurugudem | Gadaba | 8 | 5.06 | 20 | 2.58 | 22 | 2.84 | 42 | 5.42 |
| 7. | Goyyalametta | Bagata | 8 | 5.06 | 21 | 2.71 | 20 | 2.58 | 41 | 5.29 |
| 8. | Gadedalametta | Gadaba | 25 | 15.82 | 64 | 8.26 | 65 | 8.39 | 129 | 16.65 |
| | | Total | 158 | 100.00 | 390 | 50.32 | 385 | 49.68 | 775 | 100.00 |

and females) are in the children age group of 0.1-10 years, 16.39 per cent of them are in the age group of 11-20 years, 16.90 per cent of them are in the age group of 16-25 years, 15-61 per cent of them are in the age group of 26-35 years, 19.36 per cent of them are in the age group of 36-45 years, 8.90 per cent of them are in the age group of 46-50 years, 2.32 per cent of them are in the age group of 51-55 years, 1.16 per cent of them are in the age group of 56-60 years and only 0.65 per cent them are in the age group of 61 and above years. It is noted from the table that percentage of aged people among tribal population is very less. A total of 14 males and 18 females (4.13%) falls in the age group of 51-61 and above years. It is interesting to note that the life span of an individual in tribal communities is very less when compared to caste communities of plain areas of same region. The rate of infant mortality is also very high among tribal communities of Visakha Agency. Morbidity trend is also high among tribal population when compared to castes population. Fertility rate is very high especially among the primitive tribes like *Khond* and *Gadaba.* The average family size among *Khond* tribe is 6 members, because family planning is exempted to primitive tribes. In general, high rate of mortality is noticed in the *Khond* tribe. The physical characteristic features of the tribes in the study village appears to be short stature, dark brown skin colour and dark hair. They belong to the racial stock of *proto-Austroloid.*

**Table 8.2:** Age and Sex-wise Population of Pasuvulabanda Revenue Village

| *S No* | *Age Group* | *Males* | *% to Total Population* | *Females* | *% to Total Population* | *Total Males and Females* | *% to Total Population* |
|---|---|---|---|---|---|---|---|
| 1. | Below 1year | 11 | 1.42 | 9 | 1.16 | 20 | 2.58 |
| 2. | 1-5 | 38 | 4.90 | 36 | 4.65 | 74 | 9.55 |
| 3. | 6-10 | 52 | 6.71 | 50 | 6.45 | 102 | 13.16 |
| 4. | 11-15 | 31 | 4.00 | 29 | 3.74 | 60 | 7.74 |
| 5. | 16-20 | 34 | 4.39 | 33 | 4.26 | 67 | 8.65 |
| 6. | 21-25 | 41 | 5.29 | 39 | 5.03 | 80 | 10.32 |
| 7. | 26-30 | 25 | 3.23 | 26 | 3.35 | 51 | 6.58 |
| 8. | 31-35 | 34 | 4.39 | 36 | 4.64 | 70 | 9.03 |
| 9. | 36-40 | 33 | 4.26 | 35 | 4.52 | 68 | 8.78 |
| 10. | 41-45 | 42 | 5.42 | 40 | 5.16 | 82 | 10.58 |
| 11. | 46-50 | 35 | 4.51 | 34 | 4.39 | 69 | 8.90 |
| 12. | 51-55 | 8 | 1.03 | 10 | 1.29 | 18 | 2.32 |
| 13. | 56-50 | 4 | 0.51 | 5 | 0.65 | 9 | 1.16 |
| 14. | 61+above years | 2 | 0.26 | 3 | 0.39 | 5 | 0.65 |
| | Total | 390 | 50.32 | 385 | 49.68 | 775 | 100.00 |

**Table 8.3:** Occupational Background of Tribes/Caste in Pasuvulabanda

| *SNo* | *Name of the Tribes/Caste* | *Traditional Occupation* |
|---|---|---|
| 1. | Bagata | Agriculture |
| 2. | Valmiki | Barika or vetti |
| 3. | Nooka dora | Agriculture |
| 4. | Konda Kammara | Blacksmithy and carpentry |
| 5. | Gadaba | Shifting cultivation, sheep and goat reating |
| 6. | Khond | Shifting cultivation, piggery |
| 7. | Madiga | Leather work and agriculture labour |

Table 8.3 shows the occupational background of the tribes in Pasuvulabanda village. The *Bagatas* are the traditional agriculturists, Valmikis are Vettis, Gadabas and Khonds are Podu cultivators, Konda Kammaras are blacksmiths, Madigar are leather workers and Nooka doras are sedentary cultivators.

### *Ecological and Cultural Background*

*Pasuvula Banda* is located in the agency tracts of Visakhapatnam district. The district Visakhapatnam has two distinct regions of contrasting ecological and topographic features, one with plain landscape extending from the sea coast up to the foot hills of eastern *ghats* with moderate temperature and the other covered by thick forests a top elevated eastern *ghats* with cold elimate. The geographical area of the district is 11,161 sq. kms, of which the agency area covers 6298 sq. kms, i.e. 56.4 per cent of the area of that district. The entire agency area in the district is covered with thick forest growth of numerous trees and dales. Trees like gallnut, nalla maddi, jack, tamarind, teak, mango, bamboo, buruga, eucalyptus, sampangi, silver oak, etc., and tree creepers like *adda*, soap nut are common in the forest. Apart from these, coffee plantation also found under the shades of big trees. A number of wild animals are also seen in the forest. The most commonly found animals in the forest are bison, deer, bear, tiger, fox, wolf, snakes, numerous birds, wild fowls, peacocks and hares.

Social divisions like clan, lineage and family are common in each tribe. For instance the *Bagata* tribe have the totemic clans like *Hanumanthu, Surbi, Peyya, Elugu, Naga, Matsya, Surya*, and *Puli* and also the lineage names like *Sagina, Garthuru, Reemala, Murla, Bakuru, Arada* and *Veluchuri*. All the tribes observe the endogamy at tribe level and exogamy at clan and lineage levels. They follow the patriarchal system. In the local hierarchy, the *Bagata* stands at top whereas the *Valmiki* occupies the bottom most position. The traditional dressing pattern of tribal men is loin cloth as undergarment and *sari* for women. The dead are cremated. *Dimsa* is the popular tribal dance in the area in which both men and women participate. Their economy is agro-forest based and subsistence in character. Rearing of livestock is very common to each and every tribal family. Almost all the tribes collect the non-timber forest produce. About 60 per cent of the tribal families stands at below poverty line.

The tribals have superstitious beliefs and worship the nature. They take religious service from the local *Guruvu* and consult the witchdoctor or sorcerer for various diseases. The important deities for them are *Konda devata* and *Sanku devudu*. Their festivals are associated with the harvesting of crops and seasonally available forest resources of edible fruits, roots, tubers nuts and leafy vegetables. *Modu Kondamma Theerunallu* is an important and popular fair to the tribals of Visakha Agency. *Etum or Etekala Panduga* is an important festivals, on such occasion all the men compulsorily participate in small hunting game. Each tribe has its own traditional head, and a village council of informal political body which deal the cases like divorce, adultery, elopement, thefts, family and property disputes. Moreover they live in harmony and very much attached to the local religions, political institutions and intertwined with the environment which they inhabits.

### Food Resources

Agricultural products, forest resources like, edible fruits, roots, tubers, nuts, wild leafy vegetables, flesh of wild pigs, deers, hares and birds, and livestock are the major sources of food material available to the tribals of *Pasuvula banda*. They get major portion of food material from agricultural lands of dry, wet and *podu* categories. In the study village about 84.18 per cent of the families depend on cultivation, and the rest 15.82 per cent of the families on labour employment in agriculture and in forest department as well as other government construction works. The landless families actively participate in seasonal minor forest in collecting more quantity of forest products when compared with that of the land owning families. About 50 per cent of the families have kitchen gardens in which they grow vegetables like chilies, brinjal, beans, bottle gourd, pumpkin, drumstick, banana and tomato, mostly for consumption purpose. Stream and spring are the major water resources available to the residents, which they use for both irrigation and domestic purposes. They drink the polluted stream and spring water without any hesitation, in turn affected with water borne diseases. Table 8.4 shows the tribewise landholding and landless families in Pasuvula banda.

**Table 8.4:** Tribewise landholding and landless families in Pasuvulabanda

| *S No.* | *Name of the Tribe/Caste* | *No. of Land Owning Families* | *% to Total Households* | *No. of Landless Families* | *% to Total Households* |
|---|---|---|---|---|---|
| 1. | Bagata | 19 | 12.03 | 3 | 1.90 |
| 2. | Nooka Dora | 20 | 12.66 | 5 | 3.16 |
| 3. | Konda Kammara | 1 | 0.63 | 3 | 1.90 |
| 4. | Gadaba | 53 | 33.55 | 10 | 6.32 |
| 5. | Khond | 14 | 8.86 | 2 | 1.27 |
| 6. | Valmiki | 22 | 13.92 | 2 | 1.27 |
| 7. | Madiga | 4 | 2.52 | – | – |
| | | 133 | 84.18 | 25 | 15.82 |

Among the land using families only 51 families own wet category of land in addition to dry and *podu* type of lands. The wet land cultivators raise the paddy crop only in rainy season. The extent of land available for wet cultivation is very limited and such kind of land is mostly owned by the advanced tribes like *Bagata* and *Valmiki*. The tribal farmers grow the rain fed crops like millets, pulses and oil seeds in dry and *podu* types of lands and gets very low yields. The agricultural resources are not sufficient to meet the subsistence of the entire population of the village. In addition to the aforementioned resources, a few of them catch small fish in the streams, ponds and tanks for their own consumption. The rice distributed to the public through the G.C.C. is another source of food material supplied to them, which they mostly use for preparing *maddi* (rice beer) as an intoxicating drink.

### *Dietary Habits*

The staple food of all the tribes is *Ambali* (gruel), which is made up of with *ragi* (millet) flour. The rice growing families take rice at least once in a day. After introduction of free and subsidized rice scheme of government into tribal areas, even the other tribal families started to consume it occasionally. Some of them are non-vegetarians, among them, Valmikis, Khonds, Gadabas and Madigas eat beef. The consumption of non-vegetarian diet is very less in all the tribes and they have it occasionally. In the vegetarian diet, they make curries with seasonally available vegetables like water gourd, beans, brinjal, tomato, drum stick, pumpkin and pulses. The curry prepared with pumpkin is very auspicious and delicious dish for the tribes during socio-ceremonial occasions. A few literate and elite among them used to buy certain English vegetables like carrot, beet root, cauliflower, cabbage and potato in the weekly market (*shandy*) and from the *Malis* of *Chowdipalle* for their own consumption purpose. They prepare *chatnies* with the inflorescence of tamarind, tamarind fruit, chilies, *Konkadikoora*, *gongura* and redgram *dal*. They take redgram or greengram *dal* in liquid cooked from which is mixed with *Ambali* or rice. Quite oftenly they prepare *rasam* with the boiled tamarind mixed water which is added to the rice. They use *olusulu* oil (niger seed oil) as cooking medium. During food shortage periods a considerable number of families in Khond, Gadaba and Nooka Dora Tribes, subsist on *Tenka ambali* (which is prepared with mango kernel powder) *Jeelugukallu* (sagopalm extract) and certain edible fruits, roots, nuts, tubers and leaves of forest resources. A major portion of such forest resources they obtain from adda plant, mango, jack and tamarind in the form of fruits and nuts.

The oil consumption is very less in all the tribes. The consumption levels of vegetables, pulses, leafy vegetables, and meat are also very less among the Gadaba, Nooka Dora Khond and Konda Kammara tribes when compared with that of Bagata and Valmiki. In Visakha Agency area, Bagata and Valmiki tribes are economically better than other tribes. Literacy rate is also high among Valmiki and a considerable number of salaried employees are also found in this tribe. The quality of food intake is closely associated with the economic position of family and tribe. The consumption of milk products is almost nil in all the tribes. They do not have the practice of milching their cattle. About 59 per cent of the tribal families take black tea once in a day (morning).

Both men and women smoke cigar and chew tobacco. Alcoholism is very much prevalent among the tribal people. Even the tribal women take the intoxicating drinks like *sara* (*arrack*), *Jeelugu kallu* (sago palm extract) and *Maddi* (rice beer). In the past, each family used to have two or three sago palm plants but now only ten per cent of families owning such plants in the village. The intake of intoxicating drinks are more in Gadaba, Khond, Nooka Dora, and Konda Kammara when compared with that of Bagata and Valmiki tribes.

Table 8.5 shows the consumption of types of food items by the tribals of Pasuvulabanda in a week duration period. It is noted that almost all the families consumed millets twice a day, and 45 families consumed rice one time in a day and 75 families consumed it five times, 65 families taken tea once in a day and 30 families drank it three times in a week period. Rest of the food items are not consumed more than three times in a week.

**Table 8.5:** Consumption of Type of Food Items by the Families in Pasuvulabanda

| | *Number of Times Consumed in a Week* | | | | | | | |
|---|---|---|---|---|---|---|---|---|
| *Food Type* | *No. of Families* | *No. of Families* | *No. of Families* | *No. of Families* | *No. of Families* | *No. of Families* | *No.of Families (Twice daily)* | |
| (1) | (2) | (3) | (4) | (5) | (6) | (7) | (8) | (9) |
| Beef | 9 | – | – | – | – | – | – | – |
| Pork | 12 | – | – | – | – | – | – | – |
| Fish/Dry fish | 34 | 51 | – | – | – | – | – | – |
| Chicken | 6 | – | – | – | – | – | – | – |
| Milk/Ghee/butter | – | – | – | – | – | – | – | – |
| Black tea | – | – | 30 | – | – | – | 65 | |
| Eggs | 12 | 26 | – | – | – | – | – | – |
| Meat | 31 | – | – | – | – | – | – | – |
| Fruit | – | 10 | – | – | – | – | – | – |
| Vegetables | – | – | 40 | – | – | – | – | – |
| Leafy vegetables | 14 | 6 | – | – | – | – | – | – |
| Dals | 1 | 30 | 49 | – | – | – | – | – |
| Rice | 9 | 25 | – | – | 78 | – | 45 | 1 |
| Millets | – | – | – | – | – | – | – | 158 |
| Wild roots and tubers | 22 | 13 | 15 | – | – | – | – | – |

It is noted that the intake of protein food items is very less in almost all the tribes. Consumption of carbohydrates contained food items are more when compared with that of vitamins contained food items. And also all of its population do not get atleast the minimum required calories of food during the period of July to September in a calendar year.

### *Food Restrictions and Taboos*

The tribals avoid to take their concerned totemic plants and animals as food items. They do not consume the sacrificial animal blood where as it is offered to the supernatural beings. Generally the woman is restricted to take alcoholic beverages during her pregnancy. And also it is prohibited to the children who are aged below six years. After the birth of a child, the lactating mother will not consume pumpkin, onion, egg, meat and fish atleast for a period of six months. It is interesting to note that the restriction of certain food items like egg, meat, fish, to woman during pre and postnatal periods, has no scientific reason and it is a belief. Definitely these food items have much protein and nutritive values and in such periods which provides strength, good health for both mother and child.

***Nutritional Deficiencies and Health Disorders***

Food insecurity is the major problem to more than 50 per cent of the population in Pasuvulabanda. In the past, forest flora and fauna had plenty of food resources, such resources met the food requirement of limited and proportional size of population. Over a period of time, the population size has enormously increased consequently tremendous force build up on the available energy base in the natural habitat. And also in actual practice, the food habits and intake levels of tribals have changed considerably, due to the influence of outside foods, and market economy. The declaration of forest areas around the tribal habitats as reserve forest actually resulted in removing shrub jungles for growing commercial forestry. This in turn resulted in reducing the food availability in terms of roots, tubers, nuts, fruits, etc. Introduction of cash economy also received attention from the tribal peasants and in terms they have started to grow commercial crops, which resulted in the reduction of cereals production. The pressure of high cost economy and depletion of food resources has ultimately led to lesser intake of food and consequent malnutrition. Especially the shifting cultivation ecology of Khond and Gadaba tribe is vulnerable and prone for high incidence of malnutrition.

The calorie intake of primitive tribal population living in thickly forest areas of Visakha agency is deficient only by 6.74 per cent compared to Recommended Dietary Allowance (RDA). The most severe deficiency in calories was found in almost half of the tribal children and lactating mothers. The Khond food intake is deficient by 20 per cent in protein content compared to RDA. Vitamin A and Vitamin 'B' deficiencies are also more in the tribal population. The "original influence" among the forest dwelling tribes is only a myth and the modernization process seems to have added miseries to the tribals, as it is reflected in the nutritional deficiencies and health disorders. Certain diseases like night blindness, itching skin, beri beri, nervous system deterioration, cataracts, diarrhoea, dermatitis, anaemia, bleeding gums and loose teeth, scabies are common in the tribal population which are associated with vitamin deficiencies. The tribal people drink the contaminated stream and spring water and they do not take hygienic food and also not aware of the nutritious value of certain food items which are available within their ecosystem.

### *Role of Nutrition Rehabilitation Centre (NRC)*

To improve the nutritional status among children aged below three years, pregnant women and lactating mothers, under integrated child development scheme, the government has established *Anganwadi* schools in rural and tribal areas. The aims of the project are to provide nutritional rehabilitation to the target group of severely malnourished children (II and IV grades) and to obstetrical risk women i.e. those with toxemia, severe anaemia and other forms of severe malnutrition deficiencies. One such centre is also functioning at Valmiki colony of Pasuvulabanda village. At the time of study this centre had the strength of 26 children, (both boys and girls), 7 pregnant women and 9 lactating mothers. This centre is look after by a teacher and an *Aaya*. The health visitors also visit the centre at least once in a month to check nutritional and health status of children.

This centre is providing integrated nutrition and health services to at risk mothers and children who are severely malnourished with supplementary nutrition's in the form of *Upma*. Locally the centre is called *Upma badi*. Some of the objectives of this centre are:

1. To device simple, effective, less expensive dietary recipes for treatment of nutritional problems using locally available foods
2. To demonstrate to mothers the dramatic improvement in malnourished children when they are feed right quantity and quality of food at right frequency.
3. To bring about ever lasting behavioural change among mothers regarding feeding of children.

4. To impart skills to mother in making use of locally available food to prevent malnutrition in children in the family.

The work organization at the centre would mainly contains three aspects such as (i) daily routine of preparing *upma* and serving to the beneficiaries, (ii) assessment of nutritional status, and (iii) nutrition education. It is observed that the working condition of this centre is very poor due to lack of commitment and sincerity from *anganwadi* teacher and less involvement of local people. The tribal people were aware of the programme and enrolling the children, pregnant women and lactating mother. The *Anganwadi* centre at this village is not functioning effectively due to lack of commitment on the part of teacher, irregular supply of food material, no supervision, pilferage, low educational qualification of teacher, less payment to the teacher and *Aaya.* Moreover, *Anganwadi* teacher consider her job as part time and pays very less time towards the programme.

The aims and objectives of this programme are good. The basic problem lies at the implementation level. It is observed that a few nutrition rehabilitation centres, located at road side are functioning some what better than that of interior centres in Visakha agency because constant supervision and community participation. Even such centers also need to be strengthen further to achieve expected results in enhancement of nutritional status among high risk groups. Some of the following measures to be taken to strengthen this programme in the tribal areas are:

1. Enhancement of salary for both the teacher and *Aaya,*
2. Selection of at least a minimum SSC qualified teacher,
3. Checking records periodically with constant supervision,
4. Proper motivation to target high risk groups with effective communication,
5. Nutritional education to pregnant women and lactating mothers,
6. Pre-school education to the children in the age group of 2 to 5 years
7. Community participation,
8. Frequent health check up and nutritional status evaluation,
9. Regular supply of supplementary food items, and
10. Assurance of good quality of food preparation with the supplied material.

This programme should be intensified especially in the interior forest areas with people's participation. Much focus is needed on the worst affected primitive tribal habitats, which are much prone for malnutrition.

## Conclusions

The study reveals that the habitats of Khond and Gadaba tribes are much prone for high incidence of malnutrition which leads to high rate of morbidity and mortality. In general, the tribal ecology is not meeting the subsistence of its entire population. The influence of myth, food taboos and modernization process seems to added miseries to the tribals, which are reflected in the nutritional deficiencies and health disorders among them. A clear cut food policy has to be taken into consideration in order to enhance the health status of tribals. Natural foods requirement of fruits from nutritional angle should be assessed, and such foods to be made available within the purchasing capacity of tribals, so that the incidence of malnutrition, caloric deficiency can be tackled. The nutrition rehabilitation centres should be further strengthened with people's participation.

Poverty alleviation programmes should be intensified in such areas, with the much involvement of the personnel belonging to ITDA and health departments. Population control measures should be taken even among the primitive tribal communities. Mobile health clinic services, and community health workers programmes are to be intensified in the tribal areas. Conservation of natural resources, maintenance of balanced bio-diversity and enlargement of energy base are the best solutions for the problems of nutritional deficiency and health disorders. Education levels must be raised among tribal populations. Specialized training—as in food, nutrition, home economics and sanitation—must likewise be geared to improvements in general education.

Land reform is a prerequisite to solution of food and nutritional problem. It is closely related to improvements in agricultural production. Traditional agricultural practices should be encouraged with better land and water management. Increased production of agricultural commodities and other products is obviously a vital goal in the direct attack on hunger. Agricultural improvement with better quality seeds, more organic manures, better breeding, crop rotation, quality animal stock, increased skills, more land in production, more scientific research in agrarian sector and shifts among commodities such as less roots and tubers, more proteins, more leafy, green and yellow vegetables, more grain legumes are needful to tackle the food problem in the tribal areas of our country. Forest policies should not become threat to the livelihood of tribals. Market system of GCC and facilities should be improved in the tribal areas. In general economic development at family level ensures food security which in turn solves both nutritional and health problems. Good health of all people assures the progress of the nation. It is possible only in keeping good quality of environment with more cautious and consciousness.

**Policy Implications**

1. A clear-cut separate food policy should be taken up for tribal population.
2. Supplementary food material for high risk groups through NRC to be strengthened in the interior primitive tribal areas. Supplied food items should be suitable to their dietary habits.
3. Public distribution system through Girijan Cooperative Corporation should need to be strengthened, and good quality of staple food items must be distributed apart from other domestic requirements. Outside market agencies interference should be eradicated.
4. Poverty alleviation programmes should be intensified in the interior primitive tribal habitats with peoples participation, and enlargement of energy base is much essential in the malnutrition prone areas.
5. Nutrition and health education should be provided at household level with much involvement of health personnel and *Anganwadi* workers. Community health workers scheme need to be strengthened and tribal medicine should be promoted.
6. Periodical nutrition and health assessment and also evaluation studies on nutrition and health programmes should be conducted, in order to take appropriate measures, based on the results.
7. Protected drinking water should be provided to the tribal settlements where such facility is not available at present.

8. Forest environment should be protected form out side threats and locally available fruits should be made use of fully by the tribals.

## REFERENCES

Atkinson, S.J. (1992): *Food for the Cities: Urban Nutrition Policy in Developing Countries*, P.H.P. Department Publication No. 5 ISSN, London School of Hygiene and Tropical Medicine.

Mead, Margaret (1943): *The Anthropological approach to dietary problems*, New York. Academy of Sciences, Transactions series 5: 177-182.

Subramanyam, V. (1997): *The Ecology of Malnutrition in the Agency Area of Visakhapatnam: Food Resources, Habits and Deficiencies*, U.G.C. Minor Research Project Report, Andhra University, Visakhapatnam (unpublished.)

Subramanyam, V. and K.R. Rama Mohan (2001) Tribal Ecology and food Security: A study in Visakha Agency Area of Andhra Pradesh—*Journal of Human Ecology*, 12 (5): 351-356.

Tiwari, P.D. and Sharma A.N. (1989) (ed.): *Tribal Eco System and Malnutrition in India*, Northern Book Centre, New Delhi.

# 9

# Tribals of Ladakh: Ecology and Health

VEENA BHASIN

## Introduction

Health status of people of Ladakh is related to its habitat, human settlements and amenities available there. Other factors affecting health of the people are historical, socio-cultural, economic and developmental. Ladakh division in the state of Jammu and Kashmir in India, comprising Leh and Kargil districts, and inhabited by different ethnic groups, is remote, inaccessible, resource-poor high-altitude zone in western Himalayas, that witnessed little change or advancement in the operative economic and technological level over the centuries. Till recent times, the region evidently remained a model of human adaptation to an extremely sensitive environment by evolving time-tested methods to meet the challenges. The high-altitude, harsh natural environment of Ladakh is characterized by extreme cold and dryness, high radiation, strong winds, low precipitation, low humidity; and desert-like extensive barren landscape, rugged topography, steep and vertical glaciated slopes, minimal forest cover and mineral resources, few pasture lands at high elevations; and settlements in narrow oases like valleys having limited arable land and limited water for irrigation purposes [Suggesting an encapsulated environment as elaborated by Goldstien (1983)].

In Ladakh, where ecological constraints are high, socio-cultural factors and economic development have been found to have effect on the demographic structure. Natural environmental constrains dictate many aspects of traditional life, especially settlement site and agricultural system. Ladakh's steep mountainous terrain makes ground transportation difficult. The roads connecting the region to the rest of India are closed for six to eight months each year because of snow. The inhabitants live primarily in small villages scattered over a vast region. The region is extremely poor in conventional energy sources (fossils, fuels and wood) and has almost no industrially exploitable resources. Ladakh's subsistence level agro-pastoral economy, traditional social and religio-cultural systems (extra-somatic medium to counteract environmental stresses) are composite part of the cold desert's ecological system which developed as a totality and a closed system. But, certain significant developments, such as, the accession of Jammu and Kashmir to India in 1947 establishing democratic institutions, uniform laws and regulations; the communist revolution in China bringing an end to the caravan-trade in 1949 and subsequent Chinese occupation of Tibet (leading to the severance of the link with Ladakh); the Indo-Chinese war in 1962 leading to closure of the border and occupation of considerable area by China; and constant conflict with Pakistan giving the zone extreme strategic importance; resulted in a series of rapid changes—unplanned as well as planned, fast altering the ecosystem and also the population homeostasis of 'pristine' Ladakh of yesteryears, when various natural and socio-economic constraints minimized and slowed down any exogenous or endogenous initiatives, interferences towards innovations and expansions.

In recent decades continuous massive defence investment and improvement in communications; proliferation of government departments; introduction of policy of developmental activities; provisions for basic amenities; alterations in traditional subsistence economy, its commercialisation and extension of technical know-how through government departments and non-governmental organisations; changes in political and economic expectations, alterations in food habits and material possessions leading to the over-dependence on non-local food grains and industrial goods; land reclamation and afforestation, etc., are the major moves behind the changing face of Ladakh. Additionally, decline in the temporal role of religion; introduction of the 'Big Land Estate Abolition Act', the 'Buddhist Polyandrous Marriage Abolition Act', equal inheritance (among siblings) laws, individual rights; and opening of Ladakh to tourism in 1974, (which has led to large tourist influx, predominantly from Western countries), are the other major impulses symptomatic of changes in the environment, population dynamics, mobility, economics, socio-cultural values and systems, and communal harmony. The region, therefore, evidenced breaking down of traditional systems and regulations of celibate institutions like monasticism, marital systems like fraternal polyandry; estate inheritance modes like primogeniture; as well as family structure; community grouping, cooperation; social stratification; frugality and prudence.

It is also generally perceived that the region has been subjected to frequent conflicts and that the pace of development has been chronically sluggish. Consequently, often the populace have faced considerable impediments, besides being affected by environmental stresses, natural calamities, epidemics and various illnesses. The constraints and difficulties ensued not only from harsh environmental or strategic location of the region, but also from the short-sighted planning and policies, delayed implementation of projects and programmes, preoccupation with strategic matters and apathetic attitudes on the part of the authorities; which has brought about serious regional imbalances. Therefore, the changes witnessed currently in Ladakh, are in a way, deemed to be inevitable in search of development and well being an important and necessary goals for all societies and nations. Also segregating Ladakh from such much-needed pursuits is unreasonable. But side by side, the alarming facts of accelerated development processes, lure of short-term advantages, population surplus and allied issues, which are undoubtedly posing multiple problems in the 'finite' Ladakh today, must not be undermined and require urgent assessment and correction.

## PEOPLE AND SOCIETY OF LADAKH

### The People: Ladakh

The people of Ladakh are a mixture of Mongolian and the Aryan races. Ladakh Division is inhabited by followers of two major religions: Buddhism and Islam, 52 per cent of the total population is Buddhist while 44.6 per cent are Muslims. The Baltis and Muslim Dards professing Islam are inhabiting the valleys of Dras and Suru and the tract above Pashkim, which is called Purig. These are not geographically separated from the main body of Baltis, which borders on Dras. Then there is an isolated colony of Baltis right in the middle of the Buddhists area only a few kilometres from Leh at Chushout. The largest tract of cultivated land in Ladakh is in great part held by them at Chushut, on the left bank of the Indus. The rest of the Ladakh division is mostly inhabited by Buddhists.

Many languages and dialects are spoken in Ladakh, Ladakhi is spoken by 56 per cent of the population of Ladakh. The next important language is Balti which claim 37 per cent speakers. Bodhi and Tibetan is spoken by two per cent each and Brokstat (Brokpa) and Kashmiri one per cent each.

62 per cent of the population residing in Ladakh speak an additional language besides their mother tongue. The everyday language in use in Ladakh is Ladakhi, but there is a Tibetan dialect, and its correspondingly literary form is normal literary Tibetan. The Tibetan can actually be chosen as an option in Government schools in Leh, but it goes under the name of Bodi and not Tibetan. Otherwise English or Urdu or Hindi is used. The corresponding literary form of spoken Ladakhi, namely Tibetan survives only as a medium for religious institutions and for religious ceremonies. The minimum necessary is usually learned orally in so far as it is required for ritual use. A Buddhist Philosophical School at Choglamsar just outside Leh has been started by Indian Government. This is intended for young monks from monastries all over Ladakh, and courses are offered in Tibetan, Sanskrit, Buddhist Philosophy and English.

## Scheduled Castes and Scheduled Tribes

The disrict had negligible percentage (0.33 per cent) of Scheduled Castes to total population in 1981. In the year 1981, eight population groups, namely, Bot, Mon, Beda, Garra, Brokpa (Dogpa, Shinna, etc.) Balti, Changpa and Purigpa have been declared as Scheduled Tribes.

## Ethnic Composition of Ladakhi Population

Ladakh is inhabited by following ethnic groups:

A. Buddhists—
   1. Ladakhi Bodh/Bhot/Boto/Bot
   2. Gara
   3. Mon Dolba
   4. Beda
   5. Changpa (Pastoralists of Changthang)
   6. Brokpa (Buddhist Dards)

B. Muslims—
   1. (a) Balti, (b) Purigpa
   2. Argons
   3. Drokpa (Muslim Dards)
   4. Tibetans (Recently colonized in Ladakh)

Apart from these groups, Ladakh is inhabited by Christians, Hindus, and Sikhs. Some of these groups are characterized by specific occupation, dress code, language, mode of life while rest have more than one occupation. An average Buddhist village has one or two families of Gara, Mon and Beda, while the rest of the population is of Buddhist Bodhs, which are referred as Ladakhis. The word Ladakhi does not correspond to each and every person inhabiting Ladakh, it is only the privilege of Buddhist Bodhs, signifying a specific ethnic group. The Ladakhis are characterised by the high cheek bones, flat face, eyes with epicanthic folds, wide and broad nose, scanty body hair growth and straight to slight wavy head hair. The Ladakhis speak Ladakhi akin to Tibetan. Bodhi is their script. Salient features of the population groups in Ladakh are given in Table 9.1.

The ethno-historic characteristics of the various population groups represented in Ladakh are as follows:

***Buddhist***

*Bot, Bodhs (Scheduled Tribe)*

They belong to the Mongoloid (descendants of Mongols of Central Asia) ethnic stock and form the Leh district. They inhabit the area between Skara-Igo to Taru-Umla including Leh town to Achinabang, Nubra Valley, along the Srinagar Leh highway and the Zanskar region of the Kargil district. All Bots-Bodhs speak the same language of the Tibeto-Chinese group commonly know as "Ladakhi" but there are local variations in respect to some words and pronunciations. The devotion of these people to their religion consisting of four sects is profound and intense. The sects Nigmpa, Dukpa-Kargyut and Sanskia are known as Red sect and Gelugspa the reformed Yellow sect. Their main occupation is agriculture and they grow mainly barley and wheat. A few of them grow vegetables and fruits also. Buddhism does not recognize any caste system but some differentiation is made on the basis of social and occupational considerations.

*Gara*

The Gara are Mongoloid Buddhists of lower order (Rignun) and speak Ladakhi. Their main occupation is blacksmithy and they are found in almost every large Ladakhi Bodh or Bhoto village. Between Gara and other ethnic groups in the village there is a specific kind of relationship which resemble *Jajmani* (patron-client) system of caste society of plains.

*Mon*

Mons are Ladakhi speaking Buddhists, occupying a lower status (Rignun) in the social hierarchy of the Ladakhi society. They are professional drummers and musicians but few also grow barley, wheat in their small landholdings. It was stated in a recent report that the population of Mons in Leh district is 873 and forms 1.17 per cent of the total population of Ladakh. The term 'Mon' has been used for water dwellers by Tibetans. They contributed largely to the development of Ladakhi irrigation system.

*Bedas*

They too belong to the lower strata of the Ladakhi society. A family or two of these are found in every village. Bedas are pipers but have taken to agriculture on small land holdings. Bedas are 319 in number. They are Buddhists as well as Muslim and form 0.43 per cent of the total population of the Leh District (Tribal Census of Ladakh, 1991, Registrar General of India). The term 'Bedá' is derived from the Tibetan word *be* and *da*. *Be* refers to separately and *da* means reside. Local tradition maintain that the Beda came from Lahul, a long time after the Mon. All Muslim musicians are called Bedas. Muslim Bedas have permanent homes like the Mons whereas Buddhist Bedas are wandering minstrels. Muslim Bedas have some land also while Buddhist Bedas earn their living by playing music only.

*Changpa (Scheduled Tribe)*

The Buddhist Changpas are the tribe of tent *(Rebo)* dwelling pastoral transhumans of Ladakh who form an ethnic entity. The nomadic and semi-nomadic Changpa people of the Rupshu plateau are pure Tibetans and it is probably herders like them who first populated Ladakh (Table 9.1). Through experience they have mastered the art of not only living but thriving in one of the most hostile environment of the world. They inhabit high plateaus of Rupshu, Kharnak and Karzok. In Rupshu and Kharnak whole community leads transhumane life, while in Karzok 90 per cent are transhumant and ten per cent lead sedentary life. In Karzok, pastoralism, trading and marginal agricultural are the economic pursuits followed by Changpas. They too belong to the Mongoloid ethnic stock and Changkyet, a Tibetan dialet is spoken by them. They profess Buddhism but their young men do not become Lamas (For details see Bhasin, 1996).

**Table 9.1:** Salient features of the population groups in Ladakh

| *S No.* | *Population Group* | *Scheduled Tribe/Scheduled Caste/Community* | *Religion* | *Language Family* | *Occupation* |
|---|---|---|---|---|---|
| 1. | Bodh | Scheduled Tribe | Buddhism | Tibeto Chinese | Agro-pastoral |
| 2. | Gara | Scheduled Caste | Buddhism | Tibeto Chinese | Blacksmithy |
| 3. | Mon | Scheduled Caste | Buddhism | Tibeto Chinese | Carpentry, Drummer Musicians |
| 4. | Beda | Scheduled Caste | Buddhism | Tibeto Chinese (Tibetan) | Pipers |
| 5. | Changpa | Scheduled Tribe | Buddhism | Changkyet | Pastoralism |
| 6. | Brokpa (Buddhist Dards) | Scheduled Tribe | Buddhism | Brok-skad (Dardic) Linguimstic group | Agriculture, horticulture and animal husbandry |
| 7. | Balti, Purigpa | Scheduled Tribe | Islam (Shia Muslim) | Batti (Tibeto Chinese) | Agriculture, agriculure labour/horticulture and animal husbandry |
| 8. | Argons | Community | Islam (Sunni Muslims) | Tibeto Chinese | Trading/agriculture |
| 9. | Drokpa (Muslim Darda) | Scheduled Tribe | Islam (Sunni Muslims) | Shinna (Dardic) | Agriculture Linguistic group |

### *Brokpas (Scheduled Tribe)*

Brokpas (high-landers) are Dards, believed survivors of the pure Aryan race inhabiting the lower Indus valley from Dah of the Leh district to Batalic of the Kargil district. According to historians, they migrated from Dardistan in search of pastures and settled along the lower region long ago in areas which are comparatively warm abounding in apples, apricots and grapes. Some 130 kilometres north-east of Kargil, there are villages of Dah-Bema, Hano (Hano Goma and Hano Yogma), Darchik and Garkon, situated on the northern banks of Indus on the road of Baltistan inhabited by Dards. These villages are inhabited by 1920 Buddhist Brokpas (Census of India, 1991). All other Dard groups are Muslims and settled in few villages in Ladakh (Dras village and in north of Kashmir in Gurials and Tibet). The Muslim Dards from Marol in Baltistan to the Buddhist Dards in Ladakh formed a contiguous line along the Indus. They separated during the 17th century when the border between Ladakh and Baltistan was demarcated at Gur-Gud. Buddhist Dards are known as Brogpa/Brokpa in Leh District but Dogpas or Dukpas in the Kargil district. The Buddhist Brok-pa Dard villages have once again in the last few years been subjected to an arbitrary jurisdictional division as subject of Leh district and Kargil tehsil. Administratively Dah-Bema, Hano are in Leh district and Darchik and Garkon are in Kargil tehsil resulting in Buddhist influence in the earlier and Muslim influence in the later bringing changes among the growing generation. Buddhist speak Brok-skad an offshoot of Dardic linguistic group.

The Brok-pa form a distinctive cultural ethnic community nestled in central Ladakh on a offbeat track. They have preserved their language and social customs including many archaic traits of their Aryan forefathers through endogamy and oral tradition. Ethnically, they have no relationship with the Mongoloid-Tibetan strain, otherwise dominant in Ladakh. Surrounded by other ethnic groups on all sides, Ladakhis, Purigpas and Baltis, they are able to preserve certain archaic traits of language, dress and culture. Though, nominally they are Buddhist, their Buddhism does not conform with the Buddhism of rest of the Ladakh. Their acceptance of Buddhism is superficial.

### *Muslims*

#### *Balti (Scheduled Tribe)*

Balti are Shia Muslims believed to be the product of the admixture of Dards and Mongoloids. They are originally from the Skardu area of Baltistan and now inhabit the Kargil district including Kargil town.

Balti population is also found in the Leh district in certain pockets. During the reign of Jamyang Namgyal several hundred Balti Muslims are thought to have migrated from Baltistan and Purig to Chushot and Shey. The descendants number has swelled upto 6,000.

Some were descendants of the musicians and servants who had accompanied the Balti princess to Ladakh, when she came to marry Ladakhi Kings Jamyang Namgyal. Others facing poverty and hardships in their own lands, came to Ladakh between the 17th and 18th century. The Balti who were Shia, mainly *Nurbakshi,* spoke a Tibetan dialect. They were held in contempt not only by Buddhists but also the Sunnis for whom Persian was the language of culture and religion, and who did not recognize them as "real Muslim". Poor, illiterate and rejected, the Baltis were employed by the Kashmiri Muslims of Leh, or by rich Argons, in lowly ranks. They worked also as butchers, leatherworkers and shoemakers. The woman worked, especially during the harvest. The poorest among them were employed in the thankless job of sorting, carding and washing the *pashmina* and *shatush.* The goat-hair which they separated from the wool was given to them in payment. A few Sayyids or descendants of the Prophet were wealthy, powerful and became successful merchants. In Kargil Baltis speak 'Balti' language, which belongs to the Tibeto-Chinese family and preserved the archaic characteristic of pronunciation. Balti is a language without a script. There is a hazy racial recollection of the language once having had a script and this dates from Buddhist time. However the population being Muslim, Urdu, Persian characters are also used for writing. Their main occupation is agriculture and agriculture labour. Horticulture and animal husbandry are sometime marginally undertaken. They too have some occupational stratification, with chiefs and nobility forming the highest rank followed by commoners. Those engaged in menial jobs constitutes the lowest. It is suggested that they were earlier Buddhists, but long back converted to Islam when mass conversion took place, after Mirza Haider Daughlat invaded Baltistan. Baltis profess Shia faith of Islam, therefore, they are sometimes referred as 'Shias'. They are quite conservative and orthodox, and mostly do not partake any thing touched by non-Muslims. Music, dance, entertainment are still avoided unlike the Bodhs. In villages, mosques often serve as focal points. In cases of illness, calamities, 'Maulvis' and 'Aghas' are consulted. Much of the non-official activities embarked upon by individuals or groups are planned and sanctioned by these religious heads. Aghas are their religious leaders; all of them are Sayyids. The word of the Agha is the law for a Shia. The cult of ceremonial cleanliness, an essential part of their faith, as observed by them is unique. Anything touched by a Buddhist or a Hindu is shunned by a Shia-Balti. This even applied to a chunk of meat exhibited in a butcher shop. If it is unknowingly touched by a non-Muslim customer, he is severely rebuked by a owner for contaminating the things. This restriction of accepting any thing from a non-Muslim Shia is so strong that Baltis were not even accepting liquid medicines from the dispensary.

*Purigpa (Scheduled Tribe)*

The bulk of the Kargil population consists of Purigpas. Orginally, Kargil was known as "Purig" and the Purigpas, the original inhabitants and their descendant have been named after their original place. Purigs too claim themselves to be Baltis but Baltis refer to them as Purig-pa. They profess Islam. Their dialect is a mixture of Ladakhi and Balti. The main occupation of this population is agriculture and they grow barley, wheat and peas.

*Argons*

Argons are the descendants of immigrants from Kashmir valley and Central Asia who intermingled with the local Ladakhi community. The Kashmiri who came from Srinagar in the 17th century were among the first Muslims to settle in the small Buddhist Kingdom. Most were traders, but occasionally they were accompanied by men of religion. In Leh, they met the traders from Central Asia. Unlike the Kashmiris, few of them lived there. Most would leave Leh when the caravan season was over. Many of Kashmiris who settled in Leh married Ladakhi women and left progeny of 'Argons'. Most of them speak the 'Ladakhi' language but can also converse in Turkish and Tibetan language. They are found in both Leh and Kargil districts. They profess Sunni faith and are mainly traders. Few, however have taken to agriculture akin to Bodhs.

*Drokpa (Scheduled Tribe)*

Drokpas are Dard Muslims who inhabit the cold, bleak Dras valley. They are also called 'Shin' on the basis of their language 'Shinna' which belongs to the Dard group of languages in the non-Sanskritic Indo-European family. They are also believed to have the estate of their mother's brother.

Today polyandrous marriages are becoming rare and since it is not a legal form of marriage* the cohabitation of brother with a wife of one of them is purely informal arrangement of economic benefit. There is change in inheritance pattern. Primogeniture, eldest son inheriting house and farm is the thing of the past. Now-a-days inheritence is associated with neolocal areas, related families may live close by or close-together and regularly share both economic activities and meals. The breakdown of the monomarital principle and percentage decrease of monks and nuns mean that Buddhists population is on increase. In the last decade around 70 per cent increase in Ladakhi population has been recorded, however CBR 22.4 in the present study is still much less than the State and Indian average of 33.4 and 32.6, respectively.

Among Muslims, the different ethnic groups Purigpas, Baltis, Drokpas and Argons all show different fertility rates. Muslim Dropkas, seem to be comparatively less bothered about small family size, health and sanitary awareness, educational attainments, contraceptive usage thereby registering higher CBR than other groups. Muslims Baltis are more conducive and accommodating towards such issues and are adapting them gradually for their benefits. Muslim Agrons, being traders are mostly economically well off and show preference for higher educational attainment and do not see children as an economic asset. As they are mixture of Buddhist females and Kashmiri male traders, they share preference for better living conditions and lifestyle.

Ladakhis are facing rapid population explosion. It reflects a young population strucure associated with high degree of morbidity and high rates of mortality. Infant mortality rates among Buddhists and Muslims are 97.6 and 152.8 respectively against India's IMR of 104.0. Ladakhis happened for a long time to do many things that reduced their exposure to disease for reasons unrelated to any such goal. They drank hot *'Gur Gur'* tea, brewed with boiled water, and there by made water safe to drink well before the germ theory explained that harmful micro-organisms might lurk in unboiled water.

---

* As polyandry was declared illegal by the Buddhist Polyandrous Marriages Prohibition Act of 1988 (A.D. 1941). See *Laws of Jammu and Kashmir* Vol. III, pp. 878-81.

Ladakhis are engaged in a host of practices that protect them from some of the mortality risk. Recyling of human waste by means that meliorated the risk of disease is one of those. Human waste is mixed with sand and used as manure in the fields. The clinical tetanus in neonates and adults is absent among Ladakhis. Ladakhis claim that they got natural immunity against tetanus or it is acquired through the habit of keeping new-born in *Tsa-nu,* a woollen sack made up of sheep and goat skin. The sack is filled with powdered sieved dung and made warm by placing a hot stone on it. To keep children warm this practice is followed at least for six months. The same dung powder is used repeatedly after drying. Infant mortality rates among Ladakhi Buddhists are high but lower than Buddhists of Sikkim (177.8) and Buddhists of Nepal (147.4). Among Ladakhi Budhists the Crude Death Rate (CDR) is 14.3 which is higher than India's CDR of 10.0 in 1994. The economic and social factors which affect mortality are many and complex. They include education, occupation, nutrition, housing conditions, sanitation, public health services, medical services and general living standards. Definitely, the environment, the people are living in and the climatic pressures are taking toll of the lives.

The risk of death varies with the age of an individual. Furthermore, improvement in public health and medical services have been found to affect different age groups to a different extent. Age-wise mortality shows a U-shaped curve indicating a high rate up to age of 14 years and after that a very low rate and a steep rise after the age of 55 years.

Age specific death rates among Buddhists and Muslims of Ladakh show that mortality rate in the age groups 0-4 is high being 39.6 and 36.4, respectively. Mortality rates in the age group 60-64 are 69.0 among Buddhists and 84.1 among Muslims of Ladakh. In the age group 65+ the mortality rate is 111.1 per thousand among Buddhist and 160.3 per thousand among Muslims of Ladakh.

Infant mortality is considered to be fairly sensitive index of the health conditions of a region. Though it is difficult to control the endogamous causes like congenital abnormalities, the exogenous or environmental causes like nutrition, prenatal care, sanitary conditions, incidence of diseases to which infants are highly prone can be controlled and reflects the health measures taken by the community, government and other agencies. Apart from genetic and endogenous factors, biological factors like the age of mother, order of birth, prematurity and birth spacing also have a bearing on child surviving.

Low death rates have been achieved in parts of India, where primary health care procedures, midwifery, maternal education on breast feeding and weaning, vaccinations, oral rehydration of victims of diarrhoea, and antibiotics against respiratory infections have been implemented.

Health supporting utilities are supposed to have some direct or indirect affect on health status of the people. It was found that mothers do not generally panic when a child is struck by a diarrhoeal episode, especially when such cases are associated with developmental stages of the child (teething, walking and crawling). Most mothers do not seek treatment outside home until the third day. The decision making process is influenced by traditional values, distance to health facilities, availability of other pharmaceutical products and/or financial resources. However, treatment outside home is sought only when the episode persists and is resistant to home management techniques. Mother's decision to seek health care in modern facilities comes after a complicated process of choices or alternatives. Housing conditions and household attribute, represents health environment at the hosehold level. Type of construction, number of rooms, separate toilet, separate kitchen, cattle shed, bath rooms, chimney in the kitchen/rooms, drainage system/ sewerage system, ventilation, general sanitary conditions all represent health environment.

Mortality was found to be related to availability of sanitation, piped water supply, utilization of health services and host of socio-economic and demographic variables at household level.

The area of dwelling is found to have an inverse relation with mortality in general. This is also an economic indicator. The higher social classes are more likely to have larger dwelling areas and people in higher social class have more ability to take curative as well as preventive measures of health factor in bringing down infant mortality. It has been found that presence or absence of sanitary conditions affects the mortality differentials. It was observed that where sanitary conditions were satisfactory, the mortality differentials were low.

General and infant mortality respond favourably to education. It was observed that among Buddhists and Muslims of Ladakh, the educational achievements of both husband and wife affected the infant mortality differentials. The analysis reveals that educational achievements of both husband and wife are significantly associated with infant and child mortality. As expected, the probability of dying declines with age of child and education of mother. In Ladakh, the mother's education is more influential factor than father's education and occupation. In the study area in Ladakh where landlordship is an important criterion of social and economic status, the infant mortality differentials were affected by landownership. The infant mortality differentials were high among landless and were minimum among the people who owned less than 10 acres in both the the groups. Both the groups, Buddhist and Muslim, classified by income, showed that the infant mortality differentials were high among those whose income was less than Rs. 10,000 per annum and minimum in those household where income was more than Rs. 50,000 per annum. Nature and occupation of both husband and wife is strongly associated with infant mortality.

The study from Ladakh corroborates the theory that social development and various facilities available in the study area attribute to lower mortality rates. As observed that infant mortality is significantly associated with *pucca* roads, bus services and mass media. When the communication facilities index is high mortality rate is low.

The analysis of mortality rates of neonatal, postnatal, the infant and child revel that the distance to government dispensary, public health centre and hospital is significantly associated with the mortality rates. The rates increase as the distance of these facilities increases from the respondent's place. Other factors such is the *Dai* (traditional birth attendants), number of visits by fieldworkers, occurrence of natural disasters and epidemics also show a systematic pattern with mortality rates. The Maternal and Child Health Programme has not been successful in extending service to the target pupulation. In terms of immunisation, only 46.6 per cent Buddhists and 41.4 per cent Muslims have been immunised. Survey data also show that most of the women prefer to deliver at home.

In view of the difficult means of communication and distance of dispensaries from the villages in Ladakh, medical aid is not availed by Ladakhis except in serious cases. However, in areas, despite easy accessibility, survey findings show that a sizeable proportion of those who were ill did not seek treatment in health centres or hospitals. Ladakhis depend on traditional folk-medicine practitioners who besides relying upon certain occult phenomena deal with various herbs for preparing herbal medicines for therapeutic use. Throughout Ladakh, the people are obsessed with the uncanny unearthy activities of spirits, ghosts and deities. The diseases thought to be caused by supernatural, demand magico-religious remedies. Ladakhis resort to various magico-religious practitioners for relieving people of death and disease caused and delegated by the wrathful supernatural. Percentage distribution of deaths (1986-88) among Buddhists and Muslims in the present study was reported highest by respondents while availing the allopathic medicine. Though they fail to mention that allopathic medicine was taken as a last resort or in terminal cases. It was found that deaths reported by availing the services of traditional folk medicine practitioners was minimum or negligible. The reason underlying this was that their first choice was traditional folk medicine.

The Ladakhi's response to problems of health and disease has components from various systems of medicine. Components of Ladakhi medical pluralism are Lamaism, Shamanism (locally known as *Lhawaism*), scholarly *Amchi* medicine and allopathy. The study reveals a multiple and simultaneous, usage of home remedies and multiple therapy system.

The religious background, particularly the belief in the fear of evil spirits, the influence of Shamanistic healing performed according to Bon rites, means of protection against evil spirits, amulets, thread, crosses, etc., make Ladakhi medicine colourful and multifarious. The plurality enables them to switch from one type of health practitioner to another in search of the best. The Ladakhi who can avail the facility of western (or bio-medicine), do so without being familiar with the theoretical principles of medical system. Although the economic status of the households differ, they show certain similar patterns of illness behaviour. They employ pluralistic strategies not perceiving any conflict among these alternatives, nor do they seem to perceive them as different systems, but rather as variety of options, among which they can choose.

Most usage is sequential but some is simultaneous. For example, an infant who is being given prescribed medicine for diarrhoea may also be taken concurrently to a Lama for the evil eye. Although certain illnesses such as evil eye, are thought to be cured only by folk curers, this does not preclude the use of modern medicine to treat the symptoms. Gonzales (1966) reports that in Guatemala, the symptoms are treated with modern medicine, while the cause of illness is dealt with through a folk specialist. Traditional (or folk) theories of illness etiology are often multifactorial and multilevel (e.g. immediate and ultimate levels of causation), which permits the use of different treatment resources for different causal factors and levels (Cosminsky, 1977). As reported by Cosminsky (1980) for Guatemalan plantation, pluralistic behaviour among Ladakhi population groups is pragmatic, often based on trial and error, perceived effectivenes, uncertainly of illness causation and expectation of quick results. In addition to this empirical and pragmatic behaviour, however, is the role played by faith in the supernatural (or spiritual) in curing. As a person is simultaneously a body (his soma), a self (his psyche) and a social being (his polis), so are healers corresponding to three different realms of individual functioning. In other words, a person is simultaneously a body, a self and a social being. Ladakhi Shamanism "pursued a dialogic, relational remedy for its patients through receiprocal relationships that encouraged community, such as in gift giving to spirits and etiologies based on real social conflicts" (Adams, 1992: 154). Ladakhi shaman attempts to resolve sickness caused by the disorder of the "Social self". Lamas and *Amchis* on the other hand claim to cure diseases which arise from disorders of body and mind originating from individual actions and desires in craving and clinging. Excessive anger, greed and lack of discipline in attachment to the physical and social world result in body disorders. Lamas cure with prayers and rituals while Amchis cure through the site of the physical body by means of an elaborate diagnostic system and pharmacopeia. The Ladakhi healers emphasize different aspects of Ladakhis self: social (*Lhawaism/Lhapaism*), mental (*Lamaism*) and physical (*Amchis*). Bio-medical systems as a rule stand in sharp contrast to the indigenous ones, although a study done in Kerala and Punjab has suggested that there are numerous indigenous medical practitioners who used western medicine, including penicillin injections (Neumann, 1971: 140-141). Among Ladakhis, no such practitioners exist as *Lhama/Lhapa* are spiritual healers and *Amchis* are traditional herbal doctors, who do not use biomedicine.

The pluralistic medical situation in Ladakh provides flexibility and fills different needs of the population. The folk systems are open as manifested by electicism of both the clients and practitioners, who adopt and adapt aspects from an array of coexisting medical traditions. This openness of the folk systems, as Press (1978) point out, is manifested by the acceptance of inputs from other/alternative health systems, and also inputs from institutional sectors such as religion and the family. According to Landy (1974) the traditional healer role stands at the interstices of religion, magic and the social system and gain its power from the position. This contrasts sharply with the closeness of cosmopolitan medicine, which is "discontinuous from ordinary social process (Press, 1978; Mannig and Fabrega, 1973) and is unaccommodating to alternative systems.

A general quantitative survey on the utilization of multiple therapy systems among Ladakhis gave an impression that they have inclination towards indigenous type. In Ladakh, there are multiple medical systems available to people and the options available to any specific group are many. The acceptance of any or a combination of these forms of therapeutic help depends on a variety of factors.

With their age-old folk medical system, people have been able to survive and maintain the ecological balance. With the advent of western medicine a new system has been introduced and people always react differently to this transplant system. Traditional type of system, which does not allow any scientific exploration, is obviously based on myths and powers that are not within human control, i.e. for such things a supernatural elements may be responsible. Consequently the treatment of the ailment also reflects appeasement of the supernatural powers which are extraneous to the individual (patient). In such a society, adoption of new medical therapy obviously will be challanged by the existing system and hence, unlesss the new system is capable of replacing the traditional values by its efficacy and acceptability, it will not be a success.

From the interviews which were carried out in the health centre, one thing was clear that the patients were coming to health centre only after they had received treatment from their own practitioners. Disease as an area of inquiry and the attitude to curing disease has its special importance *vis-à-vis* other areas like status, political power, because of the personal equation and time factor involved. It is a matter of life and death in case of a critical disease and their range of action pattern is limited. It is a crisis response rather than a calculated response. When the human system is out of order all types of irrationalities come into play. Since the response to critical disease are *adhoc*, they do not reflect the traditional cultural norms.

People modify pre-existing practices if the economic costs are within their reach. People are pragmatic in trying and evaluating new alternatives. In case of health behaviour, the cost-benefit mode of analysis and the empirical evidence help in deciding, whether it is to their advantage or not. There is a change in overt behaviour of the people, but it does not necessarily explain or mean changes in the belief system. Among Ladakhis, it was found that although the traditional beliefs about fertility, pregnancy and abortion have remained unchanged, many births in the study area took place in the health centre or government hospital. The study of Wily (2002) also corroborate this study that there is widespread and increasing usage of biomedical services for prenatal care and birth among women in Ladakh, over the course of the past 20 years. Ladakhis have their own traditional-folk medical system with traditional beliefs and practices. But when they were offered the western or government sponsored medical services they accepted them and put them to the test even if as a last resort. They do not in all cases continue to use western medical services, but they show open-mindedness in trying them out. Among Ladakhis, the situation is like what Wagner found among Navaho. Wagner found that Navaho "have a very open, pragmatic, and non-discriminatory attitude towards various medico-religious options available in time of need. White medicine, traditional chantways, peyotism and even various Christian sects on reservation tend to merge in their minds into alternative and somewhat interchangeable avenues for being used" (Wagner, 1978:4-5). Ladakhis have a open pragmatic and non-discriminatory attitude towards the multiple medical system available to them and acceptance of any one combination of these depend on the individual or houseld decision. As far curative medical services are concerned, these are embraced more readily than preventive services, as was seen in the case of immunization. All were not ready to immunize their children as only 43.2 per cent children are immunized in study area, out of which 46.6 per cent were Buddhists and 41.4 per cent were Muslims. The reason for this is that the result of the scientific curative medicine are much more easily demonstrated than the results of preventive medicine. "Cause and effect are easily comprehended when serious illness gives way to no illness in a few hours or days, cause and effect are less easily seen when, in the case of immunization and environmental sanitation programmes, no disease is followed by no disease" (Foster and Anderson, 1978:245-46). As there are multiple medical systems available to Ladakhis to opt for, the course of action to follow depends on the situation and condition of the sick. The strategies that underline these decision-making process have come to be called the "hierarchy of resort in curative practice" (Schwartz, 1969). The way in which people structure their personal hierarchies of resort tell us about their preferences.

Among Ladakhis, a sequence of resort does not seem to exist, although the trend is to begin with home remedies to Lama to *Lhama/ Lhapa* to *Amchi* as the course of the illness proceeds and become more serious. However, there is also a back and forth movement between resources, or a shorten approach, often based on referrals and advice from relatives and neighbours and other practitioners, which seems to be associated with desperation over the perceived increasing severity of an illnesss.

In view of the extremely difficult means of communication and distance of dispensaries from the villages in Ladakh, medical aid is not availed by the people except in serious cases. The use of traditional herbs for curing disease is most common in the area. Percentage distribution of deaths (1986-88) among Buddhists and Muslims of Ladakh was reported highest by respondents while availing the Allopathic medicine which is taken as a last resort or in terminal cases. It is observed that deaths reported by availing traditional folk medicine is negligible. The reason underlying this is that their first choice is traditional folk medicine.

The area being difficult, the sanctioned posts in most cases remain vacant. Thus, medical facilities are not sufficient to cater to the needs of people. Those who want to avail these facilities often have to travel long distances. This combined with shortage of medicines, results in most of the patients remaining unattended. So the people in interior areas have to depend on their own medical treatment.

In general, the health problems in Ladakh can be grouped into five main categories: a high rate of infectious and water borne diseases, poor environmental sanitation and hygiene, unsatisfactory nutritional status, ignorance about health, and an unsatisfactory health care delivery system. The belief in the interference of a supernatural agency is strong in both the communities. It was seen from the data that when both the facilities (namely modern and traditional) were available in the area people often accepted and availed of the western medicine. Though they go to the Health Centre, side by side they also perform various traditional rituals. Unfortunately, adequate medical facilities are not available in many areas, and people are accused of not accepting these non-existing medical facilities. In areas where medical facililties are not within their reach, people depend on traditional medical care; herbs are used as medicines along with rituals to cure different diseases. The dependence and confidence on traditional medical practitioners *Lhama/Lhapa* and *Amchis*, and Lamas are the result of faith and confidence among the patients. As the traditional practitioners share the common cultural traditions of the patients, naturally the patients have more faith in them. The system of cause, effect and cure, is thus a circular and enclosed system of knowledge. The cause is a spirit, the effect is spirit possession, and the cure is controlled spirit possession. This system of knowledge provides the manifest of explanation and control in the face of disorder, chaos and inexplicable circumstances. The social function here described is adaptive, or as described by Spiro (1966:120), it (spirit possession) is the basis of "Social stability" in potentially unstable and disruptive social circumstances. It has similar function that witchcraft belief, as described by Evans Pritchard (1937:63-83), have for many African societies. The beliefs and institutions surrounding spirit possession fulfil the function as noted by Spiro (1967: 121) of providing a "culturally approved means, for the resolution of inner conflict (between) personal desires and cultural norms" (cited from Jones, 1976). Medical system's degree of productivity depends on the effectiveness of its armamentarium and the technical skills of its practitioners. However, in some cases efficacy have little or no positive effect on the productivity of the medical system. It happens in cases where improvements in efficacy are restricted to a small number of people and have a negligible effect on levels of morbidity and mortality of the total population. Improvements in efficacy are made available to population around urban centres for which they can make a difference. However, this means diverting resources needed for improving the health of a larger segment of the total population. For example, this is the situation in Ladakh where the capital absorbing medical intervention demanded by urban centres siphon resources away from the primary health care needs of a much larger rural at-risk population. The net effect is no change or even an increase in overall levels of morbidity and mortality.

Despite improvements in health facilities in Ladakh in the past, no significant improvements in health status could be achieved. Morbidity pattern in Ladakh shows that the incidence of the diseases is concentrated more among children major diseases has already started, diseases which are related with congestion, contaminated drinking water, poor hygiene and sanitation could be kept under control if educating the public on primary health care becomes a part of the local health care services. Greater emphasis should be placed on creating facilities for the treatment and control of infectious diseases which are closely associated with cramming up of family members in a room during winter months at household levels. Given the interlinkage between health, education and occupation, all are important in their own sphere, emphasis should be placed on improvement in all.

While the control of population should be among the prime objectives of the Government's development programmes, in an effort to redeem the adverse consequences of growing population because of breaking up of monomarital system or polyandrous marriages and decrease in number of monks. Greater emphasis should be on creating employment opportunities in the non-agricultural sector. Distribution of educational institutions across different geographical areas should cover, rather on the relative concentration of school age children in the respective localities. Rather than constructing new facilities, under resource constraints, maximum possible effort should be made to maintain properly the existing institutions. Greater emphasis should be placed on creating health awareness about primary health care.

Given the interlinkage between health, education and occupation, local institution could be used for multiple purposes. For instance, the existing school building could be used as health centre, or as a training institute for new technology, new crop variety cropping pattern and even for development of local skills.

## REFERENCES

Adams, Vincanne (1992): "Reconstructured relationships of production in sherpa Tourism", *Ann. Tourism Research*, 19.

Bandy, D. (1974): "Traditional Curers under the impact of western medicine", *American Ethnology*, 1:103.

Bhasin, Veena (1990): *Habitat, Habitation and Health in the Himalayas*, Delhi: Kamla-Raj Enterprises.

Bhasin, M.K. and L.P. Singh (1992): "A study of anthropometric somatotype in two high altitude populations—Bodhs and Baltis of Ladakh, Jammu and Kashmir, India." *J. Hum. Eco.*, 3:27-34.

Bhasin, V. (1992): "Brok-pa of Ladakh. A case of adaptation to habitat". *Journal of Human Ecology*, 3:81.

Bhasin, V. (1996): *Transhumants of Himalaya: Changpal of Ladakh, Goddis of Himachal Pradesh and Bhutial of Sikkim.* Delhi: Kamala-Raj Enterprises.

Blumenhagen, W.D. (1980): "Hypertension: A Folle illness with a medical name." "*Culture, Medicine and Psychinatry*, 4:197-227.

Carstairs, G. Morris (1957): *The Twice Born*, London: Hogarth.

Census of India (1991): *Series I, India.* New Delhi: Controller of Publications, India, 1983.

Comaroff, Jean (1982): "Medicine Symple and Ideology." in P. Wright and A. Treakher (eds). *The Problem of Medical Knowledge.* Edinburgh: Edinburgh University Press.

Cosminsky, S. (1977): "Impact of methods on the analysis of illness concept in a Guatemalan Community." *Social Science Medicine,* 11:325.

Cosminsky, S. and Mary Scrimshaw (1980): Medical Pluarlism on a Guatemalan Plantation, *Social Science and Medicine,* 14B: 267-278.

De young, John E. (1955): *Village Life in Modern Thailand.* Berkeley: University of California Press.

Elisde, M. (1964): *Shamanism: Archaic Techniques of Ecstasy* (Translated by W.B. Trask). New York: Pantheon.

Erasmus, John Charles (1952): "Changing Folle Beliefs and the Relativity of Empirical Knowledge." *Southwestern Anthropology,* 8:411-428.

Foster, George and Barbara Gallatin Anderson (1978): *Medical Anthropology,* New York, Wiley.

Frake, C. (1961): "The diagnosis of disease among the Subanum of Mindanas." *Amer, Anthrop.,* 63:113-132,

Furer, Haimendrof, Von. (1964): *The Sherpas of Nepal,* London.

Geertz, C. (1973): *The Interpretation of Cultures.* New York: Basic Books.

Goldstein, M.C., P. Tsarong and C.M. Beall (1983): High attitude hyporia culture and human fecundity/fertility: A comparitive study". *American Anthropologist,* 85:28.

Gonzales, N.S. (1966): "Health Behaviour in Cross-cultural Perspective: a Guatamalan example." *Human organization,* 25:122.

Good, B.J. (1977): "The Heart of What is the Matter: The Semantics of Illness of Iran. *Culture Medical and Psychiatry,* 1:25&58.

Gorer, Geoffrey (1943): *Burmese Personality* (Mimeograph). New York: Institute for Intercultural Relations.

Hackett, William Dunn (1953): *The Pa-o People of the Shan State Union of Burma,* Ithaca: Cornel University Press.

Joses, Rex L. (1976): "Spirit Possession and Society in Nepal." in T. Hitchcoik and L. Rex L. Jones (eds.). *Spirit Possession in Nepal Himalayas.* New Delhi: Vikas Publishing House.

Kleinman, A. (1978a): "Concepts and a model for Comparison of Medical System." *Social Science Med. Bull.,* 85-93.

Kleinman, A. (1978b): "Clinical relevance of anthropological and cross-cultural research: Concepts and strategies." *Amer. J. Psychiatry,* 135 L427-431.

Kleinman, A. (1980): *Patients and Healers in the Context of Culture: An Exploration of the Border Land Between Anthropology, Medicine and Psychiatry.* California: University California Press.

Landy, D. (1974): "Traditional Curers under the impact of Western Medicine". *American Ethnology,* 1:103.

Lock, Margaret (1982): "Models and Practice in Medicine Menopause as Syndrome of Life Transition." *Culture Medicine and Psychiatry,* 6:261-280.

Manning, P. and H. Fabrega Jr. (1973): "The Experience of Self and Body: Health and Illness in the Chanpas highlands in G. Psathas (ed.) *Phenomenological Sociology.* New York: Wiley.

Murthy Y.K. 1981. "Water Resources Potentials of the Himalayas" in J.S. Lall and A.D. Moddie (eds.). *The Himalayas, Aspects of Change.* New Delhi: Oxford University Press.

Netesky-Wojkowitz (1975): *Oracles and Demons of Tibet: The Cult and Iconography of the Tibetan Protective Deities.* The Hange: Mutton.

Neumann, A.K. *et al.* (1971): "Role of Indigenous Medicine Practitioners in Two Areas of India: Report of a Study", *Social Science and Medicine,* 5:13.

Nichter, Mark (1980): The Lay Person's Perception of Medicine as Perspective into Utilization of Multiple Therapy System in the Indian context. *Social Science and Medicine,* 4B:225-233.

Norboo, T. and Yahya. M. (1988): "Health Problems in Ladakh". *Voice of the Himalayas,* 1:5-9.

Peter, Prince (1963): *A Study of Polyandry.* The Hague: Muton and Co.

Press, I. (1978): "Urban Folk Medicine." *American Anthropologist,* 80:71.

Samual, Geffery (1990): *Mind, Body and Culture Anthropology and the Inteface.* Cambridge: Cambridge University Press.

Schwartz, Lola R. (1969): "The Hierarchy of Resort in Curative Practice: The Admiralthy Islands, Melansia." *Journal of Health and Social Behaviour,* 10:201-209.

Spiro, M. (1967): *Burmese Supernaturalism,* Indianapolis: Standford University Press.

Tribal Census of Ladakh (1991): New Delhi: Registrar General of India.

Wagher, Roland M. (1978): "Traditional amd Modern Medicine as Reflected in Contemporary Peyotist Practices". in B. Velimirovic (ed.). *Modern Medicine and Medical Anthropology in the U.S. Mexico Border Population.* Washington, D.C.: Pan.

# 10

# A Comparative Study of Reproductive Health among Two Primitive Tribes of Andhra Pradesh

M.P. SACHDEVA, R. CHOWDHARY, K.N. SARASWATHY, A.M. ELIZABETH and A.K. KALLA

## Introduction

In the present paper an attempt is made to compare the reproductive health of women, belonging to two primitive tribes, with the help of two major demographic indicators, namely fertility and offspring mortality. The tribes chosen for the present study are Kolam and Thoti who are mainly concentrated in Adilabad district of Andhra Pradesh. Despite sharing the same geographical area they are maintaining their respective cultural identity by not at all indulging in any inter tribal marital exchanges. According to Heimendorf (1979) both tribes are the satellite tribes of the Gonds.

## Materials and Methods

### *Kolam*

Kolams are mainly distributed in Andhra Pradesh, Maharashtra and Madhya Pradesh. The total population of Kolams in Andhra Pradesh according to 1991 census is 41,254 individuals of whom 92.4 per cent belong to the rural areas and 7.6 per cent belong to the urban areas. Kolams constitute 1 per cent of the total scheduled tribal population of Andhra Pradesh and 11.4 per cent of the district Adilabad. 97.7 per cent of the Kolam population of Andhra Pradesh is confined to Adilabad district alone. Kolams (as called in Urdu) call themselves *Kolawars*, while Gonds call them *Pujaris*. In Telugu Kolams are called *Mannevarlu*. They, like the Gonds, are organized in exogamous clans and most of these clans have names identical to those of Gond system of "seven-brother clans" and "four-brother clans". Each *phratry* is divided into a number of *Paris* or clans. All Kolams irrespective of clan or phratry worship *Ayak* (*Bheemanna* in Telugu) as principal deity of the tribe, unlike the Gonds who worship the clan deity. People belonging to the same clan or phratry are considered to be siblings and thus the marriages are always contracted outside a *Dayyam* or *phratry*.

### *Thoti*

The Thoti tribe is known by different names. The name Thoti is based on the traditional occupation of their women, which is tattooing (*Thochi* in Marathi means tattoo). The Thoti women proudly proclaim that they are traditional tattooists to Gonds. On the basis of this occupation they are also known as *Pachabotluvandlu* or *Chukkabotluvandu*. The other name *Birdu Gond* resulted from bard-patron relationship between Thoti and Gond. In the *Taluks* of Asifabad, Luxettipet and Chinnur, Thotis are known as *Pandavulu* as they narrate the stories of Pandavas, the heroes of the epic.

The Thoti tribe was recognized as primitive tribal population by Government of India in 1983. According to Guha (1935), the Thoti belong to the proto-Australoid stock having dark skin, sunken nose and low forehead. Russel (1916) had described Thoti as a sub-tribe of the Pradhans. But it is difficult to confirm this though these two tribes are identical in their traditional relationship to Raj Gonds as ritual beggars (Haimendorf, 1979).

According to 1991 census, Thoti in Andhra Pradesh numbered 3654 persons and a large percentage (49.04%) lived in Adilabad district alone. They are found in erstwhile *taluks* of Adilabad, Boath, Luxettipet and Khanpur. They are also present, however, in small numbers in Asifabad, Wankidi, Chinnur and Nirmal *taluks*. Thoti generally live along with other tribal and non-tribal communities and their villages are easily accessible. All the villages or hamlets where Thotis live are multi-ethnic ones and a majority of them are having *kacha* or *pucca* road facilities.

The mother tongue of Thoti is Gondi; besides Gondi, they speak Telugu, Marathi, Urdu and Hindi. The Thoti are Hindus by religion.

They worship Gond gods; besides these they also worship Hanuman and other Hindu gods and celebrate Hindu festivals.

The Thotis are divided into four exogamous phratries known as '*Saga*' in Gondi, each of which traces its descent from a fixed number of divine ancestors: Yerwen Saga (seven-brother folk), Sarwen or Pandwen Saga (six-brother folk), Siwn Saga (five-brother folk) and Nalwen Saga (four-brother folk).

Demographic data was collected from 20 Kolami villages and 18 Thoti villages, which fall under 15 *mandals*, the so-called *taluks* of other states. The unit selected for the study was an ever-married woman of the household. 350 ever-married Kolam women and 246 ever-married Thoti women were interviewed using extensive and pretested schedules, which consisted of questions pertaining to demographic profile of both populations, and the reproductive details of the respondent.

## Results

Demographic variables like dependency ratios, fertility indicators like crude birth rate (CBR), total fertility rate (TFR), general fertility rate (GFR) and mortality indicators like crude death rate (CDR) and infant mortality rate (IMR) were calculated using the standard formulae.

**Table 10.1:** Distribution of Certain Demographic Variables in Some Indian Populations

| *Population* | *Young Dependency Ratio* | *Old Dependency Ratio* | *Total Dependency Ratio* | *Reference* |
|---|---|---|---|---|
| Kolam | 927 | 55.90 | 982.90 | Present study |
| Thoti | 409.33 | 32.82 | 442.15 | Present study |
| Rural India | 709.60 | 131.50 | 841.10 | SRS 1998 |
| Rural ST population | 764.50 | 106.50 | 871.00 | SRS 1998 |

Young dependency ratio of Kolams is found to be higher and that of the Thotis is found to be lower than those of Rural Indian and also the rural schedule tribe populations. This may be partly due to higher fertility among the Kolams, which is reflected respectively in their higher CBR (40.8), GFR (191.78) and higher TFR (6.33) and a lower CBR (32.4), lower GFR (144.0) and lower TFR (3.8) among the Thoti. The crude birth rate of both the tribes is found to be higher than that of Andhra Pradesh (27.9).

However the old dependency ratio is quite low for both tribes in comparison with other above-mentioned populations (Table 10.1) that may be partly due to a lower longevity among the two primitive tribes. The nuclear family system prevailing in the present populations could be one of the possible reasons for the lower longevity among these two tribes as old people have lesser chances of being taken care of by their younger ones. Total dependency ratio of Kolams is higher and that of Thotis is lower than those of other above-mentioned populations.

**Table 10.2:** Distribution of Mortality Indicators

| *Population* | *Crude Death Rate* | *Infant Mortality Rate* | *Reference* |
|---|---|---|---|
| Kolam | 11.67 | 142.86 | Present study |
| Thoti | 14.07 | 108.10 | Present study |
| Rural Population India | 9.7 | — | SRS, 1998 |
| Rural Population AP | 9.1 | — | SRS, 1998 |
| Schedule Tribes of AP | — | 144 | Registrar General, 1979 |
| Savara | — | 213.23 | TRI Hyderabad |
| Jatapu | — | 102.04 | TRI Hyderabad |
| Mooka Dora | — | 88.88 | TRI Hyderabad |
| Gadaba | — | 239.43 | TRI Hyderabad |
| Konda Dora | — | 102.56 | TRI Hyderabad |
| Hillill Kolam | — | 70.59 | Murthy & Ramesh, 1978 |
| Mannel Kolam | — | 68.00 | Murthy & Ramesh, 1978 |

The crude death rate (CDR) of Kolam population is found to be lower than that of the Thoti population. (Table 10.3). However the CDR of both tribes is relatively higher respectively than those of the other above mentioned populations. However, the IMR (Infant Mortality Rate) among the Kolams (Murthy and Ramesh, 1978) has more than doubled over the last two decades.

**Table 10.3:** Distribution of Prenatal and Infant mortality among the Kolams and Thotis of Andhra Pradesh

| *Population* | *Number of Conceptions* | *Prenatal Mortality* | | *Number of Live Births* | *Infant Mortality* | |
|---|---|---|---|---|---|---|
| | | No. | % | | No. | % |
| Kolam | 1383 | 24 | 1.74 | 1363* | 173 | 12.69 |
| Thoti | 985 | 61 | 6.19 | 924 | 88 | 9.52 |

* Includes some twins.

A higher prenatal mortality observed among the Thotis may be attributed to lower age at marriage (13.59) and lower age at first conception (17.60) among the group and partly due to lack of antenatal mother child health care programmes in this region.

Higher infant mortality of Kolams should be seen in the backdrop of the fact that all the deliveries took place at home and that they were not exposed at all to the modern health care system, especially the antenatal and postnatal care. The Thotis seem to be a little better off in this respect as among them 0.8 per cent of the deliveries took place in hospitals and they are expected to be somewhat aware of the modern health care facilities.

The situation seems to be aggravated among the Kolams perhaps because they live in scattered hamlets far away from the townships and the centres of modern health facilities. This is further compounded by the 100 per cent illiteracy coupled with the fact that they cannot even converse in the state language.

The high infant mortality among the Kolam tribe may partly be explained by the earlier findings (Sachdeva *et al.* 2002) wherein it was reported that the Kolam population had a high rate of NESTROFT (Naked eye single tube red cell osmotic fragility test) positive, meaning thereby that there is a likelihood of high incidence of thalassaemia among them, which is known to take a severe toll of life at infant stage particularly in the absence of adequate medical care.

## Recommendations

The specific recommendations concerning the health issues of the Kolams and Thotis, which emerge from the present study, are the following:

1. Infant health care programmes need to be augmented effectively particularly among the Kolams with a constant

monitoring of thalassaemic status of the population, which, in turn, may be used for genetic counselling in order to safeguard against giving birth to thalassemic children.

2. Antenatal mother child health care programmes specially need to be executed particularly among the Thotis who are found to have very high incidence of prenatal mortality.

If the above two recommendations are properly taken care of, the overall health status of these populations may substantially improve.

## REFERENCES


Guha, B.S. (1935): *The racial affinities of people of India*, Census of India, 1931, Vol. I, Part IIIB, government press, Shimla.

Heimendorf, C.F and Heimendorf, E.F. (1979): *The Gonds of Andhra Pradesh*, Vikas Publishing House, New Delhi, p. 25.

Ramesh, A., Murthy, J.S. and Blake, N.M. (1979): Genetic studies on the Kolams of Andhra Pradesh, *India. Hum. Hered.*, 29: 147-143

Russell, R.V. (1916): *The tribes and castes of the central province of India*, London 1916, Vol. IV, p. 354.

Sachdeva, M.P., Elizabeth, A.M., Saraswathy, K.N., Chowdhury, R. and Kalla, A.K. (2002): Incidence of Nestroft-positives, G6PD Deficiency and HB S among the Thotis and Kolams of Andhra Pradesh. In M.K. Bhasin and A.K. Kalla (ed.) *Expanding Horizons of Human Genetics*, Kamla-Raj Enterprises, Delhi. Pp. 199-231.

Sample Registration System (1998): *Registrar General, India*, 32, (2) New Delhi.

11

# Demographic Aspects of Tribal Health in India with Special Reference to Major States

DISHA TEWARI

---

It has been truly said that health was combined in sympathy and born out of necessity and the first doctor was the first man and the first woman, the first nurse. The prehistoric man motivated by feeling of sympathy and kindness was always at the behest of his kindred, trying to provide relief, in times of sickness and suffering.

Further in ancient times health and illness were interpreted in cosmological and anthropological perspective, medicine was dominated by magical and religious beliefs, which are an integral part of ancient cultures and civilization. As the time passed, there was plethora of discoveries, which had taken place in the field of health (Park).

Mankind is proceeding towards greater and greater homogeneity, racially, culturally and linguistically. This march encompasses a variety of dimensions and some agonizing implications. Oldest cultures are either dying or are being exterminated. In such a broad category comes a great segment of primitive, tribal, indigenous, aboriginal, native and so on. Some characteristics of these groups have been simple pre-machine economy, unsophisticated rituals and social customs, lack of a script for their speech which itself is not developed, small local community organization and homogeneity (Nadeem Hasnain).

The present paper discusses the tribal health in terms of infant and child mortality and other social factors, practices like exposure to mass media, current use of any contraceptive method. Few of the health indicators like anaemia among children and diarrhoea with blood are used. Despite of all health projects and schemes, some states still show high incidence of mortality, more than the national average. This is characterized by illiteracy, sub-human physical living conditions, high malnutrition, etc.

The purpose of this paper is to rank the states, which have the highest levels of IMR and child mortality rates and the comparison of different parameters with the national average. The paper is divided into three parts; first part gives the brief account of tribals in India, second part discusses the database, methodology used with the analysis. The discussion and conclusion is included in the third part.

## Tribes in India

India has largest tribal population in the world. The tribal population of India is 67.7 million, larger than that of any other country in the world. Myanmar, with the tribal population of 44 million has the second largest population. The tribal in India constitutes 8.08 per cent of the total population. In some states and union territories they constitute an overwhelming major, e.g. Mizoram (98%), Meghalaya (90%), Nagaland (84%), Arunachal Pradesh (68%) followed by Manipur (38%), Sikkim (28%), Madhya Pradesh (24%), Orissa (22%), Assam (21%), negligible in north region (3%) except in Rajasthan and in Goa, Tamil Nadu and Uttar Pradesh (NFHS-2).

The tribals live in forests and mountains somewhat isolated from the general population. Because of this they have been called as Girijan and Vanvasi.They are overwhelmingly illiterate. The literacy rate of tribals is 23.63 per cent (1991). This is lower than that of general population (52.21%).

## Methodology used and Analysis

The secondary data used for the analysis is taken from the National Family Health Survey conducted in 1998-99. The principal objective of NHFS-2 is to provide state and national estimates of fertility, practice of family planning, infant and child mortality, maternal and child health and utilization of health services provided to mothers and children. The survey used uniform questionnaires, sample designs and field procedures to facilitate comparability of the data and to achieve higher level of data quality.

The data analysed pertains to nine states where NFHS was conducted in 1998-99, along with National level averages. Since the main focus of this paper is on the tribes, so data is taken only of the tribal populations of nine states.

The different factors that are chosen are as follows:

(a) *Infant Mortality Rate (IMR)*: It is the ratio of infant deaths (under one year of age) registered in a calendar year to the total number of live births registered in same year.
(b) *Child Mortality Rate (CMR)*: It is the ratio of children deaths (between first and fifth birthdays) to the total number of children in that age group.
(c) *Not Regularly Exposed to any Mass Media*: Percentage of ever married women age 15-49 who are not exposed to any kind of mass media.
(d) *Any Contraceptive Method Currently Used*: Percentage distribution of currently married women by contraceptive method currently used.
(e) *Percentage showing Vaccination Card*: Percentage of children with a vaccination card that was shown to the interviewer.
(f) *Diarrhoea with Blood*: Percentage of children under age 3 who had diarrhoea during the two weeks preceeding the survey.
(g) *Any Anaemia among Children*: Percentage of children age 6-35 months classified as having any kind of anaemia like mild, moderate or severe.

### *Choice of Technique for Analysis*

In order to analyse and rank the states with high rates of tribal infant mortality and other factors certain indicators are selected as described earlier. Composite values of each state is calculated by using Z-score and ranks have been given to each of the nine states and then they are categorized into high, medium and low levels of health status.

The resultant composite scores clearly reveal the levels of development in terms of health status, which is uneven among the states. The highest value depicts the lower levels of health status and the lowest value of Z-score gives the higher degree of health status.

**Table 11.1:** Gives the values of various indicators chosen to explain the health status

| *States* | *IMR* | *CHILD-MO* | *EXP* | *CONUSE* | *VACC.* | *DIARRHOEA* | *ANAEMIA* |
|---|---|---|---|---|---|---|---|
| India | 84.2 | 46.3 | 61.8 | 39.1 | 24.5 | 3.7 | 79.8 |
| Rajasthan | 94.7 | 66.6 | 83.3 | 29.3 | 10.3 | 6.5 | 80.2 |
| Madhya Pradesh | 101.0 | 87.4 | 64.1 | 32.9 | 16.3 | 5.8 | 83.9 |
| Uttar Pradesh | 83.3 | 45.0 | 65.5 | 15.1 | 19.6 | 7.0 | 72.9 |
| Bihar | 81.9 | 37.8 | 88.3 | 14.1 | 12.1 | 1.8 | 93.5 |
| Orissa | 98.7 | 44.0 | 84.1 | 37.5 | 29.7 | 4.0 | 83.9 |
| Assam | 59.3 | 15.1 | 53.1 | 47.5 | 28.5 | 1.8 | 59.1 |
| Gujarat | 60.3 | 36.5 | 54.1 | 57.1 | 18.9 | 1.6 | 82.4 |
| Maharashtra | 73.6 | 20.2 | 54.0 | 53.7 | 39.4 | 2.7 | 83.2 |
| Karnataka | 85.0 | 38.9 | 34.7 | 44.8 | 27.7 | .0 | 71.9 |

*Abbreviations used—*

IMR : Infant Mortality Rates
Child-MO : Child Mortality
Exp. : Not regularly exposed to mass media
Conuse : Any contraceptive method currently used.
Vacc : Percentage showing vaccination card
Diarrhoea : Diarrhoea with blood
Anaemia : Any anaemia among children.

## *Description of the Table*

(a) *IMR*: Table 11.1 depicts that Madhya Pradesh has the highest value of tribal IMR (101) more than the national levels, followed by Orissa (98.7). The lowest is in the Assam (59.3).

(b) *CMR*: Madhya Pradesh holds the topmost position with 87.4; followed by Rajasthan with 66.6 and lowest is in Assam 15.1. The National average of tribal CMR is 46.3, which is nearly half of that in Madhya Pradesh.

(c) *Exposure to Mass Media*: In a country like India where a large majority of women are illiterate or have little formal education, informal channels such as the mass media can play an important role in bringing about modernization. In India two-fifths of women are not regularly exposed to any mass media. Bihar with 88.3 per cent is at the first place where tribal women are not exposed to any kind of mass media whether it is radio or television, followed by Orissa

84.1 per cent. The least value is in Karnataka with 34.7 per cent of tribal women who are not exposed to any media.

(d) *Use of any Contraceptive Method*: As a social practice family planning is old, preventive and birth limiting checks were used to control the population and to space births. It is also one of the methods to limit fertility rates and the family size. In Gujarat 57.1 per cent of women use any contraceptive method followed by Maharashtra with 53.7 per cent and in Bihar it is the least, only 14.1 per cent.

(e) *Percentage showing Vaccination Card*: 39.4 per cent have vaccination card in Maharashtra followed by Orissa i.e. 29.7 per cent while Rajasthan has the least number of just 10.3 per cent of the tribal children having them.

(f) *Diarrhoea*: It is the second most important killer of children under age five all over the world, following acute respiratory infection. Deaths from acute diarrhoea are most often caused by dehydration due to loss of water and electrolytes. Because deaths from diarrhoea are a significant proportion of all child deaths, Government of India has launched the Oral Rehydration Therapy Programme as one of its priority activities for child survival.

One major goal of this programme is to increase awareness among mothers and communities about the causes and treatment of diarrhoea. Mothers are taught how to use ORS packets. Despite these, Uttar Pradesh reports 7 per cent of tribal children suffering from diarrhoea with blood followed by Rajasthan, i.e. 6.5 per cent and Karnataka does not report even a single case of it.

(g) *Anaemia among Children*: It is a serious concern for young children because it can result in impaired cognitive performance, behavioural and motor development, coordination, language development as well as increased morbidity from infectious diseases. Bihar is at the top with a very high percentage of children suffering from any kind of anaemia, i.e. 93.5 per cent followed by Orissa and Madhya Pradesh with 83.9 per cent. Assam has the lowest count i.e. 59.1 per cent.

**Table 11.2:** Gives the Z-score values of Nine states

| *States* | *Z-score* | *Rank* |
|---|---|---|
| Rajasthan | 6.1 | 1 |
| Madhya Pradesh | 5.6 | 2 |
| Uttar Pradesh | 2.7 | 4 |
| Bihar | 4.4 | 3 |
| Orissa | 2.1 | 5 |
| Assam | –7.4 | 8 |
| Gujarat | –3.7 | 6 |
| Maharashtra | –4.9 | 7 |
| Karnataka | –4.9 | 7 |

### *Explanation of Table 11.2*

It is quite evident from Table 11.2 that BIMARU states, namely Bihar, Madhya Pradesh, Rajasthan and Uttar Pradesh have the higher values of Z-score.

When the scores are divided into three categories of high, medium and low values, Rajasthan, Madhya Pradesh and Bihar come under high category, i.e. having scores above 4.01, followed by Uttar Pradesh and Orissa in the medium category with scores between 0.01-4.0 while Assam, Gujarat, Maharashtra and Karnataka come in the lowest category, i.e. below 0 scores. This gives a picture of deteriorating health conditions of the tribes in high category and good health conditions of the tribes within low category.

## Discussion and Conclusion

Health is a function, not only of medical care but of the overall integrated development of socio-cultural, economic, education and political. Each of these aspects has a deep influence on health which in turn influences all these aspects.

It has been noted by many that tribals living in remote areas have a better health status and more balanced food than those living in less remote areas (Chaudhuri 1986, Chaudhuri, *et al.* 1989). But in many cases it is noted that certain diseases may be common. It is recognized that health problems of the tribals are not the exclusive domain of medical sciences; socio-cultural tradition does play an important role in the context of health and treatment. The widespread poverty, illiteracy, malnutrition, absence of safe drinking water and sanitary living conditions, poor maternal and child health services, ineffective coverage of national health and nutritional services, have been traced out in several studies as possible contributing factors for dismal health conditions prevailing in these vulnerable population (working group report of Ministry of Welfare).

Infant and child mortality remain amongst the highest in India, the risk of dying is exceptionally high for children from households with a low standard of living, children from S.C. and S.T. households, rural children and for children whose mothers are illiterate.

The grim situation of tribal health is seen in BIMARU states, with Rajasthan at the highest level. These states have almost 45 per cent of the total tribal population (1981, primary census abstracts) and literacy rates among tribals were 8.5 per cent in 1961 and 16.4 per cent in 1981, which is very much lower than the national levels of 24 per cent and 36.2 per cent in 1961 and 1981, respectively. There is no significant change in the literacy rates as evident from 1991 census.

Since the literacy levels are low, tribal people using any type of contraceptive methods would also be affected, as less number of people are aware of the benefits of contraceptive use. Contraceptive methods are used for spacing between the children. If the spacing between children is less, they tend to become weak as mother is unable to recover fully from the previous delivery and therefore the next child born is prone to infectious diseases that increase mortality levels among the children.

As it is evident from Table 11.1, tribal people exposed to any kind of mass media is fairly low in BIMARU states and that is also a major factor of deteriorating status of child health as mothers are not aware of various deficiencies that occur in the children because of malnutrition and under nutrition.

Infant and child mortality are the direct indicators of the socio-economic condition of the people, children of persons with high socio-economic status have better chances of survival because of better sanitation and hygiene while with poor status are prone to infections because of unhygienic conditions.

Thus infant and child mortality, which indicate health of the child, should be given much more attention especially in the BIMARU states. It depicts the level of development of the states so better care, health and medical facilities should be provided to overcome the present situation. This is possible only when supportive services such as nutrition, environment and education reach a higher level.

## REFERENCES


Bhende, A. and Kanitkar, T. (1978): *Principles of Population Studies.*

Census of India (1981): Series 1, India, Part II-B (iii), Primary Census Abstract, Scheduled Tribes; Controller of Publications, Govt. of India, Delhi.

Miri, Mrinal (1993): *Continuity and Change in Tribal Society*, Indian Institute of Advanced Study, Shimla.

National Family Health Survey (NHFS-2), (1998-99): International Institute for Population Sciences, Mumbai (October 2000).

Park, K. (2002): *Text Book on Preventive and Social Medicine*, 17th Edition, Banarsidas Bhanot, Prem Nagar, Jabalpur.

Rao, K. Sujata (1998): Health Care Services in Tribal Areas of Andhra Pradesh: A Public Policy Perspective. *Economic and Political Weekly.* 33(9), (481-486), SNDT Churchgate.

Report of the Working Group on Development and Welfare of Scheduled Tribes during Eight Five Year Plan (1987, Nov.), Govt. of India, Ministry of Welfare, New Delhi.

Singh, A.K. and Rajyalakshmi, C. (Dec. 1993): Status of Tribal Women In India. Social Change. 23(4), (3-18), SNDT Churchgate.

# 12

# Women and Health among the Moyons

LANGLOM NAOMI MOYON

## Introduction

Woman is the key to the provision of health services for the family and society. Yet she has been neglected and exploited by health services. The mother is the central figure who provides child care, hygiene, nutrition, and even primary health care. Without good mental and physical health care for the mother herself, it will not be possible for her to give her best for the health and development of her child, family, society and nation. Until and unless, they are allowed to be educated, become healthy and develop positive self-image, health programmes will not bear much fruits.

The present paper is an attempt to bring forth the socio-economic and environmental factors that influence the health and hèalth care system of Moyon women. The study also focuses on the problems faced by women during pregnancy, child birth and health seeking. It also deals with the female mortality and its causes. This paper also includes suggestive measures to improve the health and health care system. The study is based on the survey of 60 households contacted during my fieldwork.

The Moyons inhabit mainly the Chandel District, which is in South-Eastern part of Manipur. They are Mongoloid and speak Naga-Kuki language of the Tibeto-Burman group. Ethnically, they belong to Naga group. The Moyons are one of the 29th recognized tribes of Manipur with distinct identity, rich traditions and cultural heritages passing down from generation to generation.

The Moyons are patriarchal, patrilineal and patrilocal. Property passes down from father to son. Elder brothers and sisters move away from the parental house after marriage but the youngest son remains at home and looks after his parents in their old age because he gets the lion share of his parental property. Nuclear family is much sought in Moyon community.

According to the Moyon legend, Moyons were believed to be emerged out of the cave (KHUR) which some believed, was somewhere in China. The people then, settled at Siijuur in China and later on moved towards the south passing through different countries and finally made their settlement in Manipur. Their first known settlement in Manipur was at Ikamphae in Churachandpur district. Then, they shifted to Taasuwnbung or Haobi Ching in Manipur. From Haobi Ching they migrated to Seekhuw, Taangleen, Kamlaangphae and finally settled at Khungjuur or Khongjon village.

## Female Infant and Child Mortality

In Moyon communities, there is no gender discrimination. The birth of a daughter is also welcomed warmly even though they prefer boys for fulfilling the roles of patriarchy like transmition of property, expansion of lineage and looking after parents in their old age. So, there is no female foeticide at all. They often believe that the birth of a child is a gift from God. So, in older days, a woman gave birth till the end of her fertility period. Now, because of modern form of media that keeps on reminding them about family planning, they have accepted family planning.

Infant and child mortality is mostly correlated with socio-economic and environmental factors. So, mortality occurs more in outskirt areas than in the main lands. This is because of the poor facilities of medical aids within the areas and also because of their poverty and unhygienic way of living, epidemics mostly breaks out in these areas. But in comparison to the neighbouring communities, infant mortality is very low among Moyon.

The mortality is higher in the age group of 0-4. These deaths are mainly on account of the poor health status of the mother during pre-natal and postnatal period. There was also a case of asphyxia-neonatorum which could not be saved due to the delivery done at home.

The major diseases noticed among children were air-borne diseases like chicken pox, whooping cough, ordinary fever, cold, cough, etc.

These were followed by water-borne diseases like diarrhoea/dysentery, jaundice, cholera, typhoid and measles. An epidemic like diarrhoea/ dysentery, jaundice, cholera, typhoid also broke out in the remote hilly areas where medical aids could not reach in time.

Environmental factor are responsible for the death of many children as they move away from parents. During these periods, they were found playing around ponds, ditches, and eating and drinking what ever comes in their way. There was also a report that some life of children were taken by high current of river during rainy seasons because they loved to swim.

## Maternal Health and Causes of Maternal Death

The mortality of women was higher in the age group of 40-54. The death occur more in the outskirt areas where there is little health care and the habit of giving birth at home because of their socio-economic problems. Most of the female deaths were related with gynaecological problems which occur during pregnancy and child birth and also because of the effects of over-burden of domestic works during reproductive periods. Women engaged in hard physical labour during pregnancy, lactating and child care period as they took part in activities like cooking, fetching water, collecting fire wood, washing clothes and cleaning houses. Because of these over-burden domestic works, she has no time to take care of herself. Due to their engagement in such work, some women often suffer from back pain, broken bones, miscarriage and fractures mostly during pregnancy.

The causes of maternal mortality are both medical and social. The main causes are anaemia, haemorrhage, infections, etc. In Moyon community, a major complicacy in child birth that leads to mortality rarely occur even though there were cases of caesarean operation. This, they believed, is because of the nature of their work that needs movements and stretching of their body during pregnancy.

Health status of a woman is also related with economic status of the family. In some families, even though the sick persons are not recovered completely, they discontinue taking medicine because they could not afford the medicine. This habit is mostly seen in women from poor economic background because, they are more concerned of their family members and neglect themselves.

## Life Crisis and Cultural Pattern on Cases of Pregnancy, Child Birth and Menopause

Most of the women in Moyon society are engaged in maintaining the household, and at income generating tasks: both of which are essential to keep the family and economy alive. The latter include a long list of activities ranging from agricultural processing, weaving, sewing, knitting, making baskets, containers and mat out of bamboo, opening a shop of grocery and miscellaneous other income generating tasks. A large number of these tasks are performed within the home. Women also contributed in family income by working in schools and offices.

When a woman is pregnant, she refrains from strenuous work but she continues her daily works from cooking to maintaining a house to contributing in the household income till the day of delivery. Even if her husband, mother-in-law and sister-in-law help her in the work, her contribution in household work is always needed.

There are certain traditional taboos that are still followed by pregnant women and their husbands with the thought that if any thing happens to their child, the consequence will be unforgivable. A pregnant woman is considered weak and she is not allowed to go out at night with the belief that she can easily become a victim of spirit. She cannot eat any climbers because that would prolong her birth pains. Any vegetables, which are lying under the wood, cannot be eaten by a pregnant woman with the thought that it will make a child physically weak. The husband of the pregnant woman is not allowed to kill animals with the thought that the baby will inherit a physical characters or a nature of that particular animal that was killed.

A pregnant woman is supposed to be taken for a check up every month but due to their busy schedule in household activities and long distance to reach hospital, most of the women neglected themselves and visited doctors or nurses or hospitals only when they needed them very urgently. Ultra sound is preferred but it does not lead to female foeticide. For the delivery doctors and nurses are called. In some places, where doctors and nurses could not reach in time, mid-wife is often called for the delivery. Now-a-days, most of the pregnant women are taken to hospital for safety, especially if she is giving birth for the first time.

If the delivery is done at home, the woman is kept in one room in which men and unmarried women are not allowed to enter.The husband remains outside and his duty is to call the doctors or the mid-wife and to bring any items needed by her while during delivery.

After the birth of a child, both the child and the mother are washed properly with turmeric-paste. If a baby cries uncontrollably for a long time, a fresh turmeric is applied on the body. In the past the mother used to lie down on a wooden bed near the hearth with the belief that it released gas out of the body. Old woman believed that because of this practice no one complained of back pain and women's face were clearer unlike the present generation. The mother was kept near the hearth till the naming of the child, i.e. 7th day. And then she was brought to her usual bed. In some places, this practice is still continuing.

Menopause usually happens in the age group of 40-45 or above depending on the individual. The symptoms are the irregular menstrual cycle and most women have fever for few days. Menopause care is neglected in Moyon community. People do not even realize that they are having menopause because of the work pressure they have in their daily life. If they have fever, they take tablets for fever otherwise they take menopause as normal in their life.

## Access to Health Care Service

Most of the Moyon people believe in Allopathy. Only a handful people of them follow Homoeopathic treatment. If a person suffers from acute symptoms, which cannot be diagnosed by doctors, he approaches visionary (spiritual leader) with the thought that the cause must be due to supernatural a agent. Even though they are not much into ethno medicines, the use of it is still going on.

When the present study was undertaken, in the area, there is no hospital, but there is only Primary Health Centre (PHC). It is run by the Government of India and was established in 1961. The Primary Health Centre has three nurses and a doctor. The centre provided Pulse Polio immunization and medicine for certain diseases. They also conduct programmes on family planning, malaria eradication, leprosy programmes, mother-child health care, etc. Free contraceptives were also provided as birth control measures. They also gave advice to pregnant women that the delivery of the first born child should take place in the PHC. The villagers, whenever they are unwell, go to the Primary Health Centre for treatment. But due to lack of provision, if the patient cannot be treated at this centre, they are referred to Kakching or Imphal hospital.

Health camp is also organized frequently in the area. In the health camp, the organizer makes the people conscious about the ill effects of malaria, deficiency diseases and the like, and also tells them the importance of good sanitation and a hygienic way of living. World Vision an NGO, also visits Moyon areas every year for free health check up and medicines are also distributed freely. Moyon Naga Baptist Association (MYNBA) also sponsors doctors and nurses for health check up at remote areas when there is epidemic.

*Anganwadi* also takes care of children and pregnant women by giving them milk, flour, wheat, sugar, etc. They also make the women conscious about their own health and their family members. They also teach the pregnant women how to take care of their children and how to keep their house and environment in hygienic condition.

Moyon people of this generation do not fully rely on ethno medicine. Even though they believe that certain herbs are good for certain diseases and ailments, they use such herbs in addition to modern medicine, if the disease or ailment persists. The following are certain diseases along with ethno medicine used.

| *Sl. No.* | *Disease/ailment* | *Ethno medicine used* |
|---|---|---|
| 1. | Cold and Cough | Paarchiip, Siing (Zinger) medicated bath with paarchip. |
| 2. | Sprain/Strain/Joint pain | Hot rice is put on the area and bandaged. |
| 3. | Diarrhoea/Dysentery | Mih (Banana). |
| 4. | Indigestion | Oiled the stomach with oil and salt. |
| 5. | Jaundice | Buchuu (Sugar cane), Brown Sugar. |
| 6. | Gastric | Savean, Sugar can juice. |
| 7. | To safe guard from evil eye. | Applied Jaenghaang (fresh haldi) on the body. |

Besides, they have faith in visionary. For a disease that is believed to be caused by super natural being like spirit intrusion, spirit of sickness etc., they approach visionary. The visionary along with pastor and decons conduct prayer meeting for the victim and pray for him. Prayer meeting is conducted for 2/3 times until the victim is fully recovered. In a Moyon community, for any diseases and ailments, they help each other through prayers.

Besides, women camp, women seminar and women workshops were also organized in which women and family health development lectures were also delivered.

## Conclusion

Moyon people mostly depend on Allopathic for health care service. There are also some people who go for homeopathy. People approach visionary for the sickness, which are caused by super natural agents. Ethno medicines are used along with allopathy if the disease persist.

Moreover, the health of women and her family depends on the socio-economic status of the family and their educational level. People who are living in main land are more educated and economically sound than those people who are living in outskirt areas. Those who are living in outskirt areas are more prone to illness like diarrhoea/dysentery, typhoid, jaundice, cholera, etc. than the main land dwellers. This is mainly because of the lack of proper knowledge of sanitation and hygienic condition.

Women are mostly engaged in domestic works from child bearing to child rearing to cooking to cleaning. If she works outside the house, it is double-burden that she carries. Because of the nature of the work, she gives least importance to her health. Her energy is more consumed in her daily life than maintaining her nutritional level.

Infant and maternal death, are also correlated with socio-economic status of the family. So, mortality occur more in outskirt areas than in the main lands. This is because of the poor facilities of medical aids within the areas and also because of their poverty and unhygienic way of living. Deaths of infant are mostly on account of the poor health status of the mother during pre-natal and post-natal period and also because of the lack of proper experience in rearing infant. Maternal death is mainly due to improper care during pregnancy and child birth and also because of the effects of overburden of domestic works during reproductive periods.

## Recommendations

1. For controlling fertility and mortality, it would be appropriate to improve educational and developmental programmes in a coordinate manner for rationalizing programmes inputs and achieving mutual benefits.
2. Marriage-cum-pregnancy counselling coupled will health education should be given especially to all girls.
3. Improvement in food choice and nutritional status of the mother and babies along with adoption of healthy child rearing

practices.

4. *Anganwadi* and Primary Health Centre needs to be re-vitalized/extended and re-oriented to improve an effective measure for the purpose.
5. Intensified efforts should be made to improve the quality of health and family planning programmes and to increase their acceptability and effectiveness.
6. To make the people understand the importance of pre-natal and post-natal care.
7. Improve nutrition, sanitation and health environment.

## REFERENCES

Abidi, Nigar Fatima, (1993), *Women Physicians*, Delhi, Manah Publication Pvt. Ltd.

Aleem, Shamin, (1996), *Womens Development*, New Delhi, APH Publishing Corporation.

Chaudhuri, Buddhadeb, (1986), *Tribal health:* Socio-cultural dimensions, New Delhi: Inter India Publications.

Kosa, John, *et al.* (ed.), (1969), *Poverty and Health,* Massachusetts, Harvard University Press.

Kumar, Ram, (1990), *Women Health Development and Administration,* Vol. I, New Delhi, Deep and Deep Publication.

Kumar, Ram, (1990), *Women Health Development and Administration,* Vol II, New Delhi, Deep and Deep Publication.

Nungchim, Donald Kosha., N-d. *The Moyons* (unpublished manuscript).

Seymour, C. Susan, (1999), *Women, Family and Child Care in India,* United Kingdom, Cambridge University Press.

# PART III

# SOCIAL AND CULTURAL ASPECTS OF TRIBAL HEALTH

# 13

# Tribal Witchcraft and Personalistic Disease Theory: Concepts and Issues

A.K. SINHA AND B.G. BANERJEE

---

It is of primary importance to the members of a community to try to maintain their health and to restore to health those who fall ill. Possibly this is because illness and death are disruptive events that impose high economic, social, and psychological cost wherever they occur.

The evidence of diseases, in general and also in particular, varies in different societies. Each society interprets and treats illnesses differently. Standards for sick and healthy bodies are cultural constructions that vary in time and space (Martin 1992). The questions about the nature of illnesses, conceived in different societies, and about its causes and its cures are some of the moot points in the subject-matter of medical anthropology. We enquire into the types of therapist that seek to alleviate illness and about their skills and social roles.

The curiosity of anthropologists about the medical beliefs and practices of the members of traditional societies they have studied is the oldest of the roots of medical anthropology. Consequently, ethnomedicine, the contemporary term of the vast body of knowledge that has resulted from this curiosity and the research methods used added to it, is of interest to anthropologists both for theoretical and practical reasons.

The term ethnomedicine is used to refer to those beliefs and practices relating to disease which are the products of indigenous cultural development and are not explicitly derived from the conceptual framework of modern medicine. It explores environmental, biological and socio-cultural factors as they impinge upon disease pattern and how people respond to it.

Interpretation of illness is a culturally informed process, one in which the patient, the healer and a community of others make use of locally appropriate disease theories to account for the misfortune at hand. These theories typically make a distinction between immediate and ultimate cause. The former provides details on the specific nature of the problem and the latter offers rationalisation as to why this problem occurred. Immediate cause would be the intrusion of a foreign object into a patient body, the ultimate cause would be the anger of a spirit or a sorcerer or a witch because of a patient's inappropriate behaviour (Banerjee, 2003).

According to Foster and Anderson (1978) all societies have disease theory systems to identify, classify, and explain illness. A perusal of disease theory systems of traditional societies world wide, anthropologists have concluded that in the explanation of illness, there are a number of causal perspectives or themes that appear with greater frequency. These themes cross-cut time periods, geographic space and ethnic boundaries. There are three basic theories about the causes of illness: personalistic, naturalistic and emotionalistic (Foster and Anderson, 1978). Although these terms refer specifically to causality concepts, they can also be conveniently used to speak of entire medical systems.

A personalitic medical system is believed to be caused by the active, purposeful intervention of a *sensate* agent who may be a supernatural being (a deity or a god), a non-human being (such as a ghost, ancestor, or evil spirit), or a human being (a witch or sorcerer). The sick person literally is a victim, the object of aggression or punishment directed specially against him, for reasons that concerns him alone.

In major category of cause as characterised by the purposeful intervention of *sensate* agents who, whatever their reasons, seek out a victim who falls ill. We can call this category personalistic in that aggression or punishment is directed against a single person as a consequence of the will and power of a human or supernatural agent or being.

Personalistic explanations appear to predominate in the traditional systems of such vast areas as Africa, preconquest America, Oceania and indigenous Siberia, They also underlie the more complex systems of contemporary Latin America, South Asia including India and China. In all these traditional medical systems we find efficient and proximate causes. In personalistic systems deities, ghosts, witches and sorcerers are efficient causes, the prime movers. But they require operational techniques such ability to steal a victim's soul, possess him, poison him, or cause a snake to bite him.

The descriptions of systems in which personalistic causality ideas predominate, it is remarkable how often one reads that all, or almost all, death and illness are caused by agents that a westerner would consider to be natural.

In all folk medical systems, belief in witchcraft was and is a part of their tradition. For example, from the beginning of black folk medicine, belief in the supernatural, magic, and witchcraft seem to have played a more important role than in Euro-American folk medicine. Snow (1974) believes that folk medical beliefs, and especially those of blacks, reflect their major worldview themes: the world is a hostile and dangerous place, the individual is liable to attack from external sources and the individual must depend on outside aid to combat such attacks. Such a worldview is congruent with a high degree of belief in witchcraft and a folk medical system designed to protect and cure a person of witchcraft and witchcraft–induced illness.

## II

The word *witch* is derived from the Old English *wicce,* meaning 'a female magician or sorceress,' but although the terms 'wizard' and 'warlock' are available for male magicians, 'witch' and 'witchcraft' are generally applied to both sexes and their magical activities. Among many peoples accidents, sickness, death, and other untoward events have been thought to be caused by witches-individuals who had magical power which they used for evil purposes (Bacon 1995: 83).

There is not always a hard and fast distinction between good and bad (black and white) magic, though there usually is a distinction between socially approved and anti-social magic. *Sorcery and witchcraft are ritual means of working harm against an enemy.* Though usually anti-social they are not necessarily so; sorcery in some societies is used to detect and punish a criminal. It may be permissible to seek revenge on an evildoer by injuring or killing him or a member of his group by witchcraft. A sorcerer is a person who willingly directs injurious magic on others. He may be able to transform himself into animal shape; he may be able to injure by the power of thought, or may have the "evil eye". Such persons may keep their power secret, or it may be known and they may derive power from it. They may be regarded as public enemies, or may be tolerated and employed to wreak evil on personal enemies.

Both witchcraft and sorcery denote the projection of supernatural evil by human instigation. Both deal with supernatural or 'mystical' power and thus are integral to the understanding or religion and cosmology. They have complex social and cosmological ramifications with important implications for socio-cultural anthropology. Explorations of both concepts have generated a tremendous literature in anthropology.

The terms witchcraft and sorcery are words taken from pre-enlightenment Europe and applied to reported occult agencies in, for the most part, non-European, small-scale or tribal societies. The distinction in anthropology between the two kinds of malign occult action is usually credited to Evans Pritchard (1937) (Willis 1996:564).

Magical practices play a significant role in many peoples' traditional response to illness. The practices include magical divination used for diagnosis, as well as various curing practices. However, magical, mystical, and empirical aspects may combine in complex ways in a particular situation. Among the Azande, divination may identify the cause of illness by mechanical, magical means or by a witch doctor's going into a trance, using psychological rather than magical procedures. Treatment may utilise plant substances selected for their homoeopathic properties. For example, the bark of a tree with reddish patches is used to treat leprosy of the skin, where similar patches appear (Bourguignon, 1995:86).

Yalman is of opinion that witchcraft and sorcery refer to practices and supernatural beings which are part and parcel of the European Christian tradition. Their use in anthropology involves an essential widening of their meaning to cover a great many beliefs and practices from other cultures which have proved difficult to classify. The conceptual categories involved in such supernatural beings and practice are sometimes so unique to particular people that the translation of concepts from one cultural idiom into another becomes a difficulty of the first magnitude. Is 'witchcraft' similar to the 'evil eye'? Is a European witch the 'same' as an Islamic *djinn* or a Hindu *yaksa?* These questions about the similarities and differences between belief systems of different cultures remain largely unresolved (1968:523).

Following Evans-Pritchard, Landy (1977) sees witchcraft as the possession of an inherited power (in the case of some peoples, such as the Azande, physiologically inherited and, in the Azande case, transmitted patrilineally), used only for evil ends (though a few societies presumably have "good" witches, too). As Marwick (1970) notes the witch's power derives from his/her mystical inheritance Marwick goes on as to motive, witches are considered to be slaves of aberration and addiction, and, thus conceived, are weird, sometimes tragic figures.

The witch embodies all the feared, despised, negative aspects of a culture and thus provides a negative role and behaviour model; the sorcerer embodies rather more common antisocial urges and is a perhaps more ambiguous negative model, and in so far as he uses his powers for benign ends, a positive model as well. The witch is thus unrelievedly evil, the sorcerer combines evil with good and is much closer to the total community.

Witchcraft can be viewed as a belief in a supernatural, mystical power that develops in some (usually adult) people and enables them to work evil directly, without magic or spiritual assistance. The witchcraft power is regarded as a distinct category of supernatural agency. It may fly about by itself but is ineffective unless it has a human host (Stevens Jr., 1996: 1227).

'Although the terms witchcraft and sorcery are sometimes used synonymously, anthropologists generally distinguish between them. As practiced in a wide variety of societies throughout the world, witchcraft is an inborn, involuntary, and often unconscious capacity to cause harm to other people. On the other hand, sorcery, which often involves the use of materials, potions, and medicines, is the deliberate use of supernatural powers to bring about harm. Some societies have specialised practitioners of sorcery, but in other societies sorcery can be practiced by anyone. Because sorcery involves the use of certain physical substance, the evidence for its existence is more easily found. Witchcraft, by contrast, is virtually impossible to prove or disprove because of the absence of any visible evidence of its existence.

Whereas sorcery involves the use of material substances to cause harm to people, witchcraft, it is thought, relies solely on psychic power (that is, thoughts and emotions). In other words, witches can turn their anger and hatred into evil deeds simply by thinking evil thoughts. How witches are conceptualised varies widely from society to society, but, in all cases, witches are viewed negatively. Witches, who are viewed universally as antisocial, are generally seen as being unable to control the human impulses that normal members of society are expected to keep in check. They have insatiable appetites for food, uncontrollable hatred, and perverted sexual desires'(Ferraro, 2001: 304).

Sorcerers are generally believed to direct their malevolence purposefully against those they dislike, fear, or envy rather than acting randomly or capriciously. In any given society, hostile relations can occur between people who have some relationship to each other–such as outsiders who marry into a local village, rivals for a father's inheritance, wives in a polygynous household, men who are competing for a political office, or even rivals in competitive sports. People are, therefore, likely to attribute their own personal misfortune to the sorcery of some rival who might gain from harming them. Thus, accusations of sorcery are patterned to the extent that they reflect the conflicts, rivalries, and antagonisms that already exist among the people in any given society.

In a publication of A Committee of the Royal Anthropological Institute of Great Britain and Ireland—Notes and Queries on Anthropology (1971) it is stated that witchcraft is distinguished from sorcery in that it is generally believed to be a power, more for evil than for good, lodged in an individual himself or herself (the witch). It may be inborn, hereditary or acquired by undergoing special rites. It may be believed to act on others without the volition of the witch, bringing sickness, death or other misfortune on the victim. In many societies evil witchcraft is regarded as a crime and proved witches are punished by banishment or death. Elsewhere it may be regarded as a sickness which can be cured by magico-religious treatment. Where there is witchcraft, there are usually special cults or ritual experts for detecting and combating witches. These cults may be elaborately organised, with priests and other servants, shrines and peculiar ritual customs, affording protection to its members against witches—able by oracular means to expose a witch. Otherwise the detection of witches may be carried out by ordeals or oracles administered by an expert, or chief.

Some other general statements about differences between sorcery and witchcraft have been made; for example, that sorcery is more commonly a male prerogative and that women are more often suspected of witchcraft; that the witchcraft power, especially in Africa, is often vested in a tangible substance in the body that develops after adolescence, is discernible through autopsy, and can be extracted by the 'witch-doctor'; that the power can be hereditary, passed on matrilineally; and that the witch may be unaware that she or he possesses the power. Sorcery seems universal, but witchcraft seems characteristic of stable societies with complex social groupings; it is notably absent among hunter-gatherers (Stevens Jr. 1996:1229).

The differences between the two fields are, indeed, so great that some authors even objected to the use of the same term. Crick (1979), for instance, warned that the term witchcraft was so saturated with implications stemming from European history that anthropologists working on other areas had better avoid the term altogether. A more substantial objection might be that despite huge variations the representations concerned revolve around basic conceptions that are surprisingly similar. In many parts of the world notions that are now commonly translated as witchcraft refer not only to hidden human aggression, but also to more specific representations about people being able to double themselves, leaving their bodies at night and flying off to nocturnal meetings with their accomplices.

Especially Anthropologists, confronted by a bewildering proliferation of imaginaries in this field, have tried to clarify things by formulating strict definitions and distinctions. The best known is Evans-Pritchard's proposition—on the basis of the distinctions the Zande, the subjects of his first book, supposedly made—to distinguish witchcraft and sorcery: the first referring to an inborn quality, the second to the use of acquired means. But even for neighbouring areas in Africa this distinction proved difficult to maintain in view of the fluidity and dynamics of witchcraft discourses. More recently, some authors (Geschiere, 1997) suggested that this search for clear-cut definitions and classifications risked to make anthropologists blind to the surprising dynamics of these representations and their chameleonic qualities which are crucial to understand how they can adapt themselves so easily to modern changes. In this treacherous field of study, researchers may have to resign themselves to working with fuzzy notions that may exhibit a common core but at the same time engender highly variable and constantly changing elaborations. The differences between the historians' and the anthropologists' versions of witchcraft arc illustrative of the widely varying implications these notions can acquire (Geschiere 2001: 16514).

The historians' view paid more attention to the dynamics of these representations. After all, a central question to them was why persecutions of witches—quite rare throughout what was sometimes called the 'dark' Middle Ages—acquired epidemic forms in several parts of Western and Central Europe, precisely at the dawn of modern times (sixteenth and seventeenth century).

Anthropologists, in contrast, for a long time continued to address witchcraft as a local issue, trying to resolve its riddles by in-depth studies of local relationships and conceptions. Yet their approaches were also subject to quite surprising turns. Evans-Pritchard's Azande study, hardly proved to be a trendsetter. Its focus was on issues of cognition—on why the Azande combined very commonsensical explanations with interpretations in terms of occult aggression. But it inspired a series of micropolitical studies in which witchcraft was analysed—in line with the functionalist ideas that dominated the discipline at the time—in relation to social order and integration. In a series of in-depth monographs of local societies in what at the time was called British Central Africa, anthropologists of the 'Manchester school' studied witchcraft accusations as a form of social control. Typical for this approach was Max Marwick's characterisation of witchcraft as 'a social stain gauge': as a measure of socio-political tensions, but also as a way to restore social order. It was this interpretation that produced the in retrospect somewhat amazing view of witchcraft as 'tame' and 'domesticated'(Geschiere, 2001: 16515).

Although witchcraft and sorcery are usually associated with small-scale societies in the non-Western world, they are also found in highly industrialised parts of the world such as the United States, Canada, and a number of western European countries (Ferraro, 2001: 304-305).

Early anthropologists sought to describe primitive "laws" of thinking that governed the techniques of magic, which were widely regarded as pseudoscience, inevitably to be replaced by more sophisticated modes of thinking. Reports of people who could assume animal or spirit form, fly at terrific speeds, and suck the blood or eat the flesh of their hapless victims—and the intersocietal suspicions and accusations generated by such beliefs—were regarded as bizarre and irrational, socially divisive and dysfunctional, and received little serious attention.

Africa, the other major area of anthropological interest, became the testing ground for theories of sorcery and witchcraft. The modern history of the scholarly concern with witchcraft is generally acknowledged to have begun with the work of Evans-Pritchard, whose *Witchcraft, Oracles, and Magic Among the Azande* (1937) has had great influence, within and beyond anthropology. This study is credited with having pioneered the anthropology of sorcery and witchcraft, with having firmly established the distinction between them, and with revealing a logic and rationality in the cosmological premises underlying these beliefs. Nearly all-subsequent anthropological and some historical studies have paid initial tribute to Evans-Pritchard.

In his 'appreciation' of Evans-Pritchard's book, Max Gluckman (1944) made his oft-quoted statement: 'If a sociologist can find where charges of witchcraft in a particular society fall, he can almost reconstruct the social relationships of the society'(Stevens Jr., 1996: 1226-1227).

"In a tribute to Evans-Pritchard, Mary Douglas (1970) called for a synthesis of historical and anthropological approaches to witchcraft. Some historians, notably Keith Thomas and A.D. MacFarlane, have utilised anthropological approaches in studies of European witchcraft, and the introductory volume to Levack's (1992) multi-volume work on witchcraft, magic, and demonology focuses on representative contributions by anthropologists. Historians still have an image of anthropology as useful only for the study of small-scale, homogeneous, pre-industrial societies. Perhaps demonstration of the universality of fears of the witch's attributes will help to change this image" (Stevens Jr., 1996:1230).

The essence of Evans-Pritchard's influential distinction is that witchcraft is an inherited ability to cause occult injury to others which, at least for the Zande, can be exercised unconsciously by its possessor. Sorcery is a conscious activity associated with the skilled manipulation of certain substances, with the intention of causing harm, a usage that long predated Evans-Pritchard and had been employed in ethnographic accounts of Australian and Melanesian peoples. The witchcraft/sorcery distinction is widely reported in other parts of Africa and elsewhere. However, it is not always made. Over much of East-Central Africa, for example, the notion of inherited ability to cause occult damage is largely absent: instead the emphasis is on the use for malign purposes of occult techniques involving 'medicines'. Middleton and Winter (1963) had interestingly suggested an association between witchcraft in the Zande sense and the importance of descent as a principle of social organisation. They suggest that where descent is not of prime significance in social organisation the occult emphasis will be on sorcery, but that where descent largely determines social status witchcraft is likely to dominate. The distinction is obviously related to that between ascribed and achieved social roles. A pioneering attempt to explain the specific forms assumed by witchcraft/sorcery beliefs is Nadel's (1952) comparative analysis of four African societies, including one (the Korongo of Sudan) where such beliefs are said to be absent. Nadel's explanation for this comparatively a typical situation is that Korongo social life is unusually free of conflict; and their mythology provides a comprehensive account of causality in terms of non-human spiritual agencies.

The approach to the understanding of witchcraft/sorcery was further developed by Marwick (1965) in a study of the Cewa-speaking people of Northeast Zambia and Malawi. In what came to be known as the 'social strain-gauge' theory, Marwick showed that in this matrilineal society, sorcery accusations were particularly likely to be levelled by a young man against an ageing or incompetent village headman who was also the accuser's maternal uncle. If the accusations 'stuck' they could be used to turn the older man out of office and to install his presumed victim. A similar process by which witchcraft accusations are used to get rid of unpopular elders has been described for the Lugbara of Northern Uganda by Middleton (1960 *cf.* Willis 1996: 562-563).

Other studies have focused on the ideas, or constellations of ideas, present in indigenous thought in the areas of witchcraft and sorcery. Marwick maintains that the witch or sorcerer is always conceived of in terms that are antithetical to local concepts of the 'good' and socially acceptable person. Thus witches or sorcerers are often associated with murder, incest and cannibalism—all actions generally held to epitomise the antisocial.

Kluckhohn (1944) seems to have been the first to note the socially levelling effects of witchcraft fears on the Navaho group of Native Americans. In Navaho society those who made themselves conspicuously different from their fellows by accumulating wealth were believed to be using witchcraft to gain their ends, and were liable to be persecuted and even killed. Similar observations have been made in Africa, for example by Monica Wilson (1959) for the Nyakyusa of East-central Africa (Willis, 1996:563).

Post-modern development in anthropology have given a new twist to the tortuous semantic history of witchcraft and sorcerer. The controversial works of Castaneda (1968) and more ethnographically substantially works have cast doubt on the past assumption that witchcraft and sorcery, however, 'real to indigenous peoples' were based on unfortunate delusions.

While talking about the practice of witchcraft there is no evidence that this form of supernatural belief is dying out. In fact, some have suggested that they have been on the rise in recent years (Singer and

Benassi, 1981; Truzzi, 1993). Interest in such forms of belief fluctuates over time, but it serves as an accurate barometer of social strain and dislocation, rebellion against tradition, and the search for alternative systems for explaining the unexplainable. Witchcraft, like other belief systems, can be empowering in that it offers a sense of control, provide an explanation for personal failure and inadequacy, and allow the individual social acceptance into a group (Ferraro, 2001: 306-307).

The anthropologists of the 1950s developed insights into the functioning of witch beliefs which seemed about as relevant to the European experience as if they came from another planet. Dangerous in Europe, the same beliefs in Melanesia or Africa appeared to be tame, even domesticated; they served useful functions and were not expected to run amuck. In retrospect, one might wish the second half of this quotation to be still true. The growing obsession over the last decades in many parts of Africa and Melanesia with new forms of witchcraft seems to reflect, on the contrary, widespread popular worries that it has 'run amuck'. Yet Douglas's observation did highlight striking differences between the trajectories of witchcraft studies by historians and anthropologists and, therefore, offers a challenging starting point for any effort to come to a more general survey of the topic (Geschiere, 2001: 16514).

After the 1960s anthropologists tended to abandon the topic to theologians and journalists. An approach in terms of social order proved to be of little help in analysing the new transformations of these local beliefs.

Horton (1970) has suggested in an ingenious essay on "African Traditional Thought and Western Science," witchcraft and sorcery, like religion, serve important philosophical and metaphysical functions for their practitioners, functions that are analogous in many ways to those served by Western science to its practitioners.

In many parts of Africa, for instance, there was increasing popular concern about new forms of witchcraft that were explicitly related to the *nouveaux riches* who were supposed to accumulate wealth by exploiting the labour of their witchcraft victims. Often people made a contrast between older forms of witchcraft in which the victims were 'eaten' and the new one of 'selling people,' that is, turning them into some sort of zombies and selling them to work on 'invisible plantations.' The fear of such new threats triggered a frantic search for new forms of protection, for instance, urgent appeals to the State authorities to intervene. The pressing character of the witchcraft issue was further highlighted by the lethal witch-hunts that marked the end of Apartheid in the north-eastern part of South Africa—young men, encouraged by *nganga* (witch-doctors) and claiming to act as local representatives of the ANC, executing dozens of 'witches' (Niehaus, 1993 *cf.* Geschiere, 2001: 16516). The half-hearted implications of State authorities in such witch-hunts in many parts of the continent made it all the more urgent to gain deeper insight into the modern dynamics of witchcraft discourses.

No wonder that since early 1990s there has been a new wave of witchcraft studies in Africa and Melanesia, notably by anthropologists, concentrating on the relation with popular views of 'modernity'—that is, the dreams of the modern, in all its varieties, that effect ever wider strata of the population (*cf.* Comaroff and Comaroff, 1993, Geschiere, 1997). This linking of witchcraft and modernity, according to some even a new paradigm, implied attention to particular aspects that could explain the continuing resilience of these local beliefs–notably their circular character, their moral ambiguity, and their striking capacity to relate local realities of the family and the home to global processes of change.

The circularity of witchcraft discourses is expressed most vividly in the paradox that the main protection against witchcraft often is to be sought in the very same field. In many parts of Africa, for instance, the *nganga* (healer) is supposed to be able to offer protection and healing only because of his (or her) overdeveloped witchcraft. In some societies there is a consistent effort to conceptually or even institutionally separate the *nganga's* (or the chiefs') occult power from the evil forces of the witches. Then witchcraft seems to be, indeed, unequivocally evil. But in practice, such distinctions between positive and negative forms of occult power are often highly precarious and controversial. In many African societies, for instance, *nganga* remain highly ambivalent figures– healers but at the same time suspect because of their dealings with extremely dangerous forces. The *nganga* is, therefore, also a striking example of the moral ambiguity of these forces. Basically these forces are certainly evil, but—as in the *nganga's* case—they can be chanalised and used in a constructive way.

The new anthropological interest in the paradoxical link between witchcraft and modernity inspires even an alternative reading of developments in what are thought to be typically 'modern' societies. Already in the 1970s, the anthropologist Favret-Saada (1977 *cf.* Geschiere, 2001:16516) highlighted the surprising resilience of witchcraft practices in the French countryside in a try innovative analysis of how words are charged with power, but also of how the researcher herself became unavoidably involved.

The broader interest of new directions in the study of witchcraft, often still seen as the archetype of the traditional, is precisely that they help to debunk simplistic opposition between modern and traditional, science and magic, transparent and opaque, or even more simply between the West and the rest (Geschiere, 2001: 16516).

The first attribute is social subversion, that is, witches embody social ideas of evil; they are enemies of society and are dedicated to the undermining of social structure and values. Witches are also preferentially nocturnal, in a class of evil nocturnal creatures. 'Night' may be a metaphor for the nature of their behaviour—dark, evil, occult, or demonic, and mystical—as distinct from sorcery, a 'day' activity. Witches can transform themselves into other human forms or into the forms of specific animals, or they can become invisible.

Witches fly, often at terrific speeds. Sometimes it is the power that flies, in any form or invisibly, leaving the body of its host engaged in routine activities, or the power carries the witch bodily in flight. The witch flies directly to its target and works its evil, which may be enhanced by the use of magical objects or potions; beliefs in the use of the methods of sorcery by the witch may partially account for the confusion in terminology. Spreading disease is the most common activity of witches; either an epidemic or a sickness that afflicts just one person in a group may be evidence of the activity of witches. A slow, wasting disease is sure evidence. A first task of AIDS workers in Africa today is to assure people that HIV is not spread by witchcraft.

Witches are universally associated with death, in any of three ways; myths may state that the original witchcraft power was bestowed in Faustian contract by the god of death; witches obtain powers from death, exhuming bodies from graves and cannibalising them or using corpse material for their 'medicines;' and witches cause death. Indeed, in some societies all deaths are caused by witchcraft.

Another variant of witchcraft beliefs is the Evil Eye, the belief that malign power may be projected through direct gaze. The power is involuntary, stimulated by negative emotion, especially envy, and can cause misfortune, sickness, and even death. Such beliefs are widespread but are most notably institutionalised in areas around the Mediterranean fringe (Stevens Jr., 1996:1228).

Witchcraft and sorcery have a time-honoured past in anthropology. Landy (1977) declares: No ethnography would be complete without a discussion devoted to these phenomena in those societies in which they exist—which appear to be the majority. And yet, the concepts of witchcraft and sorcery and their corollaries, witch and sorcerer, are often confused and ambiguous in the literature. It is not always possible to know which phenomenon is being described or if the confounding of terms and related data is the consequence of the ethnologist's inability to distinguish between them himself, of his inability to elicit distinctions from informants, of ambiguity inherent in the local belief system, or of unconscious ethnocentric bias on the part of the ethnographer. Sometimes the two terms are quite deliberately equated.

Witchcraft and sorcery, and the witchcraft's offspring, the evil eye, interest us here because they enter the realm of medical anthropology through their role in causing illness and in the role of sorcerers in curing illness as well. We discover, the interest of anthropologists in these phenomena does not end with their role in magic, in supernatural, in the social roles of witch and sorcerer, and in the part they play in the medical system, but extends to their role generally in the social system. At the macrocosmic level, witchcraft and sorcery frequently are seen as symptomatic of the strains and conflicts besetting social networks, and the divination process, uncovers not simply illness or misfortune of individuals but, by implication of social groupings.

Similarly, the therapeutic process (including diagnosis, prognosis, treatment, and cure) assists in assuaging not only the illness of the individual and reintegrating him into his social system but also works to repair the tears in the fabric of social structure and thus to reintegrate the system that was temporarily essentially an equilibrium theory which, although helping to explain the integrative functions of witchcraft and sorcery (and in an equilibrium theory all events in a system must 'contribute' towards that system's operation no matter how destructive they may seem), does not explain sufficiently the disruptive consequences of these events. The effects, in fact, may be quite destructive and may require the effective use of countervailing powers of stave off the terrorisation of the whole society. As with all instruments of social control, sorcery and witchcraft may serve important social functions, but must themselves, in turn, be socially controlled else they run rampant and control the social system they supposedly serve.

We turn now to the effect of the beliefs in witchcraft and sorcery on social relations. The direct or veiled accusation of a person or a group is a critical element in the witchcraft and sorcery complex. Wherever these beliefs occur, we may expect a great elaboration of supernatural weapons of offence and defence against witches and sorcerers and these accusations.

There have been attempts to relate overt accusations of witchcraft and sorcery to the morphology of kinship or social groups. It is suggested that such accusation of evil intent of one person by another must run along the lines of stress in the structure of social groups. There is undoubtedly much truth in this statement, and it is confirmed by the widespread feeling among people of many societies that institutions such as the evil eye, witches, and sorcery spring directly from one of the most powerful human sentiments, jealousy. This is merely a different way of expressing the strained social relations between the accuser and the accused. This is why jealousy and envy are so often given as the reason for the supernatural attack (Wilson 1951). Witchcraft accusations that reveal both secret and unconscious envy as well as overt suspicions may be regarded as particularly clear symptoms of strain in the social structure (Yalman, 1968:525).

In many theories the ideology and practice of witchcraft are related with some precision to areas of anxiety and stress in the social fabric. All these theories are based on the incidence of witchcraft accusations between individuals in certain specific social roles. But, for obvious reasons, statistical evidence of sufficient depth and range in connection with such highly charged issues is difficult to collect and evaluate.

Middleton and Winter (1963) have raised some important questions regarding both the coherence of dogma and the structural aspects of witchcraft and sorcery. Accepting the notion that witchcraft and sorcery have coherent doctrines which explain events in social life, they argue that witchcraft and sorcery beliefs are exhaustive systems of supernatural explanation.

"Since sorcery is a voluntary matter and merely a technique which can be learned, anybody may be in a position to use it for offense or defence. Moreover, depending upon the motives of the sorcerer, it is not innately evil. On the other hand, witchcraft is by definition an innate matter, usually evil, in which the alleged witch has no choice. For this reason Middleton and Winter suggest that witchcraft accusations are more characteristically made against persons who are in *ascribed* roles, such as involuntary membership in unilineal descent groups where the individual acquires his position by virtue of his birth, whereas sorcery accusations tend to be made against persons in *achieved* statuses and are more characteristic of the non-unilineal aspect of societies" (Yalman, 1968: 526).

It is difficult to generalise witchcraft beliefs at large. For there is always an ascribed aspect to social status, and it appears difficult to evaluate the witchcraft of complex communities in early New England, medieval Europe, or present-day Indian communities of Middle America and South America in these terms.

Apart from the question of tension in social relations, the psychological aspects of witchcraft beliefs are another dimension of the facts. If witchcraft beliefs are regarded as unrealistic fantasies—a weak theoretical position from the point of view of anthropology—then some similarity and connection may be seen between witchcraft, sorcery, and infantile fantasies.

The dogmas of witchcraft, sorcery and magic are also relevant to the social control and inheritance systems of certain societies. In some societies where witchcraft is regarded as an innate quality in certain individuals, there are theories of its inheritance. In some cases when the main line of descent, for purposes of family organisation, is in the male line, witchcraft is thought to run in the female line (Yalman, 1968: 526).

## III

A perusal of Indian literature on tribal witchcraft is insightful and interesting. S.C. Roy reported: 'witchcraft, an art, is rare amongst the Birhors. Such wizards or witches as exist amongst them are believed to harm a person by throwing some rice in the direction of that person's house and inciting their familiar spirit to move in that direction and afflict the person with some disease or other trouble' (1978: 174).

An Oraon, who suspects magic or witchcraft, always takes particular steps to ward off the evil eye of witches or the malicious attentions of sorcerers. The Oraon, goes to the witch-doctor to find out the name of the witch or sorcerer who has brought about the evil and then compels the witch or sorcerer to appease or provide the means to appease the spirit who has been put up to the mischief (Roy, 1985:18-19).

The methods of magic and witchcraft, practised in Chota-Nagpur and its adjoining territories inhabited by the Kharias, would appear to be generally common among Kharias as well as among their neighbours, both aboriginal and low-class Hindu. In fact, there are good reasons to believe that the methods of magic and witchcraft now practised in common by practitioners of the magic art among Hindu castes and Hinduised tribes of these parts as well as among the comparatively advanced aboriginal tribes such as the Oraons, the Mundas, the Santals, the Hos, and the Kharias, have been in great part derived from one main common source, probably the ancient Dravidian peoples of Mediterranean origin. Not that the pre-Dravidian tribes like the Kharias were altogether strangers to the art. In fact, the magic incantations even among the rudest aboriginal tribes have always been resorted to, and believed to work wonders; the occult powers of certain words, names and numbers, and even of animals and reptiles, and certain herbs, grains and other inanimate objects is dreaded (Roy, 1937: 410).

With Kols witchery and the evil eye go together and a woman is more likely to be a witch than a man. Gond women particularly, it was noted, should be suspected and kept at a distance. 'The true witch is not such through any power acquired by her, but is rather born a witch from the very beginning; the gift though, may be trained and the art developed. The witch's power frequently depends upon his or her control over the supernormal powers and spirits which are at beck and call and which can be sent out on missions of evil' (Griffiths, 1946: 204).

Not only among the tribal communities, but in other communities the notion that some people are witches and can injure them by virtue of an inherent quality. The bewitched person becomes sick. Death may also occur due to witchcraft is prevailing. Fuchs studied the Balahis' concept of disease. The Balahis, a low caste community, live in Nimar district of Rajasthan. Fuchs (1950) in his study of the children of Hari comments that the Balahis, ignorant of the immense variety of human ailments, rarely recognise the real nature of a disease and attribute death to fever as the most common symptom of any disease. Many infirmities for which they have no natural explanation they attribute to evil spirits or to wrath or certain gods or *matas* who have to be appeased by sacrifices and offerings or exorcised by magical practices. Santal's concept of disease and treatment is an amalgamation of all these concepts as it is evidenced from the studies of eminent scholars like Archer (1947) and Bodding (1925).

Sorcery in the Santal area, is practised by forms of magic as amongst the Andamanese (Bompass, 1909: 429 *cf.* Biswas, 1956: 116). The District Gazetteer records how the witches draw the picture of a person to be harmed and the image is then maltreated or symbolically killed by the process of imitative magic. They also would bury tufts of hair with vermilion or *sindur* which being in contact with the victim's body are subjected to a process of contagious magic and the victim is expected to fall ill.

Choudhuri studied vividly on witchkillings amongst the Santhals. He accounted a good number of cases of witchkilling in Santal community. Witchkilling is not even considered a sin in a Santal community. According to Choudhuri, the individuals perceived the difference between sin and offence or crime, and expressed that extinction of a witch would do better to the society; for the belief that a witch can cause harm by wishing evil is fairly strong (1984: 186-187).

In an article, Deb Burman (1986) cites a case study of witchcraft in a Santhal community to understand the concept of disease and treatment. He cites an example where an outcast managed to grab land from his own brother by labelling his sister-in-law to be a witch as reason for his fever. The author stresses that this kind of episode is common to a Santhal community. He writes: A number of cases of outcast and physical torture can be heard of. This type of belief correlates with the black magic or witchcraft. Etiology of disease is not the concern of the community. Traditional village council plays the role of social control which, according to Hoebel and Frost, consists of the entire gamut of rewards and dissuasions. All the members of the community are well aware of the practice of witchcraft. They internalise the process into their value system. They regard this sort of practice as a part and parcel of their customs. Hence, they try to perpetuate it and whenever a person suffers from any disease they mostly admit it as a case of witchcraft. They consider the disease as their own and not of one particular individual. But they do not want to realise the undercurrent exploitation in the event. With the help of a thorough analysis it is revealed that to take away one's property a person pretends to be sick. Customs and beliefs also go in favour of the pretention. As the major portion of the population is illiterate and addicted to liquor they want to perpetuate such belief without judging its implications. The educated youths have a strong view against this custom but they are, in one sense, handicapped as they have no voice in their traditional village council. Only after 30 years of age a person's view is given due consideration.

It is part of belief in life beyond death and of belief in the capacity of the human being to live without a physical body that the Dublas of Gujarat, according to Shah (1958), believe in ghost *(bhut), Chudel* or *Vantri, Dakkan* or witch. They seriously believe that these human supernatural beings do great harm to ordinary persons without any reason. The believe that witchcraft is practised by certain women, called Dakkans, whose evil eye spoils good food made for children and the sick. Though many women are considered Dakkans, they are seldom beaten to death, like the witches in the West. These women are supposed to cause harm to all persons who come under their sway; when children begin to vomit, turn pale and thin, or go on weeping for the whole night without any reason, it is all believed to be due to the influence of a local Dakkan.

It is said that Dakkans are not born, but learn their art by practising in the cremation ground (*samshan*). On the dark night of *Kali Chaudas* at midnight, fourteenth day of the dark half of *Aswin*, according to Hindu calendar, the Dakkans are believed to go to the cremation ground with burning charcoal in a *sigri*, which may be tied round the neck or carried on the head. It is believed that on these darknights, the black art is best learnt with the help of the seniors who practise it and who are called *gurus*.

While writing about Bhil tribe, Hutton (1980) in his book, Caste in India, observes that Bhils are inveterate believers in witchcraft, and their women, who have much freedom and influence, used in former times to accompany their menfolk into battle, using slings with great effect. He also mentions that Baiga and Gonds are great believers in and practisers of witchcraft.

The Korku lives in a permanent dread of his deities and spirits, and also of magicians and witches who can harm him through magic spells and curses. Throughout his life, the Korku feels himself exposed to these dangers which are very real to him.

When a healthy person suddenly sickens and dies without apparent cause, the Korkus at once suspect witchcraft or black magic (*ilom*). If they are able to put the blame for the sickness or death of the patient on a certain person, they punish him with death, or at least with expulsion from the village or tribal community. Witchcraft is an unforgivable sin (Fuchs, 1986:395).

Rizvi in his study on the Jaunsaris of Dehradun district (U.P.) observes that illness is believed to be caused by the intervention of a human being (a witch or sorcerer). He further subdivided the category according to the type of causative agent recognised by the people—

evil eye, witch and sorcerer. Further he writes that a *dankan* or *daain* (witch) is supposed to possess mysterious supernatural powers of casting an evil eye with disastrous results to the person on whom it is cast. According to Jaunsari belief, a child (male or female) born on the darkest midnight of the month of *Bhadon* is supposed to have this power. On whomsoever he casts his eye, he brings a series of misfortunes. Females born on the darkest night yield this power most effectively and it is said that it is difficult to escape from their evil spell. The person yielding such a power is not aware of this power in him/her. The pandits either managed to kill a witch or try to ward off the evil power by incantations or other rituals but such rituals are too costly and hence, cannot be adopted to cope with all cases of evil spell. The witch has a power on any person whom she loves or hates and the rest are not affected or seldom affected. An individual person usually female who has magical powers to do evil, is called sorceress (*Pishaach*). It is believed that the eyes of a sorceress are so powerful that as soon as she looks at any person, he/she feels some sort of trouble. Many Jaunsaris told (the author) about the presence of sorceress in different villages in the form of village women (1986: 241-242).

In the Nilgiri Hills of southern India one of the most primitive tribes, the Kurumba, was noted for its powers of witchcraft, and members of other tribes in the area employed Kurumba witches to wreak vengeance on their enemies (Bacon, 1995:83).

## IV

To conclude, one may infer that magic, witchcraft, and sorcery are rooted in traditional customary ideas whereby societies categorise and order the universe around them. As such, they not only are intertwined with every aspect of societies, thought, and language but also provide coherent and systematic means to influence the world in which man lives. For the anthropologist such belief systems provide essential material for the understanding of the metaphysics of traditional and non-Western societies. They may also lead to a better understanding of the structured aspects of customary thought.

Ideas regarding witchcraft and sorcery appear strange in a rationalist period such as ours, but we should recall what immense sway such beliefs have held over very sophisticated and highly intelligent men. We must be guarded in our haste to dismiss these ideas of the supernatural. Rather, we must understand the very roots which provide the strength of conviction for such beliefs.

All knowledge rests on some degree of trust and respect. In modern societies the specialised task of developing knowledge and examining the basis of knowledge is given to thinkers and scientists in institutions of learning. Those not directly involved with a particular branch of investigation—if they understand its language at all—take their conclusions on trust. The respect in which the institution is held is an important aspect of this trust. Similarly, the knowledge of supernatural powers, of gods and goddesses, of demons and demonesses, of sorcerers and witches in all small-scaled societies derives from respected traditions and institutions and from men who have proved themselves worthy of trust. Commonly shared beliefs are at the basis of communal sentiments, and hence beliefs which appear primitive and totally illogical to the Western observer not only rest on dogma but also take added strength from the fact that they are part of the moral foundations of the society in which they are found.

## REFERENCES

A Committee of the Royal Anthropological Institute of Great Britain and Ireland. 1971 (1874). *Notes and queries on anthropology*. London: Routledge and Kegan Paul Ltd.

Archer, W.G. (1947), The Santhal treatment of witchcraft. *Man In India*. March.

Bacon, Elizabeth E. (1995), "Witchcraft," in *The Encyclopedia Americana, Vol. 29,* Danbury Connecticut: Grolier Incorporated.

Banerjee, B.G. (2003), "Rationalising indigenous medicine in India: Plea for a broader perspective," in *Understanding people of India: Anthropological insight.* Edited by A.K. Kalla and D.K. Bhattacharya, pp. 298-336. Delhi: Deptt. of Anthropology, University of Delhi.

Biswas, P.C. (1956), *Santals of the Santal Parganas.* Delhi: Bharatiya Adimjati Sevak Sangh.

Bodding, P.O. (1925), The Santhals and disease: Studies in Santhal medicine and connected folklore, *Memoris of the Asiatic Society of Bengal,* Vol. 1. No. 1.

Bompass, C.H. (1909), *Folklore of the Santal Parganas*, London.

Bourguignon, Erika, (1995), "Magic," in *The Encyclopedia Americana, Vol. 18,* Danbury, Connecticut: Grolier Incorporated.

Castaneda, C. (1968), *The teachings of Don Fuan.* Berkeley: University of California Press.

Choudhuri, A.B. (1984), *Witch killing amongst Santals.* New Delhi, Asish Publishing House.

Comaroff, J. and J. Comaroff. (ed.) (1993), *Modernity and its malcontents.* Chicago: Chicago University Press.

Crick, M. (1979), Anthropologists' witchcraft: Symbolically defined or analytically undone? *Journal of the Anthropological Society of Oxford* 10: 139-146.

Deb Burman, Prasenjit, (1986), "Disease: Is it individual or societal?" in *Tribal Health: Socio-cultural Dimensions,* Edited by Buddhadeb Chaudhuri, pp. 185-189. New Delhi: Inter-India Publication.

Douglas, Mary, (ed.) (1970), *Witchcraft confessions and accusations.* Association of Social Anthropologists Monograph No. 9, London: Tavistock.

Evans-Pritchard, E.E. (1937), *Witchcraft, oracles and magic among the Azande,* Oxford: Clarendon Press.

Favret-Saada, J. (1977), *Los mots, La mort, les sorts.* Paris: Gallimard.

Ferraro Gary. (2001), *Cultural anthropology: An applied perspective,* USA: ITP An International Thomson Publishing Company.

Fortune, Reo F. (1932), *Sorcerers of Dobu,* New York: Dutton.

Foster, M., and B.G. Anderson (1978), *Medical Anthropology,* New York: John Wiley & Sons.

Fuchs, Stephen, (1950), *The Children of Hari,* Vienna: Verlus Herold.

Fuchs, Stephen, (1986), *The Korkus of the Vindhya Hills,* New Delhi: Inter-India Publications.

Geschiere, P. (1997), *The modernity of witchcraft and the Occult in postcolonial Africa,* Charlottesville: University Press of Virginia.

Geschiere, P. (2001), "Witchcraft," in *International encyclopedia of the social and behavioural sciences, Vol.* 6. Edited by Neil J. Smelser, and B. Paul, pp. 16514-17, U.K: Cambridge University Press.

Gilhodes, C. 1995 (1922), *The Kachins: Religion and Customs.* New Delhi: Mittal Publications.

Gluckman, M. (1944), "The Logic of African Science and Witchcraft: An Appreciation of Evans-Pritchard's Witchcraft Oracles and Magic Among the Azande of the Sudan" *Rhodes-Livingstone Institute Journal,* June: 61-71.

Griffiths, Walter G. (1946), *The Kol Tribe of Central India.* Calcutta: The Royal Asiatic Society of Bengal.

Horton, Robin, (1970), 'African traditional thought and western science,' in *Witchcraft and Sorcery.* Edited by Max G. Marwick pp. 342-368. Harmondsworth, Middlesex, England: Penguin Books.

Hutton, J.H. (1980) (1951), *Caste in India: Its nature, functions and origins,* Bombay: Oxford University Press.

Kluckhohn, C. (1944), *Navaho witchcraft.* Boston: Beacon Press.

Landy, David (ed.) (1977), *Culture, disease and healing: Studies in medical anthropology,* New York: Macmillan Publishing Co., Inc.

Levi-Strauss, Claude (1963), "The Sorcerer and his magic," in *Structural Anthropology,* Edited by Claude Levi-Strauss and translated by Claire Jacobson and Brooke Grundfest Schoepf, New York: Basic Books.

Mair, Lucy (1969), *Witchcraft,* New York: McGraw-Hill.

Malinowski, Bronislaw (1926), *Crime and custom in savage society,* London: Routledge and Kegan Paul.

Marwick, M. (1965), *Sorcery in its social setting*, Manchester: Manchester University Press.

Marwick, Max G. (ed.) (1970), *Witchcraft and Sorcery*, Harmondsworth, Middlesex, England: Penguin Books.

Marwick, Max (ed.) (1982), *Withcraft and Sorcery: Selected Readings.* 2nd ed. Harmondsworth, England: Penguin Books.

Middleton, J. (1960), *Lugbara Religion.* London: Routledge and Kegan Paul.

Middleton, John F.M., and E.H. Winter (eds.) *Witchcraft and Sorcery in East Africa,* London: Routledge and Kegan Paul.

Murray, Margaret A. (1921), *The Witch-Cult in Western Europe,* Oxford: Clarendon Press.

Nadel, S.F. (1952), Witchcraft in four African societies, *American Anthropologist* 54: 18-29.

Niehaus, I. (1993), Witch hunting and political legitimacy: Continuity and change in Green Valley, Lebowa 1930-1991. *Africa* 63(4): 498-529.

Rizvi, S.N.H. (1986), "Health practices of the Jaunsaris—A socio-cultural analysis," in *Tribal health: Socio-cultural dimensions.* Edited by Buddhadeb Chaudhuri, pp. 223-246. New Delhi: Inter India Publications.

Roy, S.C. (1937), *The Kharias.* Ranchi: Man in India Office.

Roy, S.C. 1978 (1925), *The Birhors: A little-known jungle tribe of Chota Nagpur, Ranchi*: Man In India Office.

Roy, S.C. 1985 (1930), *Oraon religion and customs,* Delhi: Gian Publishing House.

Shah, P.G. (1958), *The Dublas of Gujarat*, Delhi: Bharatiya Adimjati Sevak Sangh.

Snow, Loudell F. (1974), Folk medical beliefs and their implications for care of patients, *Annals of Internal Medicine* 81:82-96.

Stephen, Michele, (ed.) (1987), *Sorcerer and witch in Melanesia.* New Brunswick, N.J.: University Press.

Stevens Jr., Phillips, (1996), "Sorcery and witchcraft," in *Encyclopedia of Cultural Anthropology, Vol. 4.* Edited by Levinson David and Melvin Ember pp. 1225-32. New York: Henry Holt and Company.

Willis, Roy (1996), "Witchcraft and sorcery," in *Encyclopedia of social sciences and cultural anthropology.* Edited by Alan Barnard and Jonathan Spencer pp. 562-64. New York: Routledge.

Wilson, Monica H. (1951), *Good company: A Study of Nyakyusa Age Villages,* Published for the International African Institute, Oxford University Press.

Wilson, M. (1959), *Communal rituals of the Nyakyusa,* London: Oxford University Press.

Yalman, Nur (1968), "Magic," in *International Encyclopedia of the Social Sciences Vol. 9,* Edited by David L. Sills pp. 521-528. New York: The Macmillan Company & The Free Press.

# 14

# The World of Tribal Healers

P.C. JOSHI

Anthropological writings on traditional healers have largely concentrated upon shamans (Metzger and Williams, 1963; Margetts, 1965; Handelman, 1967; Lebra, 1969; Tenzel, 1970; Boyer, 1964; Turner, 1967, 1968; Joralemon, 1985). A majority of these have focused on the psychosocial dimensions of shaman's role. The trance-state in which a shaman usually bogs down, has been given psycho-pathological treatment (see Ackerknecht, 1943; Lebra, 1969, Lewis, 1971). Extensive use of projective techniques and personalized interviews in addition to an emphasis on the trance *sceance* and role-recruitment have been the major foci of attention. Some (Turner, 1967) have meticulously analysed the shaman's abilities in manipulating the existing social symbols with a view to reinstitute the broken social ties.

In a plethora of anthropological studies of healers, unfortunately, an examination of the whole situation from the patient's frame has not been largely attempted. How do people react to the shaman's calls and suggestions is equally important for understanding the dynamics of therapy. Furthermore, scanning through the literature in medical anthropology we also notice that other types of practitioners are either ignored or not taken account of. Barring few studies (Osgood *et al.*, 1966; Parrot, 1970; Fabrega and Silver, 1970), other types of healers have not been analysed properly. In traditional societies, shamans play a very vital role in health seeking process and are regarded 'powerful' as they control benevolent as well as obnoxious powers, but there are less researched, less mystified healers who perform equally pressing and similar tasks, of course, with different diagnostic techniques and therapeutic modes. They intervene in a variety of situations with in the framework of their respective causative theory and therapeutic practices (Joshi, 1988, 2000).

The present paper is an attempt at exploring the world of Jaunsari healers who practice in the Central Himalayas in the district of Dehradun, Uttaranchal. Like any other Himalayan community, the Jaunsari also have wide variety of shamans who act as mediators between the godly powers and the human being and thus help the latter in finding answers to their puzzles and queries. But, the shamans are not the only healers that the Jaunsari believe in. They have a very well defined regiment of healers who intervene at various stages in health seeking as well as in avoiding and sorting out of generalized misfortunes.

The healers of the Jaunsari can be grouped in the following five main categories:

1. *Baman*—Astrologer, priest and healer.
2. Mali—Diviner and shaman.
3. *Jariyara*—Pulse specialist and herbalist.
4. Female Specialist—Midwife, masseur and gynaecologist.
5. Doctor—Non-traditional healer.

The Jaunsari identify illness as caused by natural and supernatural forces. When an illness is believed to be caused by natural forces it is called *bimari* while when the supernatural agency is held responsible it is called *dos*. The *baman* and *mali* healers exclusively diagnose, prevent and treat the *dos* whereas *jariyara*, female specialist and doctor deal with *bimari* problems. From the point of view of the people, doctor is also a healer very similar to the *jariyara*. The doctor as healer would be anyone practicing from a well identified place, the government hospital, the health centre, a paid clinic, an exclusive place having doctor's paraphernalia like thermometer, stethoscope, dextrose bottles, etc. Except doctor, none of the other healer has separate space earmarked as clinic. They are ordinary householders who do healing work besides their routine household duties. An important factor, which not only singles out Jaunsari traditional healers from the doctors but also from many other reported forms elsewhere, is their inexpensive treatment terms. Mostly their services are gratis and sometimes inexpensive and as such their treatment is always within the reach of the people. In nutshell, the healer role is a 'non-profit social service' which adds to the prestige of an individual as a helpful guy. There are however very few exceptions in the form of super-specialist traditional healers. The super-specialists charge exorbitant sum for their services.

### *Baman*

The role set of a *baman* is a complex one as it includes the role of a priest, astrologer, diagnostician and the healer. It also connotes a generalized *jati* name for the people hailing from the higher caste Brahmin. The *bamnai* skills are formally transmitted in the traditional ways through a practicing *baman* to the apprentice. We find two categories of persons in the Brahmin caste. The first includes the *baman* of ascriptive status while in the second; those who have achieved the *baman* status because of apprenticeship are counted. The healing *baman* (*ganechhiya baman* or *baman* who calculates) are further subdivided into two major groups, namely, *bhat* and *pabooch*. Majority of *ganechhiya baman* fall in the *bhat* group. The *pabooch* on the other hand is an exclusive category, restricted to the Chanjoi and Khorkiyan villages of Himachal Pradesh and Punning and Dimich villages of Bawar. In the caste hierarchy, the *pabooch* is ranked higher to the *bhat*.

The therapeutic modes of both *ganechhiya* group are more or less similar. The main difference being that the *pabooch baman* abstains from sacrificing animals during healing rituals which the *bhat* most often does. However, in case the sacrifice is inevitable, the *pabooch* uses a surrogate. The *sancha*, book used in the diagnosis and healing by a *baman*, of *bhat* and *pabooch* differs only in script but shows striking similarities in the content. On the whole, it may be said that the *pabooch* is held superior, not necessarily more effective, to a *bhat* on account of his being more sanskritized for making use of the great tradition icons and verses in the healing. Notwithstanding slight differences, the interchange of knowledge is, however, not restricted. Owing primarily to marital interdependence, we often encounter a *pabooch* trained in *bhat sancha* and *vice versa.*

*Composition*: Baman's role is typically a male's job. Though, it is caste specific, we find very few exceptions to this general rule. The Jogra renunciator caste is one such exception. The Jogra are ranked much below the Brahmins, but are allowed to learn and practice the art of a *baman*. However, there are very few Jogra *baman* healers except one who was very famous for inducing trance through a ritual called *bharni.* In another instance, a Bajgi musician could be cited as another exception to the caste rule. He claims to have access to the knowledge, usually administered by the *ganechhiya baman* to diagnose certain maladies and its cure. His prime specialization was in diagnosing the cases of *bis* (ritual poisoning) which he would do with the help of rice grains and a script of few pages. His status was like a quack. His scriptures were rudimentary, incomplete and seem vestigial, conspicuous unlike the ones possessed by the *ganechhiya baman.*

*Paraphernalia***:** The diacritical mark of a *baman* is a book written in a script (unidentified, probably influenced by Sarda script of Kashmir). This book is called Kashmiri Vidhya. Vidhya is a native usage for knowledge, art and skill—a person knowing English language would be termed as mastering English vidhya and so on. The book is also referred to as *sancha* meaning 'condensed'. It is believed that the scripture is a condensed knowledge capable of interpreting and answering any question perturbing people. In looks, it consists of long sheets of white paper stitched together (in earlier times it was prepared on the birch bark) and is wrapped in dear skin. It is carefully kept in a net bag made of cotton. Containing seven chapters, tables and figures, used in the process of 'calculation and search' (*ganana-khojna*), it is always consulted by a *baman.*

With a dice called *goti*, which is a rectangular engraved bone piece having one to four dots on all the four sides, the *baman* makes calculation to identify the specific *dos* responsible for the problem of the clients. He also makes use of a yearly almanac procured from a *pabooch* or purchased from the market in order to find out auspicious dates and times for the sacred jobs. Baman's healing art is a literary tradition. However, some *bamans* who have been formally educated in the school system, now a days prefer keeping printed books of great tradition.

*Practice:* The role of a *baman* is not a full time job nor can it yield sufficient for a practitioner in economic terms. A *baman* is like any other landowning *jimidar* and works as a *ganechhiya* during spare time. Most of the rituals of the *baman* are performed in the night time and except when they go to a farther place, their role does not affect day to day routine work in any way. A baman's income is also meagre. For calculations of *dos*, he generally receives five to ten paisa and sometimes even this paltry sum is withheld. It has been observed that on many occasions, people just give the *baman* a little wool for the calculations. However, a *baman* cannot demand for the fee and he has been seen to even reluctantly accept the token amount. For performing rituals, the *baman* receives the ingredients used besides rupees one to five. Only on special rituals such as *bharni* or *diya-choi* which involve trance induction and have lot of strain on the *baman* the payment could go upto fifty rupees. On an average, the monthly income of a *baman* from practice would be within the range of rupees fifty to a hundred.

*Recruitment:* "*Bamnai* (*baman's* work) is not a profitable job these days", said an old veteran *pabooch*. In his view, *bamnai* requires visits to distant places for rituals and calculations, but, what is received in return—merely one or two rupees, which is not even sufficient to buy a handful of *biris* (packet of rolled tobacco). He strongly felt that despite spiraling prices, a *baman* is still paid in customary manner. If it was one silver coin in the past, even today he is paid one rupee as paper currency. The return has greatly declined as the silver rupee today is worth rupee thirty. Another *baman* narrated an interesting incident when asked why he learnt *bamnai*? He said that though there are insufficient manpower in his family to look after the agriculture, they are constrained to adopt *bamnai* because otherwise they would get *dos*. He further elaborated that his great grandfather had left *bamnai* which had been their family tradition because he could not spare time for it. His family had great reputation in this skill for it had the command over sorcery and black magic. The *bamnai* was discontinued for two generations. This resulted in a *dos* to his family and as a consequence there were repeated miscarriages to his grandmother. She was able to deliver successfully only when a promise was made that the family will continue again with the *bamnai* and so his father was born and thereafter the *bamnai* became part of their family tradition.

*Bamnai* is a learned role. Like in a typical ashram style, a pupil imbibes the knowledge of Vidhya from his guru. In most cases, a guru is also a close kin or affine, generally mother's brother. The pupil must be obedient towards the guru. He works in guru's fields and performs household chores in spare time. Guru initiates the learning process by inculcating *kandi* (hymns) which the pupil has to memorize. Then follows the learning of *sancha* and the actual art of interpretation (*byal*) of the verses in the Vidhya.

The pupil accompanies his guru to distant villages where he seizes an opportunity to learn Vidhya intimately. When the guru is satisfied, he writes the *sancha* and hands it over to his pupil. A person with *sancha* thus becomes a legitimate *baman*. Generally, there is one student at a time because the *bamnai* learning is very intense procedure but, a popular *baman* may train two or three students at the same time. Learning the art and skills from a famous *baman* is desirable but not sufficient to attract more clients. What counts most is the individual merit, talents and improvisations, a *baman* makes during his lifetime. We may therefore come across *bamans* who have learnt *bamnai* from very famous gurus but are not having roaring practice while the *bamans* trained by ordinary gurus excelling in their practice. There was great variation in the practicing style of the *baman* although all would take clues from the Vidhya. After all, Vidhya as *sancha* is only a condensed knowledge which needs to be elaborated and interpreted by means of finding out *byal* because it is the *byal* which is the main concern of the client.

*Baman as priest*: Priests are known as *pujgi* and a *baman* learns verses, prayers, sequence of rituals and placement of ingredients during his apprenticeship. As a priest, he performs the rites of passage—birth, marriage and death rituals. The rituals are also integral part of any auspicious occasion like building of a house, starting of new venture, etc. A very common form of community ritual is *jaaga* or *thatti* ritual. This ritual is concern with the propitiation of the sacred soil of the village which is closely believed to be linked to the prosperity and well being of the village as a whole. Every village in Jaunsar-Bawar has the sacred place called *thatti* or *jaaga,* the soil of which is not given to the strangers. It is believed that the enemies of the village can perform black magic on the *thatti* soil which can result in the destruction of the entire village. The *baman* performing *thatti* ritual always comes from a traditionally specified village. Another priestly ritual performed by a *baman* is called *pap* ritual. *Pap* are the ancestral sins manifested in the form of silver idols kept in the households. The *baman* performs ritual for propitiation of *pap* four times a year.

*Baman as astrologer:* The domain of astrology in baman's practice involves searching and interpreting man's relationship with the cosmogenetic world. Right from inception of life, there exists a symbiotic relationship between the person and the cosmic entities in the world view of the Jaunsari. The life long placement, determined by the constellation of these cosmic entities at the time of birth, is prepared by a *baman* for every male child. This chart depicting the stellar configuration is called *teep*. With the help of native or printed almanac, a *baman* takes the *teep* as a reference point to decipher anything about an individual. His marriage and other important activities are decided in terms of *teep* only. In addition, a *baman* is frequently consulted for identifying auspicious date and time for starting a major work. It has been observed that a *baman* is invariably consulted for determining the auspicious time for starting any new project or affair. For instance, constructing a house, starting of a harvest, preparation of an alcoholic beverages for marriage ceremony, are some of the occasions which seldom, if any, go without consultations. Not only in the matters of life, even the death of a person should take place within the auspicious time period. In one occasion, this occurred in an inauspicious occasion and therefore the whole village had to perform the *daka* ritual for its protection. Under this ritual, the whole village was kept within the protection of cotton thread which was tied around the boundary of the village.

*Baman as diagnostician: Ganechhiya* means one who calculates *dos* from the *sancha* book. The main technique employed by a *baman* is called 'calculation-search' (*ganana-khojna*). It is done with the help of *sancha* verses. The baman's diagnosis of *dos* is an interesting scene to observe. A client coming for a diagnosis will not give any indication as to his query. It is expected that a *baman*, if skilful, should be able to interpret *sancha* verses and give a true reflection of the *dos*. *Baman*, in the first instance, calculates the 'auspicious-inauspicious' (*subh-ashubh*) state of the client. If the *sancha* verses come out as auspicious, *baman* declares that there is no *dos* to the client and therefore his misfortune is either the 'play of fate' or a *bimari* caused due to natural forces. In case the *sancha* verses come out as inauspicious, the *baman* goes in for further 'search'. Baman's mastery over making calculations is discerned not just in reading the verses but in judging how skilfully he correlates the lines and interprets them in accordance with the problems of the client. We catalogue below few cases of baman's diagnosis.

A Rajput male has come to *baman* for calculation of *dos*. Initially, he did not gave any clue to the *baman* as to what was troubling him except that it concerned human beings. Generally a *baman* inquires the name and the lineage of the client, but in this case, as the client was well known to him, he did not ask for this information. The *baman* opened the *sancha* and held the *goti* in his hand.

*Baman:* Kal Gyani chapter of Vidhya. You are sacred. Truth

enriches dharma while lie is a sin. Speak not in the tune of time but strictly according to the question. Client Jawahar Singh of Amran lineage asks for the 'life-soul' and 'cattle'. Move correctly and speak of auspicious and clearly. If there is a *dos*, then speak as inauspicious. Is there any loss-decrement to Jawahar Singh? (Saying this the *baman* threw the *goti* over the *sancha* and spoke aloud) Two, two again, two again and one-six. Three and one. Two, three, one-six. Six and five, eleven. Two, three and one. Two-three, one-six. Eleven and six-seventeen.

The total calculations in the first attempt through *goti* over nine counts in the set of three each was the following:

| | |
|---|---|
| First count: | 2 + 2 + 2 = 5 |
| Second count: | 2 + 3 + 1 = 6 |
| Third count: | 2 + 3 + 1 = 6 |
| Grand Total: | 5 + 6 + 6 = 17 |

From his memory about the written verses in the Ka Gyani chapter of the *sancha*, the *baman* spoke of the verses given at number seventeen.

*Baman:* Devta's *dos* as is always happens. A 'thought' put up to the devta superhuman entity has to be fulfilled, then only the current 'worry' will go away.

The *baman* did not cared to give any interpretation at the very first count nor did the client asked him to clarify the meaning of the verse. Instead, the *baman* on his own intiative, started another count.

| | |
|---|---|
| First count: | 1 + 2 + 1 = 4 |
| Second count: | 1 + 2 + 3 = 6 |
| Third count: | 3 + 4 + 1 = 8 |
| Grand Total: | 4 + 6 + 8 = 18 |

*Baman:* There is a hinderance in the work. Your enemy is opposing you, defaming you. You desire for peace and joining hands, you are worried but the work being never done. It will not be done (but) the day you fulfil the promise, the work will be done. That's why you are in loss. You do not be intimate with your 'friend-brother'. There will be the *dos* of family deity.

Jawahar Singh did not get impressed with the calculations though the *baman* had raised his pitch so that the client could clearly understand that there is the *dos* of devta to him and it was this that was responsible for his current troubles. The *baman* instructed that he should make a promise to the devta who is angry by throwing wheat flour on all directions.

*Jawahar Singh:* Wheat flour has already been thrown. An earlier *baman* had instead calculated the cause to be interpersonal rivalry (*makhta*).

Here *baman's* initial calculations were not in the line of expected diagnosis desired by the client. It was clearly contradicting client's earlier query. The domain of earlier probe resulted in interpersonal rivalry (human to human relationship) as the kind of *dos* while the new cause falls in the *dos* of devta (human to superhuman relationship). But, it was just the beginning of a long complex process. *Baman's* real skills lie in making his client satisfied in the end.

*Baman:* Lord Vidhya ! Is there any magic or sorcery to Jawahar Singh?

Both these conceptual categories were within the human orbit. *Baman* threw his *goti* over the *sancha*.

| | | | |
|---|---|---|---|
| First count: | 2 + 4 + 4 | = | 10 |
| Second count: | 3 + 4 + 4 | = | 11 |
| Third count: | 3 + 3 + 3 | = | 9 |
| Grand Total: | 10 + 11 + 9 | = | 30 |

*Baman:* Thirty, there should be no trouble. This 'thought' had come in the month of *Savan* (July-August). It was a good thought. There was evil spirit of *masan* near the river banks. You thought of your friend. Your friend was with you when the evil spirit struck you. Invocate red cloth. Then you will be happy.

Instead of interpreting the meaning of the verses, *baman* wanted to probe further. But before the *baman* could start again, the client interrupted.

*Jawahar Singh:* Is this evel spirit like *masan*?

*Baman:* The evil spirit is *masan*.

*Baman* did not explain further but started a new probe.

*Baman*: Lord Vidhya! Whether there is relief if the "promise" to appease *masan* is made. If there is anything else then come as inauspicious. If there is no decrement-loss, then 'speak' auspicious. Oh Lord Vidhya! The speaker.

*Baman* now started counting. But this time he wanted to check for *dos* in a different chapter of *sancha*—the Bhota Prasang. For this, he threw the *goti* only for three times.

Bhota Prasang count: 1, 1, 2 = 112

*Baman*: In (according to) this question, you are pure in heart. Victory over the enemies. There is rivalry in your extended family and the illness is increasing. There is loss in business. Some *dos* of devta is also present. Do not fear it. There is a hypocrite in your family.

The verses in the Bhota Prasang chapter were in Hindi language rather than the local dialect. The statement read out under 112 was a multipurpose one. It talked of rivalry, loss and even of *dos* of devta. It also started with something 'auspicious'. Finally, the last sentence gives a hint to the client that there is one hypocrite in his family. This statement, a typical feature of this chapter, is stated in order to prove the authenticity of the verse. The *baman* was still not satisfied and therefore started further probe.

*Baman*: 'Priced' goat is promised to Lord Mahasu. Wheat flour is also thrown in all directions. If still there is any further *dos* then come as inauspicious. We are fulfilling the promise.

| | | |
|---|---|---|
| First count: | 3 + 4+ 4 | = 11 |
| Second count: | 1 + 2 + 4 = | 7 |
| Third count: | 1+ 3+ 3 | = 7 |
| Grand Total: | 11+7+7 | = 25 |

*Baman:* This work will not be done. There is trouble in it. Bad thoughts would creep in. Do not do this work. There is fear in it. It is like enemy. Do your Karma. Give alms which will be beneficial.

Making no conclusion and telling nothing to the client, the *baman* went ahead with his probe.

*Baman:* Any other melancholy than this to Jawahar Singh then come as inauspicious. It no melancholy then 'speak of' auspicious. Oh! Speaker.

| | | |
|---|---|---|
| First count: | 4 + 4 + 2 | = 10 |
| Second count: | 2 + 4 + 4 | = 10 |

Third count: 2 + 4 + 4 = 10
Grand Total: 10 + 10 + 10 = 30

Still *baman* preferred not to make any statement and therefore started another count.

*Baman*: If there is some loss-decrement, speak as inauspicious. If no loss-decrement, speak as auspicious. Oh! The Speaker Vidhya.

The count: 4, 1, 3 = 413

He had now made only three counts for clarifying the question from the other chapter. Till now, he was reading the verses only out of his memory. But now he decided to open the *sancha* to read out the verse.

*Baman*: Persisting worry will vanish. Have courage. Money will also flow in. Do not do business. All worry will vanish. Think of east. The cosmic constellations are excellent.

Now *baman* closed the book and faced client. He wanted to give the conclusion to the client of all the probes and queries that he had made out of the Vidhya book.

*Baman*: There is no loss-decrement. The *dos* of devta comes out. As this *dos* comes out, along comes the rivalry in the family. Therefore, you throw wheat flour in all directions and promise a goat to the Mahasu. Rest, there is nothing else to you.

The calculations made by the *baman* had now satisfied the client. In calculating queries, a *baman* skilfully plays the role of an 'interpreter'. The commonly held notion, in the mind of *baman* as well the client is that the Vidhya words are never wrong or out of context. In reality, a *baman* has to manipulate and extend verse to the level of client's satisfaction. Nevertheless, the *sancha* system is more or less the complete set of knowledge and the failure of diagnosing the actual cause or factor is related to the inability of a *baman* in deriving real meaning out of the statements.

The verses have a complex structure of statements. They can be broadly classified as auspicious and inauspicious, but, they contain multifaceted conditions indicating various states of existence. A verse, at different times means different things depending upon the skills in the area. The broad mode of calculation remains the same but the style of probing and the ability to conclude varies from one *baman* to another. There are *bamans*, who even go to the extent of fighting with their clients and do not budge an inch from the written verses while there are others who carefully read the minds of their clients before arriving at a conclusion.

*Sancha* calculation is the dominant mode of diagnosis that the *bamans* indulge in. But, sometimes they also induce trance in order to make diagnosis. However, this form of diagnosis is very rare as it involves inducing a layman into trance, one who has never experienced this state of subconscious experience. Two very commonly performed induced trance diagnostic modes are:

1. *Bharni*
2. *Diya-choi*

*Bharni* includes the ritualistic search used for uncovering the hidden ancestral curse or sorcery. Ordinarily, a *baman* is capable of calculating such *dos* with the help of *sancha*. But, sometimes the hidden super-empirical force becomes extremely obnoxious and fails to be calmed by usual procedures. Under such circumstances, *Bharni* makes it possible to get to the finer details of the cause of curse since it makes the person under *Bharni* trance to give a first person account of the reason for the curse or sorcery. *Bharni* is a very elaborate and time consuming ritual for it takes days to convert an innocent person into a medium. However, it is performed under very special circumstances, especially when other modes of diagnosis fail to reveal the details of the exact cause.

In one case, the *Bharni* session became inevitable because the *dos* was believed to be harming the entire family and no amount of ritualistic appeasement of the *dos* was resulting in any relief to the family. The family then thought that may be the *dos* is due to a very complex cause and therefore, decided to organize *Bharni* session. *Bharni* involved a *baman* and a layman, the *baman* being inducer of trance while the layman the person who had no history of getting into trance. Both the partners of the *Bharni* should have favourable zodiac constellations. Thus, a Rajput male was selected for the *Bharni*. *Bharni* involves invoking nefarious forces and therefore it is started in an inauspicious day after full moon when the moonlight starts decreasing. Furthermore, the *Bharni* session should conclude before the new moon.

*Bharni* is a sequence of rhythmic singing in the session of sittings called *bharnai.* The medium sits facing *baman.* A metal pot filled with soil is placed on the ground. Then a hollow clay pitcher is placed over it with its opening upwards. Finally, a metallic (zinc) plate is kept over the pitcher, upside down. *Baman* then produces harsh metallic sounds by means of striking the plate.

Before starting the *bharnai, baman* would, firstly, light a lamp. The medium is then ritually purified. The medium would rub cow's urine on his head and palm to become purified. Finally, the head of the medium will be covered with a white cloth. Both the partners in the *Bharni* would put off their caps as a mark of respect for the ritual.

*Baman* would strike the plate with a stick held in his right hand. He would use his left hand for keeping the plate in order over the pitcher. He will sing *ved* (memorized holy verses invoking various devta superhuman). He primarily invokes Lord Vishnu and the ten incarnations. The variation in metallic sound is skilfully maintained by the *baman* by means of raising it over the pitcher from time to time. This *Bharni* session is performed in a separate room away from the normal dwelling and the medium hear nothing but the rhythmic sounds and the *ved.* Each *Bharni* session is a tiring experience for both the partners. On the whole, only five to seven *bharnai* are performed in a day.

In the case observed, the *Bharni* session lasted for eight days and for the first two days there was no apparent change in the medium. He did shiver at times but could not be gripped by any super-empirical force. It was on the third day that he started getting the spell in him. A total of eight days and after several *bharnai* sessions, the medium was able to have the true trance experience and reveal the finer details of the cause. When under full trance, the medium, firstly, saluted the *baman* by uttering Ram. Under the influence and guidance of the *baman,* he later on revealed the 'truth' of the cause of *dos* to the family.

The medium, when contacted later, told that he was not in his senses and thus does not know what he might have said in a possessed state. An interesting aspect of the *Bharni* session was that at one time this medium abused the client and scolded him very harshly. In day to day life also this man was against the client, though, both hailed from the same lineage. The medium was actually a poor person being harassed by the client on many occasions. The abuse and anger expressed by the medium in the *Bharni* session was of the super-empirical agency towards the client for the mistake committed by the latter. But, at the same time, it was also a chance given to a poor man to express his suppression towards the rich and mighty.

*Diya-choi* is another diagnostic mode used by a *baman*. *Diya-choi* literally means the lamp and the dried gourd, the main ingredients used in this highly stylistic search of lost object diagnostic session. *Diya-choi* is actually the combination of two primary modes of searching lost object by induced trance. In first method, a lamp is used while in the second method a choi dry gourd is used. In this method, the *baman* uses his skill and competence to turn an ordinary villager into trance. The ritualistic search does not take much time like the *Bharni*.

In a choi diagnostic session observed, the occasion was when the precious mushrooms of a poor villager were stolen from his house and the *baman* was asked to find out the culprit. The *baman* selected a Bajgi musician who was having the right zodiac constellations for the occasion. A dried gourd was tied at the right hand of the medium wrapped in red cloth. The *baman* stated singing *ved* holy verses accompanied by producing harsh metallic sounds on a metal plate held in hand. It took nearly half an hour for the medium to get into trance and suddenly he started running outside with his hand held to the ground. It appeared as if some unseen force inside the gourd was pulling his hand make him run in the desired direction. The lost object could not be found because the *choi* started going outside the village boundary, implying thereby that the thief was an outsider.

*Baman as a healer:* A number of healing tasks are performed by the *baman* in the arena of *dos*. From highly stylistic homeopathic rituals to 'blow and brush' and at times the healing action may culminate in preparation of charm only. The initial action in healing is of keeping *bonth* (promise). This promise is in the form of keeping the token of actual ritual, a kind of pre-testing whether the *dos* is really there or not. Jaunsari are very particular about assuring themselves of the true nature of the misfortune before giving it any complete propitiation. The actual healing ritual may involve cost and so why waste precious resources. Although, the promise may be kept by anyone having its experience for it only involves a token of the actual ingredients to be used later, the *baman* is generally preferred to help in keeping it. Promise keeping is however not the healing per se but a positive step in that direction. Promise, though temporary, is considered to be as effective as a full-fledged healing performance. Therefore, if there is no improvement in the misfortune after the promise, people start thinking of searching for further calculations and divinations.

In a case of prolonged infertility to a Kolta lower caste person, the *baman* was asked to calculate *dos*. In baman's calculations, the *dos* was found to be ancestral sin which demanded a pilgrimage to holy place for purification of the ancestral sin idol. The *baman* kept a promise of the following ingredients:

1. 10 paisa coin—symbolizing the expenses to be borne during pilgrimage.
2. Silver chip—symbolizing silver idol of ancestral sin.
3. Water filled in a cup—symbolizing act of purification by holy water.
4. Rice in a plate—symbolizing food for the ancestral sin.
5. Coat's hair—symbolizing offering of goat to be made to Lord Mahasu.
6. 5 paisa coin—an act of respect to Lord Mahasu.

All the object were held together and the *baman* announces: "Take Lord! This person has offered silver for your idol. This is the promise for your expenses (showing ten paisa coin). He offers you silver also. If you give relief, he will 'listen-respect' (propitiate) you properly. All your expenses are also being promised." After saying this, the *baman* held all the ingredients in hand and moved them in clockwise manner for nine times.

Very often, the promise keeping is accompanied by the act of further confirmation with the use of a goat. This act is called '*bakra-dhunana*', literally meaning the shivering of the goat. It is a confirmation of devta's consent in a matter. The process of '*bakra-dhunana*' involves rubbing of cold water on the back, chest and neck of the goat, followed by sprinkling of some water in the ears of the beast. After this, the goat is left alone and people state the purpose of '*bakra-dhunana*' and urge the devta for the acceptance. If the goat shiver, it is taken as a proof of devta acceptance.

Both promise keeping and goat's shivering do not strictly fall in the arena of the *baman's* healing tasks. It is mainly because the *baman* is regarded as the most skilled personnel in *dos* related matters that people like to get these things done by a *baman*. However, experienced lay villagers may also perform these tasks with equal ease and confidence.

Preparation of a charm (*bhujri*) is another important healing act carried out by a *baman*. A charm is a blending of mystical formula (*yantra*) and incantations (*mantra*). Often the paper used for writing the *yantra* is birch bark but the charm can also be prepared in any ordinary paper. Vermilion, mustard seeds and cotton thread are other ingredients used in preparation of a charm. The *baman* prepared the *yantra* on the piece of paper and keeps the other ingredients on it and then whispers the incantations to make the charm effective.

The charms can be divided into two main types, namely protective and preventive. Although, the explicit function of a charm is to bestow an afflicted one with a protective covering, the charm worn in anticipation of an evil influence and the one where the malady is already known are to be distinguished from one another. In case of charm worn to ward off the ill effects of the planets, sun and moon, the action is an attempt to avoid the harms which have not yet manifested themselves. The main purpose of the charm is to prevent ill effects. But, the charm worn after an affliction is known serves the protective purpose by lessening the ill effects.

The third important set of healing activities a *baman* performs can be grouped under 'blow and brush' tasks. The native term for 'blow' is *jhara* and for the 'brush' is *unjh*. In the act of *unjh*, the ritual brushing is done with the brush made up of grass or a feather. It is generally performed when there is swelling on the body due to an injury. The wound, it is believed, get poisoned due to the invisible arrows of the fairies. The brushing act is believed to be able to take out the invisible poison from the wound. A very special kind of 'brushing' is employed for cases of paralysis believed to be caused by the fairies again. In performing this kind of 'brushing', cow's urine, white clay, cotton thread of white colour and some coins are kept in a plate. The 'brushing' act is performed a number of times along with the chant of hymns. The manifest action in the 'brushing' is to move the grass or feather over the affected part followed by ending the action in the plate containing ritual objects.

'Blow' healing actions are usually performed by the lay healers and the diviners. However, the *baman* also has an expertise in doing this task. 'Blow' action is employed under conditions of possession by some evil supernatural force. In making the 'blow', some ash is pressed with the right hand thumb near the forehead of the afflicted person, while the *baman* whispers incantations. The end of the incantation is marked by an action of blowing the ash over the patient.

Finally, the most important healing task performed by a *baman* is *pujan* (ritual worship). These meaningful and highly stylistic rituals can also be grouped into two broad categories, namely, healing *pujan* and protective *pujan*. The healing rituals are ones where the eveil effects have already been noticed. The ritual is therefore an attempt to remove, suppress or ward off the misfortune. In protective ritual, the mal-effect may or may not be known. The ritual is an attempt to avoid any future suffering. Generally speaking, the healing ritual succeed 'calculations' while the protective rituals are performed after the 'search'.

*Masan* fairy healing ritual is one of the very popular form of healing ritual performed by a *baman*. The masans are the evil fairies inhabiting the cremation grounds and the river banks. The time for performing this ritual is night, generally the falling in the time period when the moon is decreasing or a new moon night, signifying the 'impurity' domain of the *masan* fairies. The ritual objects used in this form of ritual are:

1. Black pulses (Vigia *mungo*).
2. Wheat flour.
3. Diya lamp
4. Round gourd.

Black pulses and wheat flour are mixed in water for the preparation of *masan* idol which is an anthropomorphic figurine. A four cornered lamp is also prepared with this dough. Some pine chips are inserted into the body of the soft gourd so as to make it into a surrogate animal—ram. Finally, some wool is kept over the surrogate. Sacred smoke is produced by means of putting some clarified butter over the burning coals. The client, one who has been afflicted by the *masan* fairy, sits in front of the *baman* who firstly declares the purpose of the ritual. He sings praises in honour of fairies which are of 64 kinds. He urges the fairies to come one by one and take away the trouble from the body of the client. One by one the ritual objects are held in hand and taken near the head of the client and the *baman* makes ritual transference of the trouble—from the client to the surrogate ram. The *baman*, while keeping the surrogate near the head of the client, declares, "Over this individual, a *pujan* of *masan* has been performed. A gourd is turned into a ram. Anything 'sticking' to the individual is urged to go away".

The patient is then asked to touch the ritual objects and in the last phase of the ritual, the ingredients are thrown at a cross road where the surrogate is sacrificed.

**Mali**

Numerically the largest, *mali* is a group of diviners who bridge the gap between the superhuman forces and the lay villagers. They are the via media of supernatural forces and thus, communicate with people under the ecstasy and spell of supernatural powers.

The Jaunsari, who pay utmost importance to the culturally constructed supernatural world, believe that the benevolent devta basically protect them. The primary motive of the devta is to perpetuate *dharma* (religious order and duties). Though invisible, they exist in the environment—in shrines, fields, steams, jungles—all around. The existence of devta is explained through the conceptualization of *hava* (air). Thus, the air of devta is constantly blowing in the atmosphere. This quality of devta makes them omnipresent. Thus, constant vigil is kept by the devta over the human beings. The devta, however, tend to sleep in the night when the evil forces rule the world. Thus, the devta not only watch the actions of the people but also their thoughts, motivations and intentions.

These devta, though powerful, cannot take human form which is a lower order existence in terms of 'purity'. But, they do express themselves with the media known as *mali*. The *mali*, who represent the devta, are carefully selected individuals, who also take care that they remain 'pure' so that the presiding devta is not defiled. Thus, the *mali* are also referred to as *dori* (vehicle) of the devta. The devta thus select their vehicle and such a person has the capability of inducing in himself the spirit of the devta at the time of need. The devta incarnates over the *mali* who goes into a state of divination—an state of altered consciousness. Any individual under the incarnation state is considered to be the devta in person and as such is addressed as the divine form.

A wide variety of *mali* can be found in the Jaunsar society. They hail from different castes and age groups as well from both the sexes. A *mali* is believed to be the one who is specially favoured by his guardian superhuman force. This explains why only some people become *mali* and not all. The divination occurs when the guardian force enters into the body and possesses it. The *mali*, because of the fact that his body houses the pious superhuman, albeit temporarily, has to live the life of a 'holy person'. The *mali* thus observes certain purity rules. The most commonly followed rules are:

1. Do not plough.
2. Do not share tobacco pipe with others.
3. Do not abuse or use abuses in conversations.
4. Do not take stale meal.
5. Take bath before a meal.
6. Leave one meal if heard of a death or sees dead cattle.
7. Stop eating meal if someone happens to utter prohibited words like cow's species, nightsoil, etc.
8. Do not eat festive food collected from the higher caste families (for lower castes).
9. Do not eat sheep, pig and chicken and eat only ram and goat meat (for lower castes).

Many of these behavioural and commensality rules are applied in the inter-caste regulations. Thus, *mali* has a socially higher status in the society. Moreover, becoming *mali* would mean getting special attention in the family and the village. Having malintentions towards *mali* would be like offending a devta guarding him. Thus, *mali* which appears to a painful and tedious role is a desirable status for the Jaunsari.

Jaunsari *mali* greatly differ from many other reported forms of shamans and diviners in the sense that they do not charge payments for their services. In certain areas, they even avoid the offerings or monetary payments. Even when they get the offerings, they receive payment below one rupee. They can never refuse services unless they are suffering from some disease. The *mali*, in general, is like other healers, a part time role. There are however very few exceptions in the form of *mali* who devote most of their time to divination and get better payments for the services. But even they never demand money. However, people give them more money simply because they are specially skilled in certain kinds of healing tasks.

*Mali—The Types*: *Mali* is primarily a male's domain. Some females also become *mali*, but exclusively for the female superhuman forces. But here again, the males outnumber females. The impact of prevailing caste hierarchy can also be traced in the world of superhuman and thus among *mali*. Though all superhuman are placed at a higher order than the human forms, but, the superhuman maintain hierarchy among themselves.

Thus, there are higher order superhuman like the principal deities such as Mahasu, Silgur, Devi, etc. and also lower order superhuman like Kali, Peer, Beer, etc. The latter are considered to be inferior in rank and therefore performing the role of assistants to the higher superhuman. The *mali* of higher superhuman are always as a rule hail from higher castes and consequently the *mali* of lower castes come from lower castes. However, there was one exception. A Bajgi musician from lower caste, in a village once started getting the 'air' of Mahasu higher devta. He did not become a full-fledged *mali*, but the very fact that he would get the influence of higher devta in his body perplexed people. This never happens in normal course and therefore the abnormality in this case was searched for. It was late found that there has been a theft in the Mahasu shrine of his village in which the thiefs had entered the shrine with their shoes on and thus defiling the higher devta Mahasu in the process. This fact was attributed to be the cause of such an unusual possession.

*Mali—the Role*: *Malihood* is a legitimate diviner's status. *Mali* can be differentiated in terms of their divinatory objects, style, language used and the area of *dos* they deal with, besides sex and caste status. Apart from this, the *mali* of one area differ from *mali* of another area in their style of divination. In the area of Kandai, the *mali* would themselves invoke the superhuman forces in order to get the possession while in Bawar, the *mali* will sit quietly and it is the surrounding crowd which will invoke the superhuman. While in trance, the Kandai *mali* would primarily move their head on both sides and their entire body will remain still. In Bawar, it was observed that the *mali* would shake his entire body in the state of trance.

*Malihood* is not an easily achievable role. One has to undergo a long process of uncontrolled possession state and one achieves *mali* status after successfully controlling the possession. The whole process has to be learnt the hard way. Once someone has successfully completed this phase, he/she gets the legitimacy from the principal shrine as well as diviner's insignia. The principal shrine where the higher superhuman *mali* receive the status is the shrine of Mahasu at a place called Hanol. The lower order diviner get the legitimacy under the guidance of a higher diviner at village shrines itself. The insignia that the *mali* carry are received from the shrine where they have attained legitimacy. Thus, the *mali* of higher superhuman carry a brass pot and a silver coin, the *mali* of Kali carry red cloth and vermilion while the *mali* of Beer carry iron chains as insignia. The process of legitimization culminates in offering of a goatling in case of Kali while of a he goat in cases of higher superhuman and Beer. In becoming of a Silgur higher superhuman *mali* one has to make the offering of a ram.

The divination of higher superhuman is accomplished with the help of rice grains called *jindav* while the divination of Kali and fairies is performed with the help of rice grains mixed with vermilion called *moti*. The divination of Peer, on the other hand is performed with the help of iron chains.

During divination, the gender of the *mali* while addressing people changes to that of the superhuman. Thus, the male superhuman address their clients as male gender while the female superhuman address them as female, even if the sex of the *mali* is male.

Every *mali* uses two languages during the trance state. One is the original language of the superhuman while the other is the language for addressing the clients. In the state of intense possession or while conversing with other diviners the *mali* generally use their own divine language, which is strange, unfamiliar and gibberish language. However, *mali* were seen conversing in their respective language with ease. The divine language, so spoken is unfathomable to a layman. The language spoken by higher devta Mahasu and Silgur is identified as Kashmiri—the place from where they are believed to have arrived. The language of Kali is called Kalcuttiya (from Kolkata)—a place linked to the origin of Kali. Finally, the divine language spoken by Devi goddess is called Kila-Kangra, the abode of Devi currently located in the state of Himachal Pradesh. The higher superhuman answer the question posed by the clients in local language while Kali, Peer and Devi *mali* would use Hindi language in interacting with clients.

The posture of the diviner while in trance state would also differ. All except Kali and Beer *mali* would sit straight under the spell of their guarding spirits. The *mali* of Kali would bow down extremely such that his face touches the ground. It is believed that the Kali, a very ferocious deity has a broken waist which has been so done deliberately by the Mahasu, for she otherwise could destroy the entire humanity.

The typical manifestation of Kali's arrival into the 'body' of the medium is utterance of *Salam* (a Muslim way of greeting) to other *mali* and the people in general. The indication of Mahasu's possession on the other hand is the whistle which the *mali* produces while entering into possession.

**Table:** Characteristic feature of Jaunsari diviners

| *S No.* | *Characteristic Features* | *Mahasu* | *Kali* | *Peer* |
|---|---|---|---|---|
| 1. | Divines with | Rice | Rice and vermilion | Iron chain |
| 2. | Indication of possession | Whistles | Salam | Weeps |
| 3. | Devine language | Kashmiri | Kalcuttiya | Hindi |
| 4. | Language for address | Local | Hindi | Hindi |
| 5. | Style of speech | Slow | Fast | Fast |
| 6. | Position during trance | Sits straight | Bows down | Bows down |

*Recruitment*: *Malihood* is an achieved status and it is believed that some kind of a divine selection operates in the making of a *mali*. But, a person does not become *mali* automatically. The whole process of becoming a *mali* is very tedious and often painful. It takes months and at times year to become habituated to the possession or tame the possession.

A legitimate *mali* is one who has the insignia (*chinh*) of the guarding superhuman. The person who has not yet attained the full-fledged *malihood* is called a *noitor* (the apprentice *mali*). *Malihood* is therefore a transformation of a *noitor* into *boidori* or *bochwan*—the legitimate *mali*. A *noitor* is one whose 'tongue has not yet opened' (*bhak khulna*) which implies that such a person has no control over the possession and also can not effectively communicate in the divine language. The *boidori* on the other hand can make a controlled divination at his/her will and also communicate effectively with the people.

Despite differences in the pattern of symptoms, all *mali* pass through a state of *bawal*—an state of mental uneasiness and instability. This *bawal* state needs to be differentiated from the state of madness which is termed as *jhal*. The *bawal* is believed to be a kind of enlightenment or a condition of special favour by the guardian spirits.

A very common symptom of *bawal* is getting of uncontrolled possession which is a kind of altered state of consciousness. The person under the state of *bawal*, does not stay normal and sometimes has no control over his/her actions. He would be seen crying, weeping, shivering or speaking aimlessly to himself. Another important and commonly experienced symptom is of having uncontrolled movements. A *noitor* would wander aimlessly in the jungles and solitary places.

There are bodily problems too, like a person may feel very weak, have joint ache and show lack of appetite. A large number of *mali* have avoided food for many days during *bawal* state. The clustering of bodily symptoms varied from *mali* to *mali*. In general, it was noticed that higher the status of guardian spirit, the greater will be the pain and rigour of *bawal* symptoms. Many lower order superhuman *mali* reported that their *noitor* period was relatively less painful. The symptoms experienced by these *mali* can well be explained in the framework of psycho-pathology and possibly as reflections of culture-bound reactive syndromes. But, in the present analysis, the emphases is on culture-specific explanatory model, exploration of the experience in an 'emic' frame of reference.

The Jaunsari believe that there is difference between the superhuman forms and the human forms. The superhuman are higher requiring propitiation and oblation from the human beings. The superhuman, being higher forms, thus do not tolerate 'impurity' such as leather touch, stale food and non-righteous actions. When such forms try to make their abode in the body of ordinary human being, they expect such person to behave with 'purity'. The human being, in our case the *noitor*, do not live always up to the expectations of the superhuman entities and thus commit inadvertent mistakes defiling the superhuman in the process. The *noitor* syndrome is explained as the manifestation of a superhuman anger falling on *noitor* when he/she defiles his respective guardian spirit. But once the *noitor* starts following purity norms, the adverse symptoms start ceasing. In the meantime, the *noitor* has to constantly keep 'promises' and pay fine for the mistakes committed by him/her.

A higher superhuman *mali*, who passed through a very difficult *noitor* phase narrated:

It was the month of *Poosh* (December-January) that I had first got the experience. I was working in the paddy fields near the stream side that I suddently felt intense pain in my right arm. I also started having fever and shivering in cold. I could not do anything there and was therefore advised by the family members to slowly climb up the mountain to reach the village. They further instructed that if it becomes difficult for me to climb, then I should stop and rest. The family members promised to carry me to the village in such instance. I was also feeling very weak and tired. With the help of a stick, I started slowly moving towards the village. I had barely climbed a furlong that I was seized with the attack of *bawal*. Suddenly I started behaving like the Bheema of Mahabharta. It was all puzzlesome for I was conscious of what I was doing, but had no control over my actions. I would raise the stick like the mace of Bheema and play music with my mouth. Afterwards, I almost lost my senses and later found myself in the village. I must have run very fast under the spell of *bawal*. Then on wards, it became a recurrent phenomenon with me. I would quite often get the uncontrolled possessions and would speak to myself and walk aimlessly.

A lower caste male was in the process of becoming a Kali *mali* and was *noitor* for the last two year. This was second time that he was passing through the *bawal* phase.

I was a Peer *mali* earlier and once in the village festival I suddenly jumped in the holy fire wherein I tried to insert my head. I withdrew and came back to my senses a little later but felt severe pain in my shoulders. My fingers were stretched and tilted. It was a strange sensation, as if someone has thrust a spear in my whole body. Initially I thought that I have been possessed by some evil force and therefore I approached a healer for the 'blow and brush' healing so that the evil is driven out. The symptoms of *bawal* then started re-appearing. Finally, a higher devta *mali* divined my symptoms to be the 'the light of Kali' in my body. I then visited the Kali shrine on the first Sunday of the month and was confirmed a *noitor*. The *mali* of Kali then instructed me my new responsibilities as a *noitor*. He gave me instructions so that I do not offend (defile) Kali by my action and get the 'clear tongue'. On many occasions, Kali has examined my temperament. I should be a cool headed person under any adverse situation. Sometimes I would find that a bee is humming near my ear. I would not be irritated but fold hands in the honour of Kali. Once I saw a cobra who had suddenly appeared from no where. I immediately folded hands and it vanished.

This noitor was passing through a very hard time. He had meagre amount of landholding but was unable to cultivate as he could not plough being in a nuclear family. He has therefore started mining for stone plates used over the roofs. His major problem has been to somehow control the possession. He had been often seen talking to himself in a strange language. However, once he has mastered to 'tame' the possession, he would become a Kali *mali* with a designated shrine.

The non-normal behavioural manifestations are 'tamed' in the process of becoming a *mali*. Thus, becoming a *mali* from the phase of *noitor* in itself is a process of healing. In a clinical context, the process is treatment of psychiatric symptoms in the cultural medium.

*Divination*: Divination *per se* is a highly stylistic drama. A very common way of going into trance is to call for the guardian superhuman force to come and reside (*vas*) in the body (*pind*) of the medium. Another form of divination is through beating of drums and singing collectively. Kali divination is accomplished by means of playing of ransinga wind instrument and drum while Peer divination accompanies group singing in praise of the Peer. The higher superhuman *mali* are also skilled at inducing a lower order *mali* by means of throwing few sacred rice grains at them.

Divination in general cases is not attained spontaneously. It always proceeds a set of actions directed towards self-purification. The place of divination has to be clean. The *mali* should have had a bath. Prior to the divination, he should have physically purified himself by washing his hands, feet and head. At times, cow's urine is rubbed, sprinkled and even drunk for self-purification.

Divination is a session of question and answers. The client comes to a *mali* for getting answers to his questions concerning *dos*. The request put forward to the *mali* is called *oraj* (derived from the word *arji* meaning supplication). The entire action is termed as *oraj lana* (putting the request). A session of *oraj* is called *chhant* meaning 'choosing'. Thus the job of a *mali* is to choose or separate out the exact *dos* which is believed to be behind the miseries of the client. At a particular period of time, a client may simultaneously be influenced by a number of *dos*—some hidden while other revealed. A *chhant* is therefore an attempt in locating the most immediate and contributory factor or force causing the trouble.

Barring exceptions like Kali, a divination is always preceded by verbal discourse praising the superhuman being under invocation. Generally speaking, in any kind of divination, names of four Mahasu is a must for they are the principal superhuman ruling the four-cornered Jaunsar region.

Divination is basically of three kinds. First, there is the dialogue based divination where a client asks questions one after another and the *mali* explains the causation or the course of events to him. This is the most commonly practiced style of divination. This style of divination is termed as *chhant-lana*. Second, there is mechanical divination called *purji-lana*. The literal meaning of *purji-lana* would be 'keeping the rice'. It is performed during divinations, generally in between the course of a *chhant*. It is specifically useful when there appears to be some confusion in the minds of the clients with regard to the exact causation or the most appropriate procedure to appease the angry superhuman force. In such situations, the *mali* asks the client to keep rice grains at two places and remember the cause these stand for. The *mali* then turns his face away, so as not to see what the rice grains stored at two places stand for. After a while, *mali* disperses the rice grains kept at one place and this is taken to mean the actual cause.

Mechanical divination is in various other forms is also practiced by the *mali* during *chhant*. Many *mali* throw rice grains in air and catch them. They then count the number of rice grains in their palm to ascertain the cause of trouble. The third form of divination is of inducing the client into trance by means of throwing rice grains at him. This is done if the client is a *noitor* or a *mali* himself. In this kind of divination the client himself speaks about his *dos*.

A typical session of *chhant* is reproduced below which involved the *mali* of Mahasu higher superhuman and a client:

*Client*: Come and possess for the 'life-soul'. Speak Oh Lord! Do not put us on a wrong path, just like that. Tell only what is actually the *dos*.

*Mali*: All right, Keep a word for the Mahasu.

*Client*: I kept a word for you.

*Mali*: Let me see the 'justice and decide'.

*Client*: Yes, you see the justice and make a decision.

*Mali*: Whatever I will decide will be based on justice.

*Client*: I have left justice to you. You make it. You will be coming to my village next year and I will serve you well.

*Mali*: Remember the words that you had kept for me.

*Client*: I remember that. Oh Devta!

*Mali*: Right now you keep your promise. In the justice which I make now, I do not see any loss or decrement. The justice that you have left to me.

*Client*: Your fame. Oh Lord!

*Mali*: You see my justice. You will feel it after six months or a year. I am not respected in the entire area just like that.

*Client*: Lord! You have come to this place. Then only I have asked (so that) my heart be in peace.

*Mali*: Take my *purji* (sacred rice). When you have left the justice to me and kept a promise then I will see it myself.

*Client*: Please do that.

*Mali*: For your protection, I am your companion.

*Clinet*: Yes Devta! I need a protector. I do not have anyone else than you.

In divination, a person comes with a problem or a set of problems. He has an idea about the kind of *dos* he might have or which have been there in his family. The sum total of perpetuating past information which a person will always has is called *saunkh*. This *saunkh* becomes very important as nothing is hidden to the superhuman who is omniscient. Thus, for any divination, as a rule, the most experienced and knowledgeable person of the family is sent to a *mali*.

*Mali's chhant* is a meaningful conversation, *Mali* generally starts with naming the *dos* which leads to further elaboration of how and why of it. In the course of *chhant*, the client raises his doubts and suspicions. He may say that the *dos* was properly propitiated but continuing. *Mali* would tell about the mistakes committed during propitiation and so on. On the whole, in a large najority of the *chhants*, it so happens that the client supplies *mali* with information and *mali* builds up the course and nature of *dos*. Thus, people prefer to get the divination from a distant *mali*, one who has not first hand knowledge of the life of his client.

*Mali as a Healer*: *Mali* is primarily a diagnostician and not a healer. It is only on very special occasions that he performs certain healing tasks. At first, a very common form of healing action performed by the *mali* consists of giving *jindav* (sacred rice grains). The *jindav*, in function, act as prophylactic which is commonly turned into a charm by the people. Some people prefer to swallow the *jindav*. In this instance, the *jindav* believe to function as medicines.

Another commonly prevalent form of healing action performed by a *mali* is of brushing away the dangerous ghosts and demons causing 'fright' in a person. Although any *mali* has the capacity to perform the brushing task, but the lower order superhuman *mali* are believed to be particularly effective in doing this type of healing. Thus, a Peer *mali*, during divination may hit the person afflicted with the demon's 'fright' with the help of the iron chains.

Finally, the most important healing task which a *mali* performs is related to the *ottro* (possession) behaviour. A large majority of possession behaviour is manifested by the *noitor*. The weird experiences and bewildering phenomenon encountered by *a noitor* are properly explained in divinations. Even if the possession is not related to the divine light but due to intrusion of evil spirit, a *mali* is considered to be the most appropriate healer to approach.

## Jariyara

*Jariyara* is derived from the Jaunsari word *jori*—a term used for medicines in general. Thus all medicinal plants are termed as *jori*. Even the medicines supplied by a doctor is called *jori*. Therefore, *jariyara* is a person who has knowledge about the use and dispensation of medicines. In this sense, even a doctor will also be a *jariyara*, but since his role and the therapeutic style drastically differs from the traditional healers, he has been grouped into a separate category. Thus, people consciously differentiate between doctor's *jori* and household *jori*. *Jariyara*, though similar to doctor, differs greatly from the other traditional healers like *mali* and *baman*. A *jariyara* deals primarily in the domain of 'human'. His explanatory model includes humoral disturbances causing *bimari*.

The skills and expertise of a *jariyara* is specifically evaluated in his manners of perceiving of pulse. The belief that every *bimari* is caused due to disturbances in the humor reflected in the pulse of a person—its size and movement—is very strong in Jaunsar. A knowledgeable *jariyara* is expected to know, by merely touching the pulse, regarding what kind of diet or weather conditions have caused a *bimari*.

Besides having expertise in the feeling of pulse, *jariyara* are also familiar with some medicinal herbs, learnt from other *jariyara* under an oath of secrecy. The mechanical manipulations like massage and bodily excercises are also associated with the skill of a *jariyara*. Finally, it is also required of the *jariyara* that they should have a sound knowledge of the humoral properties of the food items. Any remedy for a *bimari*, always as a rule, is associated with a particular diet which is prescribed. There are certain food items which are forbidden (*perhej*) in the course of a *bimari*.

The skills of *jariyara* are not equally distributed. Among themselves, they are differentiated not only along the line of expertise but also for the kinds of *bimari* they can successfully control. A very widely prevalent form of *jariyara* is the *sonu* healer. *Sonu* are the intestinal worms, which the Jaunsari believe as beneficial for the digestion of the food. Every human being, in Jaunsari conceptualization, is believed to be born with his stocks of *sonu*. The *sonu* reside inside the intestine in harmony. But, the *sonu* themselves are highly sensitive to humoral disturbances. Infants in particular get the disturbance of *sonu* since they keep tasting new things. Thus, infant diarrhea is mostly attributed to *sonu* disturbance. The *sonu* healers are called the 'calmer of sonu' and they constitute the dominant category of *jariyara* in Jaunsar.

*Recruitment*: Like other traditional healers, the role of a *jariyara* is also not a full time role. People practicing this art do it in their spare time and never charge for their services. Taking payment for the services is considered a sin. It is also believed that receiving payments in exchange of services may adversely affect the efficacy of the herb.

The knowledge of herbs is a closely guarded secret and it is not revealed to others. A person may not even tell about it to his own family members. Under special circumstances, somebody may learn about the herbs by seeing a *jariyara* at work. But, such cases are very rare. In a large majority of cases, a father transfers the knowledge about herbs and other associated skills to his son. The however occurs only when a father is impaired enough to serve the people.

Herbal medicines are thus perpetuated in a family for generations together. Another characteristic feature of herbs is that these are always associated with a sacred value. A herb is not equivalent to the pills of a doctor. There are always certain ritual procedures which must accompany a herb. In many instances, there are incantations which are whispered when a herb is applied. For instance, some herbs require incensed smoke before application. In other cases, use of sacred number accompanies the application of herb. For instance, the herb is applied for seven times in a sitting.

The transferring of the knowledge of a herb to an apprentice is a very sacred act. The day of such knowledge transference is calculated by a *baman* who gives auspicious day a time for such action. Both the teacher and pupil accomplish this task in the early hours of the morning. Before imparting this knowledge, both of them would not ear or drink anything.

A number of factors like altitude, colour and most importantly the smell of the plant is used for identification of a potent herb. The herbs are never collected in advance but a healer generally has a fairly good ideas of its availability in the surroundings. For maintaining the secrecy, he always administers the herb in its finished form. He may give small piece, the root or a crushed stem or in the form of paste or juice.

*Diagnosis*: The diagnosis of a *bimari* is generally made with the help of the pulse. It is highly variable as to how many pulse are there in the body. However, it is generally held that there is one life-pulse which pulsates as long as a person is alive. The knowledge about the rest of the pulse varies from *jariyara* to *jariyara*. Some *jariyara* say that they perceive *bimari* through feeling the movement and size of one pulse only, whereas others, claim to know of two such pulse, for hot and cold, respectively. One *jariyara* even went to the extent of claiming that all major *bimari* are reflected through special pulse.

Despite great controversy in the knowledge of pulse, the physical condition of the patient plays a very significant role in identification of the humoral quality of the *bimari*. High body temperature is identified as due to 'hot' but when it accompanies shivering if is considered a reflection of 'cold' humour. Similarly, body swellings are considered as conditions caused due to excess of 'air' humour.

A *jariyara*, in the first place, is required to make an independent diagnosis by feeling of the pulse. In fact, the clients withheld any information that they have about the symptoms in order to give *jariyara* a chance to arrive at independent judgement. The true condition for the pulse to give exact information is believed to be when the patient has not had any food or drink, has taken proper rest and finally, has also not taken any medicine or injection. Once a *jariyara* makes the remark that the *bimari* is due to 'cold', 'hot' or other factors, he is immediately supplied with the related information by the patient. He is then informed about the history of dietary intake and the development of symptoms. As a skilled person, a *jariyara* is required to explain the actual course and development of the illness. Finally, he would prescribe a diet for the patient and list the forbidden foods.

**Female Specialists**

Female specialists are traditional skilled healers who intervene in abnormal cases of delivery. They are in addition to the birth attendants, a task which is performed by any experienced female of the household.

A very common abnormality treated by them is termed as *pet-tolle* meaning displacement of the womb. *Pet*, in general reference is the abdomen. Jaunsari do not have any special word for the womb. It is believed by them that both men and women have womb. The sack like womb of a man is rudimentary while it is larger in size among the women.

Female specialists are particularly skilled in doing massage. Although, their therapy is associated with specific diet and at times mixed with some herbal medicines, they primarily rely on massage therapy. The four fingers of the hand are very important in the skills of a female specialist; for it is only with the help of these that a female specialist can actually perceive the nature of internal dislocations of the womb.

Female specialist is a sex specific role, as the term also suggests. It is generally confined to the lower castes, especially the blacksmith caste. In terms of age, these females are mostly old or middle aged. Mode of learning the skills for this healer is highly personal and informal. Most female specialists have been initiated into this skill by their mothers but only after they had undergone the experience of child birth themselves.

Apart from helping in displaced womb, a female specialist knows all about the abdomen, especially if the cause for the pain is internal pull. The native theory explains infertility as caused due to dislocated abdomen. Thus, a women having dislocated abdomen will not be able to conceive properly.

Navel dislocation is another sphere of the female specialist. The abdominal cramps are believed to be caused due to stretch in the abdomen and the female specialist have the ability to skilfully treat this condition by their massage. The role of female specialist in general is a non-profit task. They themselves do not charge anything. But, because they generally belong to lower, dependent caste groups, they are offered grains for their services, specially if their intervention has resulted in a successful delivery.

The actual practice of a female specialist is very stylish. She has a working knowledge of the pulse through which she diagnoses the positioning of the humoral imbalance in the body. The massage involves treatment by stroking, pressing, tapping and kneading of the affected part. The message is accomplished with the medium of butter, oil and at times with hearth ash depending upon the humoral conditioning in the body. Ceremonial thanks giving is always performed after the healing session under which the healer and patient fold and touch hands together.

**Doctor**

The doctor is an exogenous term given to the healers who make use of non-traditional ways and means for the therapy. More specifically, the doctors are identified as people making use of thermometer, stethoscope, etc. in their diagnosis and giving tablets (*botti*), injections (*sua*), capsules and syrups as medicines. A large majority of doctors are outsiders and trained in the Ayurvedic systems of medicines. However, in their practice, they generally tend to favour giving Allopathic medicines. In the entire area at the time of my study, there were only three doctors trained in Allopathic systems of medicine—two in the Primary Health Centre (PHC) and one having a private clinic. In the public sector, most of the positions of doctors were lying unoccupied and therefore in sub-centres the lower functionaries such as pharmacists, ward boys and at times even sweepers were substituting as doctors.

A very important feature of the Jaunsari patients is that they genrally preferred visiting private clinics despite easy access to the well-equipped PHC in the town of Chakrata. The main reason for this behaviour was that the PHC did not had sufficient medicines. Patients had experienced it many times that they would be seen by a PHC doctor but would be referred outside for medicines. Another factor contributing to this fact was the unfriendly behaviour of the PHC doctors. The PHC doctors, when interviewed stated that the area was very backward and the people were highly superstitious arriving at PHC only after exhausting all traditional options.

There remained a big gulf between patient's expectations and PHC doctor's dispensation in Jaunsari clinical encounters. Consequently, many patients told me that despite taking medicines they were never sure whether they had taken the right medicines or not. A doctor, especially in the PHC, would never give an instruction in terms of 'hot-cold' domain for he thinks it to be very silly and un-scientific. As a result, the encounters of doctors with patient in PHC were generally confusing for both fail to understand each other properly.

An instance, in which I had accompanied a child and his mother to the PHC, is described below. This child was initially taken to a private doctor who wanted to get an opinion from the child specialist of the PHC on the condition of the child. Thinking both of us to be from the village, the doctor showed his anger after seeing the child. He told the mother that she had been very careless and had not looked child her child well. He further informed her that her child was underweight for his age. The mother tried to narrate the symptoms, but she was stopped in between and told that her child would have died in a few days. This was immediately followed by his instructions to the mother that she should give her child, high protein diet such as meat, egg, milk, pulses and green vegetables. Thinking me to be a villager, he told me whether I understand how the high protein diet was essential for the child. He was very rude and angry in his overall behaviour. However, later when I introduced myself as researcher, he apologized and said, "I am sorry, I thought you to be a *mama* (a term he used for the natives)".

The overall behaviour of doctors, especially those who are not familiar with the local ways is markedly different from the traditional and normative conduct of a healer. A healer is required to be very calm and patient in his diagnosis. Along with it, he is also required to be skilled in making diagnosis without asking any questions. Both these factors are lacking in the PHC doctors and for this reason they are not praised much by the Jaunsari.

The private doctors on the contrary, have tuned themselves to the requirements of the people and as a result lots of people visit them for consultations. Almost all the private doctors have spared a room for the impatients. Two of them even provide facilities for the delivery. All, except one are the natives and are well versed in the native dialect. The all make it a point to feel the pulse before making any diagnosis and discuss the problem in a very cordial and personal way. As is the norm, they always pay great emphasis on the diet. Finally, they are also sympathetic to the local healer and often give advise to their patients to consult other healers like *mali* or *baman*.

## Specialist Healers

Specialists are those healers who by virtue of their therapeutic skills and curative powers have mastered a particular healing task. They are also known throughout the area and see a number of cases everyday. Such healers differ from ordinary ones for they charge a much larger amount form their clients. In all forms of therapeutic mode, we may find such specialists. The best analogy for understanding specialists would be to draw a comparison between a general practitioner and an MD. Thus, specialists do retain some elements of the general healers but specialize and master over a part of it.

The practice of specialists demands them to be more stylish than an ordinary healer. The ability to induce instant relief aids in the process of building their reputation. The people who are successfully treated by them become their spokesmen which encourage others to visit them for their complex problems. Such specialists are very few and differ greatly in their explanatory model and the therapeutic style from each other.

*Bis specialist baman*: *Bis* is a very popular and lethal cause for a number of symptoms, the primary symptom being blood vomiting by the patient. *Bis* which literally means 'poison', however is a state of illness, and not being poisoned in the actual sense. It is a strong belief, prevailing in this region, that some women have the evil power to offer food items containing their 'poisonous wish'. The *bis* specialist was originally a *baman* healer but was considered very effective for the treatment of *bis* cases. A number of people, some even outsiders, have vouched that they have been cured of their *bis* when even the best of the doctors have lost hopes in their case.

The *bis* specialist was a middle aged man, very talkative but quite simple. He treated *bis* cases with the help of a charm and ritual. For ordinary case, according to him, the charm would be sufficient but a ritual will become imperative if the case was serious. Why and how he was so effective was not even known to him. He said that the charm was a family secret of their own which was somehow efficacious. "It is all due to thoughts in ones mind. One feels that there is *bis* and get cured after wearing a charm prepared by me", he said. He however would not reveal beyond. "It is a secret of my family and I will not tell about it even to my very close relatives", he remarked. "If I do so, the affectivity of the charm will be lost", he added. But the people in general think differently. They do not deny the immense power that the charms prepared by the specialist contain, but they associate it to the fact that the specialist has acquired control over some evil supernatural agency. However, they were least concerned about how the healing powers were achieved, they came running to him always as a last hope. Apart from treating *bis* cases, the specialist was also performing the role of a *ganechhiya baman* in the manner of a typical low-cost healer to his traditional clientele.

*Bis specialist enchanter*: This specialist was a Rajput landowner by caste. He had recently earned a great reputation as a *bis* healer. His therapeutic mode was very different for he used to give enchanted water as a cure. The healer was nearly 76 years old, healing *bis* patients for the last seven years. "My father had the knowledge of *bis* mantra. He wanted me to learn it but I refused, thinking it to be nonsense", said the healer. He further added, "I was not a believer in *bis* myself. I used to think it to be a superstition. But once I suffered a severe asthmatic attack and developed acute shortage of breath. I went to many famous doctors for treatment but none could help me. Somehow, my body started repelling to the doctor's treatment. If a doctor would give me injection, I will get asthmatic attack at that moment itself. I also consulted many *baman* and *mali*, but, no body was able to help me. As a last resort, I thought of trying the mantra of my father. I searched for it in the house and very reluctantly used it. To my great surprise, I got instant relief. I then tried it on others and they too got good results".

The specialist was initially treating the *bis* cases in his house. But, when patients started coming to him in large numbers, he rented a room in a nearby town. We must note here that such a thing is very uncommon with the native healers. The specialist opined that not only the local people but even the outsiders have also benefited by his treatment. A doctor in the town started vomiting blood which he tried to treat with drugs but could not get any relief. But, when he tried the enchanted water given by him, he made remarkable recovery. In another instance, a shopkeeper of the town fell severely ill. The specialist was called as the last alternative. On learning this, said the specialist, "I became very angry and scolded them for not going to a doctor or a good clinic. I half-heartedly gave the patient the enchanted water and to my great surprise found that the patient improved with the water".

The specialist, like the earlier one, has no clue to the fact of why his treatment is effective. The main ingredients used in the preparation of enchanted water are:

1. Barley seeds,
2. Rhinoceros's horn.

The barley seeds are specially sown by him in the rainy month of *Bhado* (July-August) on a new moon night. The seeds of such barley are then mixed with some ordinary barley seeds for the purpose of preparing enchanted water. The horn of rhinoceros has been procured by him from Hardwar. Any patient coming to the healer is first diagnosed by the healer. For this some barley seeds are put in a glass of water. If the seeds stay at one place in the glass, it implies that the person has actually been afflicted by *bis*. But if the seeds are dispersed, then it means that either the person is not suffering from *bis* or the treatment given by him will be ineffective.

The healer takes a white paper over which a magical figure (*yantra*) has already been drawn by him. This paper is folded and wrapped along with some barley seeds and chip of rhinoceros horn. Then after, it is tied with black thread to be used as a charm.

The healer also performs 'brush' action on his patients. The 'brush' is made with the help of a small knife. The charm is held in the right hand fist and he whispers mantra into it. Simultaneously, the knife is tipped in a glass containing water and taken near the body of the patient in a brushing manner. The healer undertakes three kinds of brushing on his patients, namely, right side, left side and 'soul' side. While doing the 'brush', the healer sprinkles some water on all directions over the patient. This enchanted water is given to the patient to drink. The charm so prepared is wrapped in a red colour cloth to be worn by the patient in the neck. Special efforts are made to wear the amulet so that people could clearly see it.

The charm and amulet are to be greatly protected against defilement. The main source for their defilement are the menstruating women. Thus, a patient wearing *bis* charm should take special care in not taking any food or drink from the hands of a menstruating woman. If the patient is a female then she should keep the charm aside while under menses.

The clients of the healer generally come from distant places, specially Uttarkashi and Himachal Pradesh. The healer stated that he never charges money from the patients but it has become conventional to pay him six rupees and twenty-five paisa for the charm. The patients coming to him generally has the physical symptoms such as abdomen pain, swelling, vomiting, etc. All his patients come to him after they had gone to doctors and other healers and have not received any relief.

*The Pokhu mali*: The Pokhu priest, who is also Pokhu *mali* was the most expensive healer of this area. Pokhu is a very ferocious devta of this region. 'Sticking' of Pokhu means quick and total destruction. Not only the family for which the 'curse' of Pokhu is 'put' by some oppressed soul, but also those who are in close kinship ties can get the nefarious effects of Pokhu. Therefore, 'sticking' of Pokhu to someone also means a great social loss, for people break away their relationship from such a person.

The Madaikey family was one such unfortunate victim of Pokhu. It was one of the most prosperous family of the village. But, the 'curse' of one of their female ancestor mediated through Pokhu started showing its mal effects over the family. One after other the able-bodied members of the family started dying. The *dos* was found to be of Pokhu and therefore the family had to invite the Pokhu *mali* for removing this *dos*. The *mali* stayed in their house for one day and two nights. He consumed one he-goat and 25 bottles of home brew during his stay. The other expenses that the family had made included:

1. One he-goat.
2. One ram.
3. One blanket.
4. One cushion made up of goat's hair.
5. One metal pot.
6. Two metal plates.
7. Rupees 1500.

*The specialist jariyara*: This *jariyara* was in Himachal Pradesh. He was nearly 70 years of age. His specialization, according to the people, was in feeling pulse. It was believed in the area that there was no one compared to him in feeling of pulse. He had given his skills a dramatic turn. He claimed that he can diagnose the *bimari* of a person even if he feels the pulse of the sibling provided they are of the same mother.

When I visited his village, I was directed to a room above his house. This was his clinic. It bore the name S.S. Chauhan in English. The room was about four square metres in area. A very neat and clean room, it had a table, a bench and nearly 20 bound books on Ayurveda in a shelf. He had a very clean bed over which he was sitting cozily.

He informed me that from the very beginning he had an interest in feeling of pulse: Once, a *sanyasi* visited his village who had good knowledge of pulse. The *sanyasi* became his guru and he himself became a *sanyasi*. But, later on, on advise of his guru, he returned back to serve the people.

The *jariyara* told me that he relies on three principals in healing, namely, ask, feel and touch. However, he pays special emphasis to touch and feel. "I do not ask any question because the pulse can tell me everything about the *bimari*", he said with great confidence.

The *jariyara* then said that he would demonstrate his skill by feeling my pulse. He held my right hand and pressed three middle fingers at the wrist. He asked me to sit at ease in order to make a proper diagnosis. His first diagnosis was that I originally hail from the hills but had stayed for most of my life in the plains (he was right here). He explained that the difference in the pulse of hill folks and the people of the plains was the former have more of 'hot' while the latter have more of 'air' in them. He further opined that I get sudden involuntary jerks in the body and have irregular sleep. His final conclusion was that I have constipation in me.

## Conclusion

Prevalence of multiple therapeutic modes makes Jaunsar a medically pluralistic setting. Pluralism is apparent in the therapy style of *baman*, *mali*, *jariyara*, female specialist and the doctor. Different healers subscribe to distinct paraphernalia, etiology, diagnosis, preventive measure and treatment mode. The pluralism can also be seen within a particular therapeutic mode. The personality, experience and past success contribute greatly to the fact of why a particular healer is appreciated more than the other. The doctor's arrival in Jaunsar is not very recent but their number has certainly increased in the post-independence. Through state owned dispensaries and PHC, people are exposed to the new styles of therapy. On many occasions, for the same problem, the *baman*, *mali* and doctors are consulted side by side. One may quite reasonably expect that this will lead to a drastic reduction in the number of the traditional healers. But the facts available from the area do not support such a view. It was seen that despite doctor's easy availability, people continue to see a *jariyara*, *baman* and *mali*. The reason for this may be found in the people's perception of illness and the 'meaning' they assign to its etiology.

Presence of pluralistic traditions *vis-à-vis* alternative choice may led one to believe as if there is some kind of a competitive healer's network existing in the area. However, it has been the situation so far that there are exclusive classes of symptoms which are associated with a particular healer. Therefore, the myriad healers emerge only as complementary to one another rather than obstacles in each other's therapy. The traditional healers greatly admire the powers of the doctor's medicines and have been seen encouraging patients to visit them. They however firmly believe that a doctor can only be successful if it is a *bimari* caused by natural factors and is helpless if the cause is *dos*. Some of the doctors have been found complaining of the irrational healing ways which their patients have undergone before coming to them. However some sympathetic doctors have been found, at times, referring patients to *mali*, *baman* and even a *jariyara*. They even appreciated the success of such alternative therapies.

## REFERENCES

Ackerknecht, E.H. (1943): Psychopathology, primitive medicines and primitive culture, *Bulletin of the History of Medicines*. 14:30-67.

Boyer, L.B. (1964): Further remarks concerning shaman and shamanism, *Israel Ann. Psycho*. 2:235-257.

Fabrega, H. and D. Silver (1970): Some social and psychological properties of Zinacanteco shamans. *Behavioral Science*, 15:471-486.

Handelman, D. (1967): The development of Washo shaman, *Ethnology*, 6:444-464.

Joralemon, Donald (1985): Altar symbolism in Peruvian ritual healing, *Journal of Latin American Lore*. 11:3-29.

Joshi, P.C. (1988): Traditional Medical System in the Central Himalayas. *The Eastern Anthropoligist*. 41(1):77-86.

Joshi, P.C. (2000): Relevance and Utility of Traditional Medical System (TMS) in the context of a Himalayan Tribe. *Psychology and Developing Societies A Journal,* 12 (1):5-30.

Lebra, W.P. (1969): Shaman and client in Oxinawa, in *Mental Health Research in Asia and Pacific*. W. Caudill and T. Lin eds. Honolulu: East-West Centre Press.

Lewis, Gilbert (1971): *Ecstatic Religion: An Anthropological Study of Spirit Possession and Shamanism,* London: Penguin.

Metzger, D. and Williams (1963): Tenejapa medicines: The curer, *Southwest Journal of Anthropology*. 19:216-234.

Osgood, K. *et al.* (1966): Lay midwifery in southern Appalachia: The case of mountain country in Eastern Kentucky, *Arch. Environ, Health*. 12:759-770.

Parrot, D. (1970): Maenage remedies and conception of disease, *Ethnology*. 9:68-84.

Tenzen, J.H. (1970): Shamanism and concepts of disease in Mayan Indian community. *Psychiatry*. 33:372-380.
Turner, V.W. (1967): *The forest of symbols: Aspects of Ndembu ritual,* Ithaca, New York: Cornell University Press.
Turner, V.W. (1968): *The drums of affliction: A study of religious process among the Ndembu of Zambia,* Oxford: Clarendon Press.

# 15

# Healing Practices among the Tribes of Uttaranchal

A.P. SINGH

Folk medicine can be studied as medicine in a primarily spoken, not written, tradition. This study take two directions—one towards what non-western cultures know about disease and healing, the other towards popular medicine wherever it is found (Hunter, 1976). The most important fact about folk medicine is the way in which it is integrated into a whole or a pattern and it is in such pattern that folks medicine differs from tribe to tribe and community to community. Many objectively effective factors are found in folk medicine, which make it successful. They include baths, cauterization, surgery, from fracture treatment to trophining, inoculation against smallpox and snake bite, and an enormous pharmacopoeia including opium, quinine, and many other useful drugs; of course treatment is not done rationally but in an entirely magical sense accompanied by spells, incantations and even prayers, or by weird dances. Renowned anthropologists like River (1924) and Clements (1932) have made significant contributions in the field of concepts of disease and healing. Clements had tried to trace worldwide distribution of five basic concepts of disease, viz., sorcery, breach of taboo, object intrusion, spirit intrusion and soul loss. A number of other valuable studies include field study of the Ga people (1973) and Spencer's study of disease, religion and society in the Fiji Islands (1941). In the Indian Cultural setting, numerous studies on the etiology, diagnosis and therapy of disease have been carried out in different communities by various anthropologists like Gould (1957), Khare (1963), Hasan (1967), Madan (1969), Rizvi (1991), Bhat (1986) and Das (1986).

A recent appraisal of folk medicine show that this is not a queer collection of errors and superstitions, nor is to be explained by simply stating that in the medical field, primitives use spells, blood-letting, human fat and spittle. What counts is not the gain but the place medicine occupies in the life of primitive people.

For the present study villages and informants were selected on random basis. Interview, observation, case study, free listing and group discussion were employed for data collection.

Uttaranchal is the new state of India and consists of Kumaon and Garhwal regions apart from "Terai" belt. This state has thirteen districts and is inhabited by five Scheduled Tribes, viz. Jaunsari, Bhotia, Bhoksa, Tharu and Raji and the other rural and urban people.

## The Witch Doctors

There are special functionaries among these people who take care of their crimes and diseases normally attributed to malevolent spirits. As the witch doctor of the Tharus, the "Bharra" can trace out the cause of a disease, spell out name of the spirit responsible for it and suggest its cure. He can ward off epidemics by taking preventives spiritual measures. He protects the village from evil spirits by propitiating the deities and invoking "Bhawani" who is capable of keeping the malign spirits at bay. He can wield his magical powers to bring rain, to remove adverse influence of an evil eye and even to perform the magic of love. His main instrument to accomplish these deeds is the "mantra".

The "Sayana" or the wise one operates among the Bhoksa people. As medical facilities are still inadequate and the Bhoksas have periodic visitations of epidemics like cholera, chicken pox, the "Sayana" is still very much in demand. He prescribes charms, amulets and "mantras" to neutralize or destroy the evil influence and cure diseases.

The rest of the people gladly accept the spiritual hegemony of the "Brahman" who is emerging as their most influential religious caretaker.

## The Role of "Mantra" in Curing Disease

There are different "mantras" for different occasion. For example, the following "mantra" is recited by the "Bharra" to expel an evil spirit that has descended on a person:

Mother Earth Piety is thine
Chief of the devils thou seteth the rule
Thou art a demon
If thou leaveth
I will propitiate thee with cloves and flowers
And sing song in they praise

The "Bharra" adopts the following procedure to find solution to a problem or to identify the spirit. He places some grain, usually rice, on a brass plate reciting "mantras" suited to the occasion all the time till a solution is found. Alternatively, he swings a "*guria*" or doll consisting of a red coral and white glass beads strung in a twine. Only when the "*Guria*" swings clockwise, the spirit possessing a victim can be identified. Anticlock motion signified either absence of any spirit or ineffectiveness of the "mantra".

Similarly, the "Sayana" uses the following "Vachana" or "Mantra" to expect spirit and cure disease:

I begin in the name of Allah.
Who is great and merciful?
By accepting godhood of God,
By accepting kingdom of Mohammad
By accepting Fatima Bibi
By accepting Dul Dul, the Horse,
Let "mantras" prove effective,
For my master's word is true. (Hasan, 1971)

## The Disease Concepts and Herbal Remedies

Herbal treatment was practiced even in Biblical times. Moses taught the Israelites the use of herbs to heal the body and the mind. King Soloman's herb garden was famous and doubtless the Queen of Sheba borrowed from it. The plant hyssop is mentioned in the scriptures. Perhaps nowhere was herbal treatment so much used as in India and China. The Indian herbal remedies date back to the "Vedas". India had in "Ayurveda" a hoary tradition in medicine. India has also given the world *Rauwolfia serpentina*, the Himalayan herb, which brings down blood pressure. China was the first country to use opium, rhubarb and gingseng, the herbs with remarkable rejuvenating properties. "Ayurveda" and other medical systems like "Unani" make use of the whole plant from the leaves to the bark to process salves, lotions, ointments, powders and essences (Bans, 1979).

Herbal medicine is still regarded as an art and not as a science. Written records of plant prescriptions are hard to get and most herbal lore has come orally. Ethnological details of some of the herbs practiced by the primitive people of Uttaranchal Himalaya as based on the case study by the author are given below:

1. Mr. S.W. Ambilwada lives in Gharhwal—Srinagar (India) and runs a painting shop called Alaknanda Kala Kendra. He originally belongs to the southern part of India and migrated to Garhwal a few decades ago. Bearded saint, as he appears to be, he has a good knowledge of various regional herbs and their applications to different diseases.
   He told the author about the herbal medicines to be applied for the patients of piles. "Kalmi Sora" (Potassium Nitrate) and "Nisot" (legmues of *Impomaea turpethum*) when taken orally or applied locally in the morning and evening in little quantity in the ketchup form removes irritated and chronic piles.
   Another effective herb found in Garhwal for the piles is "Nagkesar" or "Sanhinjana" (*moringaoleifera*). This was taken along with "Misri" (a kind of sugar) and butter or "Ghee" orally for six months in the morning and six month in the evening in a little quantity almost stops the bleeding of the heaemorrhoids. To some extent, the oral application of black "Til" (*Sesomum indicum*) with butter, or of "Suran" made to pulp (*Euphorbia royleana*) with curd in the morning in a little quantity relieves the irritation of the piles.
2. In the higher altitudes of Uttaranchal Himalaya many herbs useful to various diseases and general health are found. These are put in one category called "Astavarga" comprising eight different herbs, namely, "Jeevak", "Rishivak", "Kokoli", "Chhirkakoli", "Meda", "Mahameda", "Ridhi" and "Vridhi". These herbs are of medicinal value to patients of asthama, bronchitis, fever, general health loss, etc.
3. Mr. D. P. Joshi lives in Garhwal—Kaliasaaus (India) and run a herbal dispensary. He told the author that "Arusa" or "Basinga" (*Adhatoda vasica*) and "Tulsi" (*Oscimum*

*sanctum*) leaves when taken orally with honey in a little quanity regularly in the morning and evening are effective in curing pulmonary tuberculosis.

4. Some of the medicinal plants of Garhwal Himalaya useful in various ways have been enumerated by Gaur (1977) as follows:
   (a) "Bel" (*Ageic mameolus*): The pulp of the fruit is used as an astringent in diarrhoa and dysentery.
   (b) "Kharik" (*Celtis ericarpa*): Fruits are used in enorrhoea and colic.
   (c) "Bairola" (*Cordia vestita*): The geletinous and ellipsoidal drupes are demulcent and astringent.
   (d) "Kapasi" or "Bhotia badam" (*Corylus colurna*): The nuts are used as tonic and as substitute of almonds.
   (e) "Ban ka Phal" (*Fregaria vesca*): Fruits are astringent and diuretic.

Seen thus, the Himalayan herbs have a great medicinal value. Das (1894) and Vaishya (1963) have given the details of various herbs found in India in their voluminous books.

The folk medicines are women into the social web of India's rural and tribal life and in the near future they are likely to be more effective. The need is to train the indigenous practitioners not in magic or quackery alone but in the scientific use of indigenous pharmacopoeia.

## REFERENCES

Bans, R. (1979): *The Illustrated Weekly of India* (The Times of India Press, Bombay.

Das, R.B. (1894): *Vaidyak Rasraj* (Mahodadhi Bhasa in Hindi, Sri Venkateshwar Press Prakashan, Bombay).

Gaur, R.D. (1977): *The Himalays* Vol.

Hasan, A. (1971): *A Bunch of Wild flowers and other Articles* (Ethnographic and Folk Culture, U. P., Lucknow).

Hunter, D.E. and P. Whiten (1976): *Encyclopedia of Anthropology* (Harper & Row Publisher New York).

Majumdar, D.N. (1973): *Races and Cultures of India* (Asia Publishing House, Bombay).

Vaishya, S. (1963): *Bhawprakash* in Hindi (Venkatesh Press, Kalyan Bombay)

# 16

# Psychosocial Well-being of the Elderly among the Nagas

D. CHAO, N.K. CHADHA and P.C. JOSHI

## Introduction

Growing older, in any living being with only few exceptions, is related with drawing nearer towards unwanted consequences. However, to a human being, unless he enters into the consequential stage he or she seldom bothers for himself or herself that she is on that way or hardly concern for those who are already in the well of those harsh realities. Unfortunately, these harsh realities are irreversible in nature, accompanying degenerative characteristics such as decline in health, reducing physical strength, minimizing in vitality, lowering economic conditions, and social status, weakening social supports and reduced social networks. These starch conditions automatically promote the feeling of isolation, alienation, loneliness, experiencing hopelessness, and letting to relative perception of a disintegrated social environment.

To many, 'old' is a strong, confusingly, unwanted and negatively projected image word. It is something that most of us would prefer not to be, although, there is a general assumption that 'old is wit'. Without much considering the better side of the ądvantage being old, including maturity of being aging, their understanding, and realistic thoughts, our perceptions are always driven by negative aspects of being as a disadvantaged old persons. The advantageous effects of the elderly presence in any society in the old age which act as monitoring instruments of unwritten law and orders were entirely neglected and unrecognized. For the reason and so as to build better social order, understanding the conditions and positions of the elderly is considered very much important for the betterment of our future life. But to identify who are the old person in any community is another big herculean task for any individual including a gerontologist because some one would probably readily accept when address them as elderly in spite of not being in their advanced age, whereas some others would respond otherwise. Therefore, the term aging is difficult to define as a globally accepted term. In many cases, for many purposes, aging remained an uneasy topic for discussion (Birren and Schroots, 1996).

However, the importance of understanding the aging process came with a greater impact by the turn of the 20th century, with the postulation of the term gerontology-systematic exploration of the aging process.

## Concept of Aging

Aging, though its importance of studying was conceived just a century before has been discussed from the ancient time as one of the most important problems in our lives. The concept of aging begins with the first breathe and the lusty cry at the time of birth, as if to born is to start the journey of death.

The term aging is mean to denote determinate patterns of late life changes. Changes eventually occur in all people though varying in rate of change (Singhal, 1990). Old age, thus, is characterized by the gradual change in appearances such as graying of hairs, loss of hair, and teeth, elongation of nose and ear, fat losses (particularly around the face), sagging skin, wrinkles, impairment of sensory functions such as vision, audition, smelling, tactility, feeling, etc., and progressive structural changes that may result in shortened trunk with comparatively long arms and legs, and sicknesses increasing fragility accompanied by grievance and emotional negativism. Cognitive processes such as attention, intelligence, memory, language and speeches, perception, learning, concept formation, thought processes, problem solving, spatial and time orientation, and motor and behavioural control markedly decline. These changes could be aggravated due to other age related crises like widowhood, marital problems, sexual problems, retirement, sensory loss, susceptibity to disease, pains, hardiness of joints, loosening of muscles, physical inactivity, immobility, etc. These problems further promote to aggravate stereotypic attitudes. The problems are further accompanied by social changes like role changes as a consequence of retirement, widowhood, divorce, etc., that call for the role loss and economic and psychological deprivation. Thus, old age is dependent on an intricate balance of physical, emotional, economical and social forces, anyone of which can upset or evolve into others.

There are three types of patterns of changes or identifiable clusters associated with aging. They are: (a) Primary aging: refers to the changes of the aging processes that are ultimately irreversible; (b) Secondary aging: refers to the changes of the aging process that are caused by illness correlated with age but may be reversible; (c) Tertiary aging: refers to the changes that recurred precipitously in old age.

## Types of Human Aging

Birren and Renner (1977), differentiated three aspects of human aging. These are: (a) Biological aging: It is an estimate of individual's present position with respect to his or her potential life span. A person with a young biological age has a long life expectancy with regards to the species potential life span. (b) Psychological aging: It refers to the adoptive capacities of the individuals in comparison with the average. (c) Social aging: It refers to the role and social habits of an individual with respect to the other members of the society.

## Problems of the Aging

Problems of the aged can be broadly classified into three headings:

1. *Economic Problems*: (a) Income deficiency and economic insecurity, and (b) Loss of jobs retirements.
2. *Physical and Psychological*: (a) Falling of health, (b) Nutritional deficiency, and (c) Housing problems.
3. *Psychological and Environmental (Social)*: (a) Loss of importance in the family, (b) Loneliness, (c) Feeling of unwanted, (d) Feeling of being inadequate, (e) Obsolesce of skills, educational, and experiences.

In spite of numerous problems, the aging population in continuously on the rise. This continuous rise of elderly population is attributed to low rate of mortality, achievement in biological and medical sciences, improvement in sanitation, public health and living conditions, elimination of infectious diseases by vaccination, new drugs, better nutrition and a general improvement standard living. The demographic picture of the world elderly population is depicted below:.

**Table 16.1:** World Demographic Picture of the Elderly

| | *Both Sexes* | | *Male* | | *Female* | |
|---|---|---|---|---|---|---|
| | *Total* | *%* | *Total* | *%* | *Total* | *%* |
| 1950 | 205034 | 8.12 | 91237 | 7.24 | 113795 | 8.99 |
| 1955 | 224468 | 8.13 | 100383 | 7.29 | 124085 | 8.97 |
| 1960 | 245542 | 8.11 | 109186 | 7.22 | 136357 | 9.00 |
| 1965 | 274083 | 8.19 | 121164 | 7.24 | 152919 | 9.15 |
| 1970 | 310483 | 8.38 | 136515 | 7.36 | 173968 | 9.41 |
| 1975 | 347836 | 8.52 | 152377 | 7.43 | 195459 | 9.61 |
| 1980 | 380670 | 8.55 | 166113 | 7.43 | 214557 | 9.69 |
| 1985 | 428037 | 8.83 | 187175 | 7.67 | 240682 | 10.00 |
| 1990 | 486864 | 9.21 | 215657 | 8.10 | 271207 | 10.34 |
| 1995 | 541823 | 9.52 | 242048 | 8.44 | 299775 | 10.62 |
| 2000 | 602773 | 9.89 | 270493 | 8.81 | 332280 | 10.99 |
| 2005 | 658686 | 10.14 | 296615 | 9.07 | 362071 | 11.23 |
| 2010 | 745105 | 10.81 | 337597 | 9.73 | 407508 | 11.91 |
| 2015 | 869772 | 11.93 | 396540 | 10.81 | 473232 | 13.07 |
| 2020 | 1007407 | 13.13 | 461182 | 11.95 | 546225 | 14.31 |
| 2025 | 1170273 | 14.55 | 537331 | 13.30 | 632942 | 15.81 |
| 2030 | 1345167 | 16.06 | 619422 | 14.74 | 725745 | 17.38 |
| 2035 | 1508059 | 17.39 | 695679 | 16.01 | 812380 | 18.78 |
| 2040 | 1640775 | 18.37 | 756727 | 16.92 | 894048 | 19.82 |
| 2045 | 1783009 | 19.46 | 823063 | 17.96 | 959946 | 20.96 |
| 2050 | 1938204 | 20.69 | 896633 | 19.15 | 1041571 | 22.22 |

*Source*: Sex and age distribution of the world population: The 1996 Population Division, Department of Economics and Social Affairs, *United Nations Secretariat*, New York, 1998.

From the table, it is clear that the elderly population in the world in 1950 was 205 millions, growing to 486.8 millions by the year in 1990, and 603 millions in 2000, and expected to reach 1.93 billions by the year 2050.

**Table 16.2:** Elderly population by sex and age in India (1961-2016)

| *Year* | *Total* | | *Males* | | *Females* | |
|---|---|---|---|---|---|---|
| | *Total* | *%* | *Total* | *%* | *Total* | *%* |
| 1961 | 25,566 | 5.82 | 13,224 | 5.83 | 12,342 | 5.80 |
| 1971 | 32,700 | 5.97 | 16,874 | 5.94 | 15,826 | 5.99 |
| 1981 | 43,167 | 6.49 | 22,023 | 6.41 | 21,144 | 6.58 |
| 1991 | 56,682 | 6.76 | 29,364 | 6.75 | 27,318 | 6.77 |
| 2001 | 70,571 | 6.97 | 36,208 | 6.91 | 34,363 | 7.03 |
| 2011 | 95,921 | 8.14 | 48,859 | 8.05 | 47,062 | 8.23 |
| 2016 | 112,962 | 8.94 | 57,362 | 8.84 | 55,600 | 9.05 |

*Note*:
1. Excludes figures for Assam in 1981 and Jammu and Kashmir in 1991 where the Census was not conducted due to disturbed conditions.
2. Figures for 2001 onwards are based on Report of the Technical Group on Population Projection, August 1996.

*Source*: Paper presented Dr. M. Vijaynunni, IAS, Registrar General and Census Commissioner of India, on *Greying Population: 1991 Census and its Impacts*, 1997, New Delhi.

India too portrayed similar pictures. In 1961 the elderly population in India was a mere 25.5 lakhs, and increased to 70.5 lakhs in 2001 and expected to reach 112.9 lakhs by the year 2016.

Even a small state like Nagaland shows tremendous effects of elderly population growth.

**Table 16.3:** Elderly population by sex and residence in Nagaland: 1991 Census

| *Age-Group* | *Nagaland* | | | *Rural* | | | *Urban* | | |
|---|---|---|---|---|---|---|---|---|---|
| | *Total* | *Male* | *Female* | *Total* | *Male* | *Female* | *Total* | *Male* | *Female* |
| 60-64 | 22775 | 13248 | 9527 | 21150 | 12196 | 8954 | 1625 | 1052 | 573 |
| 65-69 | 13562 | 7815 | 5747 | 12822 | 7339 | 5483 | 740 | 476 | 264 |
| 70-74 | 10644 | 6202 | 4442 | 10007 | 5814 | 4193 | 637 | 388 | 249 |
| 75-79 | 6043 | 3541 | 2502 | 5815 | 3394 | 2421 | 228 | 147 | 81 |
| 80 + | 10756 | 6610 | 4143 | 9790 | 5940 | 3850 | 963 | 670 | 293 |
| Total | 63777 | 37416 | 26361 | 59584 | 34683 | 24901 | 4193 | 2733 | 1702 |

*Source*: Census of India-1991: Totals finale by Dr. M. Vijaynunni, Registrar General of India, Government of India-1997.

From the above demographic pictures, it is clear that aged (60 years and above) segment in any society, any nation or otherwise all over the world represents an important subset of the aggregate population. Therefore, there is an urgent requirement to re-orient policies and research efforts towards the elderly people.

## Psycho-social Status of the Elderly

The patterns of change among the aged may not simultaneously occur to everyone at the same age or period or stage neither at the same rate. The changes are further accompanied by social changes like role change as the consequences of retirement, widowhood, divorce, etc., that call for the role loss and economic and psychological stereotypically described as dependent and querulous, frail, suffering from anxiety, grief, depression, descript group of individuals near death, paranoid, moody, bad tempered, impatient, falling behind time, slow to react and understand, withdrawn and inadept of financial management by its social members.

The process of aging-encompassing these factors, is highly individualized and there are social, cultural and individual variation in the patterns of aging. In every culture and society, to age is accepted as the period of decline of psychological, role, minority status, and desire for rejuvenation. These social reactions and responses to the aged promote them to decrease participation in any major life decision-making processes such as in administration and economic consideration. As a result, a significant decrease of social importance, social contacts and social networks occurs with aging. These social changes probably affect their psychological well-being.

The elderly behaviour itself manifests certain roles and stereotyped like stooped walking without any physiological basis. The possible outcome of these types of behaviour would be reducing the ability to resolve the psychological crises—the disintegration of ego or the lack of unification of the personality style, which required a numbers of factors, the relevance's of social roles, lifestyles, and physical health. Ego integration enables to unite personality characteristics which further promotes the feeling of well-being. The disintegrated egos among the elderly lead to fear of death, a feeling of unfulfilling desire and wishes, which automatically lead to unsuccessful aging.

As the elderly started losing the role in the society, they withdraw from the society as they recognize their diminishing capacities. This prompt them to disengage from the society. The social labelling of the aged persons as old had serious impact to affect the perceptions of the aged towards themselves as also the youth's attitude towards them.

This brought the elderly to the position of sub-culture group within the larger society (including every member of the society). As societies are becoming modernized, older people are becoming more and more marginalized, becoming less important and less useful in the society. High rate of residential mobility, establishment of household by younger generation away from home of the extended family household, and the rise of individualism that accompanies modernization, etc., tend to reduce the power and status of the elderly in the present society. The consequence of these happenings, led to depletion of resources socially, physically, and psychologically. Thus, the old people find themselves unable to maintain their relationships adequately and perceive themselves inferior, to others. Therefore, the elderly social-psychological well-being is of multifaceted nature affecting all the factors from a particular status.

In spite of these facts which are globally apparent, the meaning of age and its well-being varies dramatically across culture, from virtually irrelevant in some to being highly elaborated in others (Keith, 1990). The values attached to the aged and its quality also vary with culture and peoples. Review of historical and anthropological evidences indicate that in many societies, elderly retained status, authority, and active social environment. But these characteristics are mostly modified by economic stresses in the present capitalist oriented society.

For instance, the Indian traditional view of elderly life represented by the last stage of a man's life on earth called—*Sanyas*—the stage of total disengagement or total renunciation, the designated age group for this stage is mostly 70 years to 100 years. Regarding this, it is also viewed that traditional Indian concept of life recognises a withdrawal from the society as an approach towards old age.

## The Nagas

The people known as the Nagas, comprised of many tribes, are of Mongoloid stock. The areas the Nagas inhabited in large part of North East India, including the states of Nagaland, Manipur, Arunachal Pradesh, and Assam, and Western part of Myanmar. These lands lie roughly between the parallels of 93 and 96 degrees longitude. The areas extend from that of the noblest of all Indian rivers, the sacred Brahamaputra on the west to the Patkai range in the north to the Jhaungdut state in the south and from Assam frontier in the west to the Chindwin river in the east in Myanmar. There are different estimates given by the different people of the area in question, ranging from 20,000-30,000 sq. miles.

Of the various tribal groups people who make up the Nagas, the following names have been mentioned—Angami, Chakesang, Ao, Konyak, Khiamniumgam, Sema, Lotha, Rengma, Chang, Zelianrong, Phom, Damsa, Yinchunger, Sangtam, Poumai, Mao, Maram, Thəngal, Tangkhul, Maring, Kom, Chiru, Anal, Mayong, Mongsang, Lamkang, Nocte, Tangsa, Wancho, Singpho, Khamti, Hemi, Htangram, Rangpan, Para, Kalyo, Kengyu, Pochuri, etc.

Many scholars would probably subscribe Naga society as an animistic society in its early stage for its characterising very low in the scale of humanity (to the externality), and thence ascends deeply modified in its transmission, from first to the last preserving an unbroken continuity into the midst of high modern culture, and independent, with a unique characteristic of sharing-giving and taking without any documented law, but of a binding principle. The concept of sharing, according to the nature of Naga tradition, is stretching and requesting helping hands without much reservation when needs arise be it economical, emotional, mental, physical, social, and others. The equation of "Taking and Giving" does not relate to bartering of what fixed amount taken be back when necessary events arise, but of accommodative in nature.

In the familial institution and its functional hierarchical structure, the decision making, for any major decisions powers, were exercised by the eldest male in the family. The male members in the family usually performed the outdoor activities like in any other patriarchal society, while the female members are also not simply confining and performing the domestic and core activities, but equally shared in farming and food gathering processing. For instance, cutting down the fire-wood is male's duty but gathering is woman's duty. Interestingly, woman folks performed most of the domestic works. Division of labour existed for sexes for two dominant reasons, one, to work according to the available resources, and two for the convenient and the practicality. Though sounds discriminatory through the western activists' perspective, but it is purely for the complementary and supplementary to each other's roles and duties, without any form of underestimation and neglects. There were definite tasks and roles for each sex according to the Naga culture. Women's roles are much larger and greater in household management and the men's roles are mostly overt and external activities. Handicrafts are differentiated for both but differentiated in terms of different crafts, e.g., making basket for men and weaving and knitting are for women. Construction of houses is absolutely a men's duty. Certain activities and roles of women were condemned when done by men and vice-versa. Similarly, certain instruments for performing differentiated duties are strictly condemnable when touched by any gender other than their designated personal instruments. This native tradition, though biased in many areas according to the western traditions, led the entire social enterprises peacefully without any dissonance for years. But in the present days, the so-called western oriented politically established concept of equality without any concern for the fabrics responsible for peaceful co-existence, or in other words, without any practical concern—diverting professionalism from the traditionality, stressing to re-orient liberal and individualistic principles and disruptive to the peaceful fabric of the society. Gender segregation, though existed, was for the goodwill and for the practically convenience of the local and neighbourhood administration, and carried without much mental prejudices. When in term of giving opportunities for education to the children, male child was given preferences because of the outcome of limited resources available and the analysis of the cost effective to the family, we witness the change.

From decision making related to properties in the family to the entire responsibilities for the administration of the village and community is concentrated to the hands of the men folk. However, most in familial decisions are not arbitrarily taken by the men folk without the consultation of their women. In fact, many local administrative agendas were not shared with women. It has been carried down for generations and was not at all to undermine their selfhood. But it was purely for the village or neighbourhood security. Because in the olden times, as there was no police systems (means to refers instruments for safeguarding public and not for the extortionist and partial system of the present department), and the villages were under the mercies of the well planned and prepared and sporadic attacks and plunders by the powerful and stronger villages or groups. Women, therefore, in such situations were not disclosed all the information related to the local administrations, because as inter-marriages were existed, so as to play safe from spying (in order to save their kin) by the outside women. However, present social order does not have any avenues to maintain such standard. Instead women are too invited to share any administrative processes. In totality, men exercise more powers in external functioning.

Residentially, Nagas are mostly inhabitated in the hilly areas which manifests the rural characteristics. However, the urbanization led thousands to migrate to towns and cities leaving behind their aged parents and the lands and other properties. In spite of different residential locations (i.e., both in towns and the villages), the nuclear family always prevailed. In the family, elderly are normally and usually looked after by either the eldest or the youngest son. But the elderly have choice to whom they want to stay and live with feel comfortable. Among the rural Nagas, one of the advantages for the elderly was that all the paternal relatives or descendents concentrated in the particular location within the village or the community neighbourhood. The advantage is mostly for those who are disabled. However, the advantages are slowly losing its meaning because the urbanization processes strongly allured youngsters, whereby the youngsters with their bleak future in the rural area (villages), started concerning more for their future than their elderly parents or grandparents. Consequently, the elderly suffered from multiple problems. Unfortunately, the advantage of neighbourness of all the relatives is not available and enjoyed by the Nagas settled in the urban areas.

Economically, Nagas are mostly concentrating to farming. Farming for the Nagas was not for the commercial purpose but for their subsistence. People have limited knowledge of commercialization as the region itself is disabled for the process of commercialization due to its inconveniences in transports and other factors. Surplus of any product from their farming, except the paddy, is shared with the neighbours. Due to its non-commercial nature, income from all sources cannot be easily determined in numerical values. Educationally, most of the rural elderly Nagas were illiterate as the spread of education was galloping only in the recent decades. There were many reported incidences that Nagas in the early times ostensibly refused to study or to hold any governmental jobs offered by the government. They just wanted to remain contented with what they have had from their humble nature. Every Naga elderly usually has land to build house and cultivate. No matter how low the value of price and unyielding the properties are, almost everyone or household (if not given to their children because of their inability to utilize) and every Naga elderly owns non-commercial properties.

Employments among the Nagas elderly in any organized sector were comparatively insignificant. For these reasons, almost all the elderly person do not receive pensions. Very little section of the elderly persons enjoyed governmental old age pension in papers but hardly the meagre amount reaches the target persons. Usually the agents, middlemen, children or the government officers taking advantage over the illiterate elderly, completely hijacked the amount. The government does not bother to check such gross violation of misuse. There were very low rate of divorce and separation. There were also very few numbers of unmarried aged. However, when compared between male and female elderly, the female unmarried elderly were relatively more in numbers.

As far as the status of the aged is concerned, the Nagas elderly persons in the early days reportedly enjoyed much higher and respectable status. Mr. X, an eighty-six years old from a village called Zakhama, (a subject in the study) describe about the present scenario "while I was about teenage, (about is probably used because no birth record is available), I saw my father and his friends hardly displayed any disrespect to their elders. They won't freely cross the frontal passage of their elderly. There used to be no incidence of defiling the elderly commands. They were always there to serve their elderly in any festivals. Their class seemed to be different. Their manners, thus, taught me to follow their footsteps. To our times too, if anyone of our grandpas called us by name, we approached them with full respect without any delay or hesitation or excuse. We obeyed whatever they asked or commanded to do. We just enjoyed doing anything for them. On some occasions, we used to go to the elderly people to inquire if any help was required by them. After doing anything, the elderly persons blessed us "may my child happily live without any disease, top over all the friends, and be able to do anything what others could not do." This relationship inculcated the feeling that we should do anything for the elderly whatever the circumstances, if commanded by any elder. There were no rebellions, dissidents by any individuals or groups of youth in any decision making led by the elderly. The decisions of the elderly persons for the village and community administration were used to be final and binding. Any treaty or memorandum of understanding or any sort of discussions for the local administration were to be made by the elderly at their disposal and wisdom. During our free times, elderly persons used to teach us administrative mechanisms and techniques prevailing in the community through the generation and we also used to keenly listen and tried to learn whatever they taught us. But now the situations has changed drastically and such environments completely vanished. Now agreements are made arbitrarily by the so-called educated youths without the concerns and knowledge of the elderly. Youngsters now are the idle lots, without any respects, regards, and very difficult to humble down. I don't know where they learn all this. Does today education teach to disobey, idle, egoistic, etc.? Earlier education taught how to adopt good behaviour. It seems today's education taught how to disobey, idleness, shamelessness, and the other anti-social activities. Now you see life is full of chaos, we the elderly are useless lots in the eyes of the youngsters. Regardless of the elderly sex, the youth used to dare not defile any of the elderly words. Though it was not a written law but it is practiced as stricture as a law that young children should go to the grandpa and grandma's place for their services. The native superstitious belief that "if any one defiled the elderly commands or received the curse of the elderly due to disobedience or negligence he or she would die with big gashes on their body" served as a binding for many young Nagas in the olden days".

According to some reliable narrations of many elderly persons, before the advent of Christianity and education, in each locality or village, there used to be groups of boys and groups of girls of the same age groups—consisting of ten members or less. Each group would sleep together in big dormitories. The dormitories were separate for the boys and for the girls. No members would be left alone in any festivals, events, sharing of meals, etc. They sleep together till they get married. Each group was called by the name of the family who hosted or provided the dormitory. The groups were indirectly competing with other group in terms of good manners and other constructive works or activities so that their group name would be popular. Such social environment thus, nurtured strong ties of friendship according to age. However, the importance of such culture decreased with the advent of the Christianity and education. And now those last group members become as the oldest people in certain village or the community. As most of their fellow friends passed away, the living members are facing high level of death anxieties because they had nurtured strong feelings of belongingness, togetherness, by the system, in their times. And now, even those who remained alive do not live peacefully because they live as if they are waiting their time to die. As a result death anxiety seemed to be strong among the many Nagas elderly. With the advent of Christianity, almost one and half century ago, especially in the rural areas, people started looking for education. But those who were once rich not go for education because of their complacency and due to their contentment with what they have had. The spread of education was becoming powerful only in the recent decades. Now only those people who got education and job enjoyed the pensions and could be able to maintain certain standard of living. Those who could not earn education due to their complacency with their riches, they become poor and now suffer economically.

As the consequences of many situations, the social systems changed drastically with the passage of time. In the name of outside standard and modernisation, the young Nagas started devaluating the in-built knowledge, advice, and wisdom of the elderly. With quantitative educational qualifications and standards, the youngsters started arbitrarily neglecting elderly wisdom to a great extent. There are over populous educated youths but without knowledge. Moral responsibility of the youth towards the elderly has completely vanished. Not only neglects and socially isolated, the elderly persons experienced different realms of problems in today's Nagas society. Geographical ruggedness also added more problems as infrastructures and its facilities are not at all available. As the children usually migrated to towns and cities, many elderly parents are left all alone in the villages, as they are not able to move with their children. When to communicate with their dear and near ones in the cities and towns, especially in the times of trouble or needs, problems are pyramidally cumulated because of its residential areas, geographical and locational inconveniences, physical disabilities, economical problems, lack of knowledge with today's gadgets for information and communication systems, etc. These problems of the elderly in the rural areas have cumulated the disabilities of the elderly to a great extent.

As compared to the rural areas, the Nagas who settled in the towns and cities under compulsion due to their children and other reasons, experienced new realms of inconveniences, with high degree of social non-importance, lack of concerns, and physical isolation and loneliness, as the social milieu is totally different from where they were nurtured. The sacred tradition of the Naga embedded in collective selves—sharing, which instilled and imparted the sense of feeling at home is totally absent in towns and cities environment. In other words, the benign Nagas tradition which moulded or nurtured its natives to share the feeling of belongingness with everyone in the native locality is nowhere found in towns and cities. Readjustment to the entirely different environmental patterns of lifestyles in a completely different environment of different culture, social order, standards, and expectation, with inflexible minds and body, the elderly persons living in towns and cities faced tremendous stresses. Couple with the pace of change, they face more and more anxieties and stressful events. Some of the elderly persons residing in towns for years are too not in their volition but through the conditions such as physical disabilities, to maintain themselves in the villages, no one to stay along in the villages, request of their children or grandchildren and other reasons. Although many children requested their parents or grandparents to stay with them in towns and cities, and they simply satisfy only their basic needs such as shelter and food as per the needs of youngster, but without any concerns of their adjustment and other intrinsic problems. Such lack of concerns by their supporters simply precipitate more anxieties, and tensions. Living in such unwanted and inhospitable environment, the aged develops and promotes several negative dimensions of life, e.g., feeling of loneliness, higher level of anxieties, and others psychological problems.

Today, while over the world people continuously strive to enhance the standard of living with qualitative aspects adding a new lease to living standard, the Nagas elderly seems to find no place to qualify their quality of life in this generation. Today some of the elderly parents encountered another realms of subjective and psychological problems. With the youth towering without jobs and could not progress much in any field, they keep on depending on their elderly parents. Elderly parents instead of supported by their children after several years of so much cares and sacrifices for their children, in spite of their aging conditions, could not afford to refuse the excessive and exorbitant demands of their children. Because on one hand, they as the society nurtured them to have a very close emotional attachment, whereby they cannot bear to see their children suffered under poverty. On the other hand, as the anti-social activities are sky rocketing, they are apprehensive of their children. As the Naga parents used to have lots of children one among many always used to be a black sheep. The parents supports till their last child of the family deprived them to get chance to relax, rest, etc., from the active physical work till they are nailed to their coffin. Not only extra dependence, today children brought numerous problems, troubles, and difficulties through gambling, drugs, elopement, and other unexpected behaviours. Some parents never enjoyed peace of mind ever since their children grown up. One Veiselie, 61 years old, (a subject of the study), reports "while my children were in schools, I could not wait for them to be in college. Now in college, life is becoming more burdensome in terms of expenses and the nature of their life. Now their employment and settlements are in the midst of uncertainty caused me to worry immensely. As the situation becoming more fragile, I don't know when I'm to hear that my children committed any anti-social activities or adopted unwanted behaviour." Parents on one hand, doing their best that their children get the best of the knowledge and wisdom, some children on the other hand, irresponsibly exaggerating without knowing their parental desire and expectation from them. Some children do their own wishes to the extent of getting married without the consent of their poor parents. Even after marriages, not only had disgraced their images before the society, but go to the extent of going back and demanding from their poor parents. It is always, especially for the elderly parents, find difficult to live in peace, until their children are not properly settled. To some instances, when the parents cannot help their children any longer due to their physical inabilities, they just succumbed to the psychological impact due to their children behaviour and leading a deplorable life. Thus, for the Nagas elderly, living in this transitional stage of the society is a blessing in disguise unless children are there to support as the real supporters of psychological, emotional, and physical needs.

## The Present Study

The present study is an attempt to understand the status of the elderly in all dimensions of life through an integrated method—both qualitative and quantitative. Several studies have been done within the domains of needs, problems, adjustments, in of social, psychological, physical, economical, and many aspects of life. Studies are also carried out on the evaluation of plans, policies, and schemes for the elderly, but studies on their life quality required special attention and trust for the global or collective intervention programmes. Many elderly especially in the developing countries are still unable to fulfil many of their long desired dreams such as proper food, shelter, security, and better social supports, where as some elderly in many developed countries concern not only their basic needs but about the quality of the facilities they ere provided. Within the elderly communities, there may be variation among the various demographic variable such as, sex, age, the level of educations, marital status, and many others.

Sex is the most important status identifing a person's carrier through out the lifespan. The importance of sex stratification variable can be seen in probability statement concerning the differential life changes (such as life expectancies, health status, mental health, etc.), and differential personal resources and prestige (e.g., income and marital status) likely to decline in male and female as they, grow old. Similarly, after identifying a person's sex one can suggest certain model lifestyle and life experience as the person is more likely to follow through the course of life. So, it would yield benefit in understanding difference between male and female elderly status.

**Justification of the Study**

1. Meaning of aging varies dramatically across culture, therefore, studying aging and the elderly quality of life among the Nagas is seen as important to ravel newer information as Nagas have a unique tribal tradition enduring generations altogether, but strongly impacted by the wave of modernization, and urbanization processes in the recent decades, where no researches in the field were known to have ever done.
2. As one of its first kind in almost over the North East India which considered most important tribal belt of the country. So it would be new information for further research in the field of gerontology.
3. Studying the psychosocial well-being through integrated method, i.e., qualitative and quantitative methods would provide better picture of the topical concerns.
4. Comparing various demographical variables such as gender differences may help to indicate the differential affectors of elderly quality of life and psychosocial well-being.

**Samples**

A sample of 200 elderly persons (60+ years) was taken from the district of Phek, Kohima, Dimapur, Zunhebuto, Workha, and Senapati. The sample includes male and female, urban and rural, age categories as young-old = 60-69 years, old = 70-79 years, and old-old = 80+ years.

**Tools**

1. For quantitative methods:

(a) Information schedule.
(b) Health awareness schedule (Easwaramoorthy & Chadha, 1995).
(c) Disability in daily activities (Jamuna & Ramamurti, 1990).
(d) UCLA Loneliness Scale (Russell, *et al.*, 1980).
(e) Leisure activities schedule (van-Willigen & Chadha, 1990).
(f) Adjustment inventory for elder people (Social) (Ramamurti, 1968).
(g) Social network schedule (van-Willigen & Chadha, 1989).

2. For qualitative methods:

(a) Case Study—10 cases.
(b) Life History—10 elderly people.
(c) Key Informant Interviews—15 key informants.

**Results**

After scoring the data from all the 200 elderly individual responses, including 15 key informants, 10 life histories, and 10 case studies, the raw data from the questionnaire method were analysed on the basic of the statistical techniques.

t-test was employed to compare the means scores for the significant differences on some psychosocial well-being indicators for the male and female categories.

When compared between male and female elderly persons with respect to some indicators of psychosocial well-being, the results indicated significant differences between the groups. The differences existed in deprivation (t-2.65, $P<0.01$), loneliness (t-3.41, $P<0.01$), happiness (t-1.88, $P<0.05$), health awareness (t-2.39, $P<0.05$), adjustment (t-6.48, $P<0.01$), and self-rated quality of life (t-4.12, $P<0.01$).

**Table 16.4:** Comparison between Male and Female with Respect to Some Psychosocial well-being Indicators

| *Sl. No.* | *Indicators* | *Male (104)* | | *Female (96)* | | *t-value* |
|---|---|---|---|---|---|---|
| | | *Mean* | *SD* | *Mean* | *SD* | |
| 1. | Deprivation | 3.00 | 1.72 | 2.35 | 1.77 | 2.65** |
| 2. | Loneliness | 46.58 | 7.55 | 50.07 | 6.97 | 3.41** |
| 3. | Happiness | 4.31 | 1.11 | 4.04 | 0.87 | 1.88* |
| 4. | Health Awareness | 5.12 | 1.44 | 4.69 | 1.05 | 2.39* |
| 5. | Disabilities in Daily Activities | 21.75 | 5.74 | 20.76 | 4.37 | 1.38 |
| 6. | Adjustment | 11.31 | 2.51 | 8.82 | 2.89 | 6.48** |
| 7. | Leisure Activities | 8.83 | 4.73 | 3.86 | 1.99 | 9.81** |
| 8. | Self-rated Quality of Life | 5.84 | 1.68 | 4.94 | 1.40 | 4.12** |
| 9. | Social Network | 48.73 | 20.54 | 46.97 | 11.04 | 0.76 |

*Notes*: ** denotes pairs of groups significantly different at 0.01 levels.
        * denotes pairs of groups significantly different at 0.05 level.

Comparing the mean scores of the two groups with respect to the above indicators, it is observed that male elderly are more deprived, less lonely, happier, better health awareness, better in adjustment, larger leisure activities, and social supports, rated their quality of life better and subjective well being.

Depending on their habitual work nature outside the family, the male elderly seems to have experienced another realm of unadjustable life when they become physically inactive and unable to work any longer. And this probably results in more disabilities among the Nagas male elderly in their late life leading to feeling of more deprivation.

> "...After experiencing of working so hard especially of external heavy works such as hunting, cutting woods, carrying and building river beds, with so many friends along, we feel so deprived, as now as we could not work any longer. Unlike before, the level of physical permit made us so uneasy, especially when we hear people organize such collective works..." *Key Informant—No. 9.*

For women on the other hand, deprivation mostly leads to the physical disabilities, rather than socially constructed isolate world.

"...Since my childhood, I did not use to have much time for collective or partying works competitions, life change used to be rather gradual. Of course year after years if I systematically observe, changes always occur. Pains in joints, stomach problems, backbone, etc., becoming significant. And these physical problems are main problems..." *Life History—No. 6.*

Loneliness for the female elderly is mostly triggered by the absence of significant persons in their life such as due to death of their spouse as women have better chance of getting widowed and mass migration of children towards town for jobs.

"...Ever since, my husband died ... and after that ... two of my eldest sons found death from bed within or span of two years. Since then living in the village is a great difficult experience with all alone. To live with the children in towns is also an uneasy experience..." *Case No. 9.*

As the Naga tribal society was a socialist type of society, happiness mostly derived from the interpersonal relationship and social contribution by the individual and the personal image hold strong for the male elderly.

"...What type of enjoyment a person get who expects if he could give feast the whole village; build the house and other subsequent performances? Yea, these days because of children behaviour parents are unhappy lots. But if children are good...?" *Key Informant—No. 4.*

Women derivation and experience of happiness resulted from a different perspective. It could be emotive response to the function of heart rather than mind, female elderly extract happiness through the circle of their socially expected designed domains of duties.

"...I had a very happy life, because if always used to obey elder's commands in childhood days, seniors used to love us. I think people care most to those who care others. And this is the happiness, I enjoyed..." *Life History—No. 10.*

Health awareness, for the elderly, is mostly from or though social interaction rather than medical practitioners advice and prescriptions.

Peer groups, family members, and through people informal gathering places, and also from personal experiences. As male elderly have larger social network they usually have better knowledge about health. However, even if they heard of pharmaceutical medicines, they cannot remember easily, as they are very much relying on the natural medicines.

> "...Last year I had a serious loose motion. I could recall some one talk about the name of medicine for that disease, while I was gossiping in a public gathering, but as I am an illiterate I could not remember the name as I didn't use to write or whatever, so, I took natural herbs fluids or fluid extracted from any medicinal trees..." *Life History—No. 8.*

Self-confidence and self-esteem through social interaction seem to determine better social adjustment. Male elderly seems to have better adjustment due to lesser responsibilities and their habitual experience of social interaction than female elderly.

> "...I wish I could actively participate in any discussion and sharing, as our place is a public-place people used to come in numbers after dinner, and discuss various things, issues, etc. Now as an old man the adjustable nature is almost loosing. I cannot remain talking to people who visit and share..." *Life History—No. 2.*

Females are more of timid and avoiding the people with their knowledge being limited for social world.

> "...Lot's of people used to come to our place. My children or grandchildren will entertain them. Sometimes as an old woman, I cannot remain like the children. So, sometimes I throw my elderly tantrum even in their gathering..." *Life History—No. 10.*

Leisure activities are few and many Naga elderly do not truly conceptualize and subscribe to it in a true sense. In which the women suffer worse. It could be resulted due to the fact that limited time, couple with lack of facilities and without standard set as per its importance.

> "...She woke up around 4:30 am fetched water two to three trips from a distance of 25 km, prepared food. After the food around

9:00 am she would go to farm/field. Around 4:00 pm returned home from work. Then started preparing food for dinner, till around 6:30 pm. Then spends some one hour on cleaning and other works. Around 7:30 to 9:00 pm went to bed..." *Case No. 6.*

For the Naga male elderly as they do not use to do much of the household jobs, after they finish the external work outside the kitchen, they get free time to go for gossiping and chatting with either neighbours or friends.

"...Men are comparatively free, because for them, if they are physical active, once they finished outside kitchen works, they just go to neighbours, friends, or anywhere, but for us works are endless..." *Key Informant—No. 1.*

However, male elderly too, when they are no longer physically active, their area of social interaction with other community members reduced significantly, which could be triggered by inflexibility of physical body resulted from excessive physical labours, in their youthful days.

"...He could not go here and there any longer for quite some time now. Therefore, he could not actively maintain his social environment. All he could do is taking sun bath during the day time, and retired to room, even facilities are provided by his children he could not play, because he does not know how to play. Consequently, the interest and enthusiasms to interact with others are slowly decreasing..." *Case No. 1.*

Supports are mainly deemed in the form of physical help, cares, and attentions. And supports are of expectations, from whom one rendered help and obliged. Female elderly are of in altruistic nature with certain level of concerning the helps, or attention they rendered to others.

"...How much more that I can expect supports from others as I myself did not give much to others. Even if I wished to help others, and be enjoyably part with others, conditions are not always congenial being poor, woman, and above all not active like other..." *Life History—No. 6.*

On the other hand male elderly are more optimistic and expect more from others to give supports anyway.

> "...As the elders of the family, of the community, the society should or ought to render helps to the elderly. No matter, whoever or whatever the situations, I am convinced that youngsters should help and are bound to help. Yea, of course, because of others helps, love, care, etc., from the family, society, and community. I could live happily till today, if not of their help, I would not be able to live thus far like this..." *Key Informant—No. 9.*

Life satisfaction and personal evaluation of life and considering its quality of life mostly determined by the social environment and the personal resources as compared to its social standards, and expectation with corresponding to certain expects of life. Male elderly Nagas viewed the concept of good life mostly from the perspectives of the social expectations.

> "...What an elderly can expect more than having understanding and well settled children around, along without any socially tainted remarks. As we are living in such a unique society, a person, especially elderly person suffers most when he carries bad reputation from the past life. And usually people of bad reputation do not have understanding children..." *Key Informant—No. 14.*

Female elderly tended to view better quality of life from the personal characteristics and its well-being. They usually internalized any happiness with their immediate surroundings such as family, relatives, and neighbours. And these surroundings seem to determine their life well-being.

> "...Congenial family atmosphere (without any disturbance or unruly nature in the family), with loving spouse, and caring children, the elderly will not find problems though. Understanding children are the greatest treasures for their parents. If children are doing well, and leading a good life, then the elderly parents forget all their worries, anxieties and can speak boldly among the friends and before the community members. In the family, the mother has a great responsibility for her children. If she is not a responsible one then the children usually become bad. And if the children are

not of understanding nature, then the elderly parents life is under threat..." *Key Informant—No. 13.*

When an elderly is asked to describe about the subjective well-being of an elderly person he replied "...man is not an isolate being, in which Nagas are a typical people, with so much affluence and difference, everything around us involved to interpret our well being. Even if one has riches, but if he is not socially regarded, then what good life he has? So also a healthy man, if he is not co-operative, then his life would be less meaningful. Being an elderly, health is very important; if health allows us to work we can earn social supports, attentions, cares, and at the same time can live independently and joyfully. But as the health for the elderly is always weak, therefore, it is the main causing factor to our poor live. Only when we grow old we wish that if we could work. As it saying, 'when a thing is missing or when a man is becoming poor, he slowly become poorer and poorer, so also we the elderly when growing old we become poorer in our social world, physical health, economy, and usually religious faith also becoming unfocused. But in all, having strong faith that the Almighty helps us to maintain enjoyably our old age poor life is a big consolation..."

Old age social-psychological well-being is not to be compared with general well-being. Being old always carries negative aspects of life. Among the factors determining psychosocial well-being of the elderly, elderly men are affected differently by different aspects. So also the women. Thus, Nagas elderly too, with its different social cultural factors affecting their lives which also shows the difference between male and female elderly.

## Discussion

The elaboration and explanation of the analyses and its interpretation in the presented results show that male elderly have better quality of life than their female counterparts among the Naga tribal community. However, as there is no frame of reference, the interpretation would be of natural explanations of the values brought out by the study. The study further explored the comparative structure of the elderly males and females with respect to various aspects of life, probably to integratedly represent the quality of life, a psychosocial well-being, of an individual. Analysis of the responses in the filled questionnaires and the subsequent reports, experiences, and life histories of difference individual elderly persons, it is therefore, to consider confidently that the psychosocial well-being of the Naga elderly differed between sexes.

The findings in the inferences statistics indicated that male elderly have score higher in happiness, health awareness, adjustment, leisure activities, social supports, and subjective well-being. Elderly male also found to have been less lonely but more deprived than their female counterparts. As compared to female elderly, male elderly have more disabilities in daily living, better social network and more spiritual. It may be explained that gender differences are resulted by the fact that Naga social cultural set up, where its strong ties based on the segregated roles, status, and many others obvious characteristics mingled and endured through the generations.

The factors responsible for the male elderly indicating more deprivation due to old age, lesser feeling of loneliness, but happier, may be explained that male elderly, as concerned with respect to Naga social set up, enjoyed the position of importance in the family even after they retired from their active life. However, as accustomed to their extrovert type of lives they enjoyed during the active days, the physical disability resulted by the aging might probably cause them to feel differently which possibly hold responsible to impact them perceive more deprived. Customarily, Nagas males enjoyed wonderfully happy lives in the olden days, in terms of celebrated and competitive types of works, such in terrain constructions, building houses, and many others. The impact of such celebrated competitions remained as part of the fantasy of fanfare, and when such events are perceived as out of their reach, they felt more deprived. On the other hand, the important role played by the male elderly, in the family and in the villagers, may cushion them to keep away from the blues.

The feeling of more loneliness by the female elderly be explained by the universal phenomenon rather than through Nagas perspective alone, that women are more likely to have better chance of be widowed, as they live longer. The emotional attachment with their spouses, and the resultant effects of their spousal death along with children no longer beside them, as children migrated to town and cities, might impact them tremendously to feel more lonely and experience the life of emptiness. The physical absences of the children also impact them to feel more lonely. Several studies (Kleshman and Weissman, 1977) also subscribed to the point that more depression and other negative effects in women than in men are due to their longevity. Elderly women also likely to have larger amounts of life events as they live longer and therefore have better chance to have more disabilities. Negative life events probably lower the satisfaction level and happiness. The findings which showed elderly men have greater happiness as compared to elderly women can be assumed as an extension of what have been found by many researchers.

Results also indicated that elderly women have lesser knowledge about their health. Several factors could be responsible for these effects. In most traditionally framed mores, especially in the developing societies, women were provided less opportunities for education due to various reasons including cost effective analysis of the given poor economic status. As the results, the long-term outcome is that, they are deprived exposure to information on various aspects of good living, including health care systems. As the health care systems not abundantly available in the olden or present Naga inhabited remote areas couple with lack of opportunities to get acquainted with day-to-day living, the women remained lagging behind their counterparts, in this area.

Concerning adjustment, results showed that male elderly have better adjustment than their woman counterparts; personal comfortably presentation among members probably plays pivotal roles for better adjustment. The general problems of the women in personal mobility and personal cares such as in walks, baths, works, eatings, etc., and secondary activities hold responsible for the poor adjustment for the elderly women. Thus, expressed ideas in the qualitative data reflect the nature of many women who did not accustom to entertaining people, face more problems in later life. On the other hand, the elderly man, as they accustomed the various social interactions in the daily basic while in active life, they continue to carry through with better understanding of their social world. But usually, when elderly become helpless in demands due to their disabilities, serious problems of adjustment developed. Role changes from the traditionally framed division of labour of internal assignment and domestic pressure as being, mother, wives, sisters, might probably play a role to shrink many avenues of adjustmental resources and where by now require some resources to integrate in order to restore better adjustment in their old age.

Complications on the personal level also cropped up due to absence of skills and knowledge of finance among the women especially after the death of their husband, or after their retirement from the active work, could be responsible for their poor adjustment. Personal adjustment of the elderly women is mostly influenced by marital status, income level, physical health, and the feeling of alienation, self-regards, satisfaction with role activities, and assessment of general health. Personal involvement with any social activities imparted to determine the level of adjustability in the old age.

Women in the Naga society are duty bound until they could not stand and work any more. This conditions is perhaps responsible for not being truly conceptualizing the meaning and importance of leisure activities. This could be resulted by the multiple factors such as limited time available, lack of facilities, and without any set standard for the pursuits. The comparison between the males and the females indicating male elderly enjoying more leisure activities among the Naga elderly persons be explained by the fact that males are comparatively free, after days work, whereas women remained engaged from the morning till late night-from kitchen, to farms, and back to kitchen. Thus, the opportunities afforded to women are lesser than to men. Education also probably play the role as Naga elderly women are comparatively less educated along with limited free times also found responsible for the lesser amount of leisure activities.

The findings indicated difference between the men and women with respect to their leisure activities. It is not surprising and also unexpected since many researchers too come with similar and parallel findings. However, it is not inborn active and voluntary determinant of gender difference in leisure activities, but rather a socially constructed outcome, as the women are stereotyped as biologically inconvenient to involve in determining the various activities. Lawton, *et al.* (1986) and Kelly's (1983) observations and findings substantiate to consolidate, the basic generally apparent outcomes with the background by indicating that women participated in several recreation activities and within the activities, women are less involved in team sports and more involved in the passive activities such as reading, and other sociable expressive and artistic activities. Men elderly, however, are more free than women in terms of basic chore duties, better chance of availing the facilities provided, and the accustomed nature of outgoing helped them to enjoy leisure activities. However, the number of activities which the elderly enjoyed is mostly unprofitable which may or may not help, in promoting their psychological or social well-being.

Male elderly are more optimistic and more open in terms of expecting and receiving supports. The constructed social system in which women were being considered with certain level of reservation in relation to active social interaction impacted to live that their social world is of inside as Chadha, Aggarwal and Mangla (1990) observed. This socially established social reality could have influencing the women world of expecting and receiving social supports. One of the reasons could be that males are more likely to live along with their spouse and children, and have better chance of getting more supports, whereas the women usually live longer and have better chance to be widowed and have lesser chance of getting proper support systems. So, this better chance of living with spouse and children have helped them to have more social supports than women who are likely to live alone.

Life satisfaction and personal evaluation of life and considering its quality of life are mostly determined by the existing and prevailing social environment and the personal level as compared to its social standards and expectation witch corresponding to certain aspects of life. The different perspectives of men and women looking towards quality of life may be explained that masculine expectation of respect, honour, prestige and other factors with the social systems provides as it endures in nurturing for the generation on one hand. The resultant of the present system would probably pull down of their perception if it continues in the near future. Female elderly, on the other hand view the better quality of life from the socially created atmosphere such as society, neighbours, and the families of understanding rather than the personal attributes of attaining good life. Personal relational resources and inherent expectation and its fulfilment are of very important but female elderly seem to down play it. Thus, the wave of social change among the Naga tribal communities, effectively impact upon the existing social norms, whereby, the fairer sex, and also who holds on and relying to find peace and rest on the society are mostly affected.

When subjective well-being is concerned in comparison between the male and female elderly, male elderly have better subjective well-being than the Nagas females. The sicky nature of women resulted from poorer awareness of their own health, more physical distress with greater prone to be sensitive to illness symptoms (Verbrugge, 1985) and lesser control of their own life and becoming more vulnerable to psychological distress, poor physical health and lack of social resources and inadequate financial resources (Prakash, 1991) could be the determinants of poorer subjective well-being among women. On the other hand, male elderly, when their better subjective well-being over the women elderly be reasoned that with their ability to master critical situation, as the Nagas male elderly practically experienced through the demands of the situations over the years, and the supportive attitudes—as they accultured through the ages, being the social system enforced down the ages, etc., may have played its role to yield to the advantage side of the male elderly.

## Conclusion

The overall view of the elderly social-psychological well-being depicted a multifaceted issue involving many factors, with a degenerative symptoms showing as people grow older, within the aging community, gender difference prominently show that women elderly than men have poorer social-psychological well-being, among the Naga elderly. This poorer social-psychological well being among the women may be due to various integrated factors like poor educations background, which is directly responsible for poor awareness, of their poor nutrition and health care, weaker in their economic status, and also resulted due to socially constructed roles, statues, and other stereotypical attitudes, which restrict their activities and limited them to household activities thereby reducing their subjective well-being—joyfully, meaningfully and purposefully living in the twilight years. Their poor status could also be attributed to the failure of formal and informal social supports system to act as a buffer.

Male elderly on the other hand, though relatively better than their female counterparts do not have enough proof to mean that their social-psychological well-being is perfectly fine. Their relative better social-psychological well-being be attributed to the factors such as their mastery over the critical life events, which prompted by the established social system in terms of roles, and status assigned better network system which the social system encouraged directly or indirectly down the ages, and factors on the siding of the male elderly advantage. Thus, the social-psychological well-being of the Nagas elderly, with respect to male and female comparison concluded to infer that male have better social-psychological well-being than their female counterparts.

## REFERENCES

Birren, J.E., and Schroots, J.F.J. (1996): Concept, theory, and method in Psychology of aging. In J.E. Birren and K.W. Schaie (Eds.), *Handbook of Psychology of Aging*. San Diego, California: Academic Press.

Birren, J.E., and Renner, V. J. (1977): Research on psychology of aging: Principle and experimentation. In J.E. Birren and K.W. Schaie (Eds.), *Handbook of Psychology of Aging*. New York: van Nostrand, Reihnold Company.

Chadha, N.K., Aggarwal, V., & Mangla, A.P. (1990). Social networks and aging. *Spectra of Anthropological Progress,* 12, 15-32.

Easwaramoorthy, M. (1995): *Quality of life of the elderly in Tamil Nadu,* unpublished Doctorate Thesis, University of Delhi. North Campus.

Jamuna, D. and Ramamurti, P.V. (1990): Old disability scale. *Journal of Psychometry*, 3(1), 21-26.

Keith, J. (1990): Age in social and cultural context: An anthropological perspective. In R.H. Binstock and L.K. George (Eds.), *Aging and social sciences*. 3rd Edition San Diego: Academic Press.

Kelly, J.R. (1983): *Leisure identities and interactions*. London: Allen and Unwin.

Kleshman, G.L., & Weissman, M.M. (1977): Sex differences in intimate friendship in old age. *Journal of Marriage and Family*, 38, 739-747.

Lawton, M.P., Moss, M., and Fulcomer, M. (1986): Objective and subjective uses of time by older people. *International Journal of Aging & Human Development*, 24, 171-188.

Prakash, I.J. (1991): Psychological profile of aging women. In I.J. Prakash (Ed.), *Quality Aging: Collected Papers*. (234-245), Varanasi: Association of Gerontology.

Ramamurti, P.V. (1968): An adjustment inventory for the aged. *Indian Journal of Psychology*, 43, 27-29.

Russell, D., Paplau, L.A., and Cutrona, C.E. (1980): The revised UCLA Loneliness Scale: Concurrent and discriminant validity evidence. *Journal of Personality and Social Psychology*, 39, 472-480.

Singal, S. (1990): Human aging: Some psychological perspectives. In R.C. Singh and G.S. Singhal (Eds.), *Perspectives in aging research*. Houston: Scholarly Publication.

van Willigen, J., and Chadha, N.K. (1990): Techniques for the collecting social network data. *The Indian Journal of Social Work,* L(4), 615-621.

Verbrugge, L.M. (1985): Gender and Health: An update on hypothesis and evidence. *Journal of Health and Human Behaviour*, 26, 156-182.

# 17

# Health Care Practices among Tribes of Manipur

OINAM HEMLATA and PEBAM KRISHNA KUMARI

The present paper is an endeavour to highlight the health care practices among the tribes of Manipur so, it would be appropriate to begin from the basic, i.e. health. The World Health Organisation (WHO), in its constitution has defined health as 'a state of complete physical, mental and social well-being.' (WHO, 1958. Annexure1) Going by this definition then, health is a basic requirement to lead a normal life and all efforts revolves around it. Health is the epicenter of happiness. Thus, the cliche "Health is Wealth" goes true. However, the concept of health, diseases, treatment, life and death is as varied as the culture of one tribe to another. To know the health care practices among tribes of a Manipur it is better to know about Manipur and its tribes.

## A Brief Sketch of Manipur

Coming to Manipur, it is situated on the lofty heights at the eastern frontier on a branch of the eastern Himalaya range which protruded towards the south along the Indo-Burma border stretching between 93.03°E and 94.78°E and latitudes 23.80°N to 25.68°N. This abode of 22,88,634 (2001 census) people is a cauldron of diverse social formation, culture, religion and dialect. The state of Manipur represent a miniature replica of the larger picture of the entire north-eastern region where numerous different social and ethnic groups merge and dovetail. Geographically divided into hills and centrally situated valley there are thirty Scheduled Tribes fortifying the plain inhabitants. Lush green valleys and cloud kissed hillocks adorn this 22,327 sq. km land. These various tribes are usually divided into two types—the Nagas and the Kukis, each having a number of sub-tribes according to the differences in dialects, customs, mode of living, etc. However, there are some tribes like Anal, Moyon, Monsang, Lamgang, Tarao, Chothe, Chiru, Koireng and Kharam who have linguistic affinity with the Kuki-chin and cultural identification with the Naga. They are in the words of B.K. Roy Burman bridge and buffer communities between the Nagas and Kuki-chin who are attracted towards the Naga ideologically and who accepted the Naga identity.

## Health Care Practices

Nestling in the nature's bountiful art treasures, the tribals in Manipur are sustaining in an impoverished, malnourished and unhygienic state. The surrounding forest ecology gives them their source of sustenance, provisions of food as well as the jest to survive. However, their hand to mouth survival are responsible for poor sanitation and unhygienic life which leads to the cause of disease. Their hard life which keeps them busy all the time make it difficult for them to take care of health.

## Spirit-man Interplay in Context of Health and Disease

Among the tribes in Manipur, the belief in the interference of supernatural agency is particularly strong in the context of health and disease. Different deities and spirits are believed to be connected with the different types of diseases. The fate of individual and the community depends on the relationship with unseen forces which intervenes in human affairs. They attribute all sickness to the designs of evil forces, whether it is a mysterious sickness, sudden appearance of boils, loss of speech, poxe or fever they consider all these the inevitable consequences of the breach of taboo which infuriate the spirit. They believe that if men offend these spirits, the mystical power punish by sickness, death or other natural calamites. Thus, the usual theory of disease among the tribes in Manipur is that it is caused by the breach of taboo or by hostile spirits. Sickness is the routine punishment for every lapse and crime meted out to them by the spirits. According to the nature of sickness, sacrifices and offerings are made to appease the concerned spirit. To drive home this point examples can be shown of some tribes in Manipur. Mao Naga, in an advent of large scale sickness of the villagers or spreading of epidemics like cholera, diarrhoea, small-pox, chicken-pox and measles the entire village will perform a black bull sacrifice to the spirit *Tho*. The Jangkhul Nagas approached *Kamyou* by sacrificing a fowl. The Kabui Nagas propitiate *Khongrui Kraan* by sacrificing pig, fowl, fruits, sweets and a jar of rice-beer. The *Khunbu* the *khullakpa* and the *Maiba*, the medicine man who is called *Pandam* take the responsibility of propitiating *Khongrui-Kraan* for seeking protection from disease. A rope made out of *Kangen* (a type of creeper) is stretched along the main road from one end of the village to the other. It is believed that the rope endowed with the blessing of the *Khongrui-kraan* would prevent the spirit of disease from coming near the residential house. Every house on both sides of the road is supposed to be covered by the rope. For sudden dizziness and miserable sickness, the Hmars make sacrifice to *Phunga Khawhring* for sanctification of the village from the influence of evil spirits. Similarly, rituals are performed where there is fear of epidemic like cholera, small pox by *Thempu* (village priest) during which no one was allowed to enter or go out of the village. The Rongmeis offer oblations now and then to *Bhamboo* and occasionally they propitiate the guardian deities in their traditional way to protect them from epidemics, diseases and disasters. The Thadou Kukis made a sacrificial ceremony to ward off epidemic diseases like small-pox, cholera, etc. to *Pathei*. In this, a gibbon is cut into two halves and blood is mixed with some plant, roots, etc. and anointed the mixture to the forehead of the villagers. The Moyons too propitiated *Lae*. They believed that all the sicknesses, diseases, deaths, accidents, etc. are caused by these evil spirits. *Gamlahlen* is considered as a male spirit who causes disease and sickness to the people. It resides in the jungle and to appease it, an effigy of a buffalo made of clay is offered along with 'zu', cock and unboiled rice. Thus, an interplay of spirits and man can be seen with special reference to health among the tribals to Manipur.

All tribal communities in Manipur have a group of sacred specialist—the priest or magician or medicine men, the services of whom are taken depending on the etiology of illness. They act as the mediator between the people and the mystical powers. By propitiation and prayers they tries to maintain a good relationship between the people, on one hand and the mystical power on the other which intervene human affairs. Mention can be made of *Siamphu* (village priest) among the Paite which is appointed by the chief of the village. He make sacrifices to spirit on behalf of ailing person. When a person is in critical stage *Nuphi* is conducted. In this, a goat, a dog, a pig and a chicken are sacrificed and offered to the spirit. The owner of the house and member of the household along with the *siamphu* dance around the house. Each of the participants carried one flask of wine. They also carried the animals on the back. After encircling around the house for three times, the animals are thrown on the roof of the house. In the meantime, the village priest will held one horn of Mithun which he beats with a horn of a goat. The malevolent spirits which causes epidemics, floods, drought, famines, diseases, etc. are controlled by *Thiempu* according to Thadou Kukis. *Thiempu* was supposed to identify the spirit causing trouble and illness and will tell the type of sacrifice which is needed to get rid of the evil spirit. Among the Moyon it is the *Ithiims* or village physicians. An *Ithiims* was supposed to propitiate evil spirits that caused the sicknesses and diseases to a person. In case he did not recover from the sicknesses after performing the act for a number of times, the final act was performed at the confluences of two streams or rivers by the *Ithiims* by cutting off the neck of a chicken and throwing it into the spot simultaneously uttering a few magical words, calling on the spirit to do as it pleased for it was the last and final sacrifice. It was also believed that when an evil spirit took possessions of a person, the latter suffered from sickness. The *Ithiims* released two chicken at the spot where the evil spirit was believed to have taken possession of the spirit of the person commanding it to leave and take possession of the chicken instead. Among the Mao Nagas, if a person is seriously ill, a member of his family will go to the house of *Ngumei* (those who know the past, present and future) or a *Pousumei* (those who know the whereabouts of spirits and their liking or demands). He shall explain where the person had gone and how the illness started and since when. The *Ngumei* without taking much time and after performing his own prayer will reveal how he was attacked by the evil spirit and prescribe the nature of offering or sacrifices. In case of *Pousumei* he cannot drag *Tho* if he does not remain chaste the previous night. The *Pousumei* will prescribe what is to be done by the patient party. The bull sacrifice, pig sacrifice, dog sacrifice, cock offering and other offering are the important acts performed by Mao with a view to saving life by appeasing the evil spirits.

Among Anals, there are two types of *Athim* (physician)—*Larni* (some are possessed by spirit) and *Patakang* (without any spirit possession). *Athim* is the mediator between man and spirit. He make sacrifices to the spirit *Zohring* is a type of sacrifice done by *Athim* which involve releasing of the chicken in the jungle representing the soul of a sick person. *Hrungtha*; performing a village purificaion ceremony in the village gate annually, *patha peting,* bringing back the soul of sick person from the hands of spirits and *Ahman Piitho,* driving away the evil possession from man, etc. are all initiated by *Athim.*

## Plants in the Life of Tribals

In addition to magico-religious method of treatment, tribes in Manipur explore their vegetative world and got a broad based knowledge on the different plant species which are used as medicine to cope ailments. For some lighter ailments like stomach ache, dysentery, diarrhoea, headache, dizziness, etc. herbal medicines are used which they prepare themselves with the help of various plants found within a few furlong.

## Modern Health Care Practices

Looking at the maternity and child health care aspects, no special care is taken of a pregnant woman. She consumes routine diet during the entire period of pregnancy. There is no respite from heavy works to pregnant woman, she works till the day of delivery. In most cases there is no system of utilizing maternity and child health services. During pregnancy they never consult a doctor in order to have MCH services, they approach the doctor only in case of complication or abnormality. Most of the deliveries are conducted at home.

The health services which are available are not fully utilized by them. The building of Primary Health Centre stands in solitude functionless. Generally people do not prefer to go to hospitals or health care centres as their first means of treatment. The tribal people in Manipur do not seek out for any treatment in the initial state of sickness. Therefore, in most of the cases, the sickness becomes chronic. When the ailments becomes acute only then do they seek for some treatment. They lay hand on domestic remedies for a couple of days but when the medicine fails to give any relief and when the ailment become acute taking a chronic form, they rush to priest or middle men as according to them this is an attack of an evil-spirit. When the priest/medicine men fails to provide any relief they consult either a doctor or again try herbal medicine. There are few countable tribals who believe in consulting the doctor immediately after the occurrence of any disease.

However, the advent of Christianity pumped up the rate of education which in turn open up new vistas in their mode of thinking. People are becoming more conscious of health care practices such as sanitation, hygiene food and nutrition. People have now started consulting doctor for the treatment of various disease. The change is, however, confined to few elite and educated section of tribes. Tribals residing in the interior and remote parts are still living ignorant of such facilities. People still resort to traditional medicine and prefer it. It is high time to find out the reason why these people are abstaining from modern health care services and the modern health care services should be ameliorated in such a way that these people will find it acceptable and convenient. So, to implement public health care services amongst these people successfully, a specific understanding of experiences between the tribals and doctor is a must. In this attempt the interaction between indigenous patterns and modern principle of treatment are necessary. If the two works as a conflicting factor no effective change can be obtained. Carstairs (1955) has shown how the differences in the context of belief and practices and techniques of curing resulted in misunderstanding between them. Therefore, there is an urgent need to explore the well-knit system of relationship between man and medicine in the tribal health perspective which could be adjustable within the socio-economic condition of these hill people of Manipur.

## Conclusion

To surmise, though education has open up new vistas in their mode of thinking, tribes in Manipur still hark back to their traditional health care practices as this proves to be convenient and easily accessible to them. The interference of supernatural agency is predominant in the context of health and disease. They give first preference to the traditional health care practices. Moreover, the modern trend of health care practices could not be reached adequately among them. Their lack of awareness and poor economy are still a hindrance in improving their health status. To make an amen of such situation it is high time to ameliorate the health care programmes and implement it according to the needs and desire of the tribes.

## REFERENCES

Athickal, Joseph (1992), *Maram Nagas—A Socio Cultural Study,* Mittal Publications, New Delhi.

Chaudhuri Buddhadeb (ed). (1986), *Tribal Health: Socio Cultural Dimensions,* Inter-India Publication, New Delhi.

Das, Rajat Kanti (1985), *Manipur Tribal Scene-studies in Society and Change,* Inter-India publication, New Delhi.

Das S.T. (1986), *Tribal Life of North Eastern India,* Gian Publishing House, Delhi.

Ethnobotany (1993) pp. 143-147. Published by (Society of Ethnobotanists). Deep Publications, Paschim Vihar, New Delhi.

Gangte, Thangkhomang S. (1993), *The Kukis of Manipur—A Historical Analysis,* Gyan Publishing House, New Delhi.

Hodson, T.C. (1989), *The Naga Tribes of Manipur,* Low Price Publications, New Delhi.

Kamkhenthang, H. (1998), *The Paite—A Trans Border Tribe of India & Burma,* Mittal Publications, Delhi.

Landy, David (1977), *Culture, Disease and Healing—Studies in Medical Anthropology,* New York, Macmillan.

Sachidananda and Prasad, R.R. (1996), *Encyclopaedic Profile of Indian Tribes,* Discovery Publishing House, New Delhi.

Sanajaoba Naorem (1995), *Manipur Past & Present,* Volume 3, Mittal Publication, New Delhi.

Shakespear, J. (1912), *Lushei Kuki Clans,* Cultural Publishing House, Delhi.

Shaw, William (1929), *Notes on 'The Thadou Kukis,* In Hutton J.H. (Ed.) Govt. of Assam Publication.

Statistical handbook of Manipur, 2002.

# 18

# Disease and Illness and their Ethnomedical Treatment among the Rathwas of Suskal, Gujarat

MITOO DAS

## Introduction

Disease, a biological and cultural universal, is the most predictable of human conditions. Sick people as cultural beings, have over time developed social institutions, etiological theories and therapeutic techniques to enable them to cope with the social and other dislocations occasioned by illness induced disability. All cultures, have a set of ideas for defining and treating disease, ways of prescribing cures, or easing pain and for making statements about the probable outcome of disease. Disease and illness are individual biological responses directed and shaped for the most part by cultural ideas learned in the course of being socialized. Medical beliefs and practices in India as in the rest of the world play an important role in every culture. Human society has created an "adaptive strategy" to counteract disease. Man in trying to learn how to treat disease has gained, a "vast complex of knowledge, beliefs, techniques, roles, norms, values, ideologies, attitudes, customs, rituals and symbols that interlock to form a mutually reinforcing and supporting system". This constitutes a medical system which includes all the clinical and non-clinical activities, the formal and non-formal institutions, and any other activity, that however tangentially, bear on the health levels of the group and promote optimum functioning of society. To be more specific, every society gives a theory of disease and also provides effective (if there is enough knowledge) treatment for the disease.

This is carried out by a medical system, which is very much a part of society. The set of medicines consists of these cultural practices, methods, techniques and substances, embedded in a matrix of values, traditions, beliefs and patterns of ecological adaptation, that provide the mean for maintaining health and preventing or ameliorating disease and injury in its members (Landy, 1977).

Of the many systems of medicines available, ethnomedicine is one which is widely made use of by different cultures, be it adivasis or other sections of society. Ethnomedicine deals with indigenous medical contributions and is generally termed as "folk medicine"; "popular medicine" etc. It includes myriad aspects of folk taxonomy of diseases, magico-religious and other therapies, its indigenous features, the role played by the ethnomedical experts and the relationship between medical phenomenon and socio-cultural setting. Folk medicine was practiced during the *Ayurvedic* period and is still practiced in the contemporary times. Traces of the use of this medicine are found in ancient manuscripts such as *Atharvaveda*, Kautilya's *Arthasastra* and even in *Ayurvedic Saṁhitas* of Charaka and Susruta. The folk sector of the health care system comprises non-professional, non-bureaucratized "specialists". Folk healing can be divided into sacred and secular subsectors, indicating its roots in both religious (e.g. Shamanism) and empirical (e.g. Herbalism). The folk practitioners are part-time, non-registered practitioners functioning within the context of village organization. The curative and therapeutic aspects are not just limited to the specialists but can be practiced at home as initial medical treatment. These are "Home Remedies" and are a section of folk medicine with a limited number of drugs which are readily prepared from materials available in the kitchen or in one's backyard. Another form of treatment which may be included in ethnomedicine is treatment done with the administration of herbs and hence known as "Herbal Treatment". A vague idea about herbs which have curative effects, are known to almost everybody in a society. This knowledge can be gained either from one's own family or from village elders. But a herbal specialist, who has a wider knowledge of the treatment through herbs is an essential necessity in such a curative system. It is also a part of the medicinal institution in societies where the medical importance of plants has been recognized.

With the above concepts as the backdrop, I now proceed to discuss the presence and use of ethnomedicine, among the Rathwas (a scheduled tribe) in a village called Suskal, Gujarat.*

**Concept of Health and Disease in Suskal**

Health and hygiene of the people of a community is directly related to its socio-cultural and natural environment. The type of life one lives conditions the health status of an individual. In this portion we explore the various ideas about health and disease in Suskal which lets us know about the native concepts of health and disease. This is an attempt to find out how do people distinguish good health from bad health? What causes illness and how much do they attribute to supernatural reasons for falling sick?

It is the socio-cultural and natural environment which shapes the health of the people in a community. The health habits and beliefs of people in any culture form a total system rather than being a separate part that stands in isolation. The way in which a person lives his life affects his health. The health status of an individual can be determined by the food he ingests, his sanitary habits, personal hygiene etc. The Rathwas of Suskal have their own ideas, knowledge and views about health and hygiene. They elaborately provide, views on how to keep oneself healthy and free from illness but the real picture is quite grim. The Rathwas are in a poor state of health (this opinion is from an etic point of view). Physically they are thin and undernourished. Barring one or two households, the children suffer from malnutrition. The most common ailments in Suskal are fever (*Tau*), Acidity (*Jalan*), Body Ache (*Dukhao*), Cough (*Khasi*) etc. The acute ones are Tuberculosis

* The Rathwas of Suskal are an agriculture based tribal society settled in state of Gujarat, on the western Coastal region of India. The Rathwas form the majority of the adivasi population in Baroda district. Almost the entire population live in rural areas. They are mainly found settled in eastern bordered 'Talukas' of Chota-Udaipur, Navsari, Pavi-Jetpur, Sankhera etc. in these Talukas, predominant population Vasav (Dungri Bhil), Naikas and Bonias are also found among the Rathwas. It is said that the Rathwas originally belonged to Chota Udaipur taluka also known as 'Rath Pradesh', hence the original inhabitants of 'Rath' are called Rathwas. According to the Baroda (Vadodara) district gazetteer, the Rathwa is an offshoot of the original Bhils. However, most of the Rathwas do not endorse this fact. The reason for this could be the fact that they consider the Bhils as belonging to a socially lower rank. Instead they claim to belong originally to the Koli tribe which enjoys a higher social status.

(*Timri*), Malaria (*Tadeo Tau*) and Jaundice (*Kamra*). Water used for drinking is not usually clean, which has led to many illness among the people. Problems arising due to snake bite are also quite common here. Besides these afflictions, disorders suffered by women are sterility (*wanjhiapanu*), white discharge (*safed pani*), menstrual camps (*Masik medukhao*), irregular menses (*animit masik*) and heavy menstrual flow (*satat masik*). Among these, white discharge (*safed pani*) is the one to reckon with as it leads to primary and secondary sterility and irregular menses. There are social and physical reasons for such abnormalities. The physical ones are poor sanitation, careless attitude towards cleanliness and well-being, habits like smoking and drinking, poor diet etc. The social reason for women having such disorders is because of early marriage which leads to early sexual life. But of course the villagers beg to differ.

## Dietary Habits

The kind of food a person consumes is directly associated with his health. If proper food is not available, it can lead to malfunctioning of the body and the mind. Regarding food, the adivasis of Suskal consume *Makai Ki Roti* which they call *Rotle* (Chapatis made out of maize flour, *Tuwar Ka Saag* (a cooked vegetable), *Dar* (lentil) and *Bhat* (rice). Sometimes they prefer to take *Valore* or *Papri*, a preparation made of *Gehu* (wheat) along with their meal. Among the vegetables, they consume the seasonal ones but the most popular is the *Bataka* (potato). At night they do not take rice. For breakfast, before going to the fields, they have a cup of tea with *makai ki rotle*. Thus this is their main item.

A young infant survives only on mother's milk till the fifth or sixth month after its birth. After this, the baby is given soup made out of lentil (mostly *tuwar ka dal*), boiled potatoes, boiled bananas and loose *khichri*. After the seventh or the eight month, the *khichri* preparation is made harder. On reaching the ninth month, along the already mentioned diet, the baby is also given pieces of chapatti mixed with milk and sugar. By one year, the baby is given normal food as taken by everyone but in small quantities. The mother too is made to maintain a particular diet for the time period of breast feeding. This is to avoid any irregularities or problems that might creep up in the child's health. They believe the mother's diet gets mixed with her milk and thus she has to eat a proper diet accordingly. Hence mothers are made to eat a special diet called *Kachali* made of coconut, ghee and milk, which is supposed to be good for the health of both the mother and child. One interesting point here is when a baby is growing inside the mother's womb, there is a belief that the mother should lessen her amount of food intake with the swelling or growth of her stomach. This is because the Rathwas think that more food, particularly rich food like milk will suffocate the child which is growing inside, as the food will occupy more space. The major problem which is quite apparent among the children of Suskal is malnutrition. Besides being poor and hence not being able to get proper food, the parents too are careless and ignorant. For example, the Rathwas feel milk is enough to keep a one year old full without any other food with it. The Rathwas, think that to be in the 'right condition of body' is to have proper health. The local term which they use fòr good health is *Saro Swast* or *Tandarust Swast* but when asked to define what *Swast* is, they were unable to so. They do not understand where good health ends and bad health begins. As long as they are able to work and be active, they think they are in good health.

Economically better people have the means to take good quality food. The amount of food that such people consume is also high. This is obviously to maintain good health. But not every family in Suskal can manage to possess all the food mentioned above. Different food is required for people of different age groups, or people performing different works and again special conditions like pregnant and lactating mothers. But I observed that most families in Suskal are only able to have *makai ke rotle* with some vegetables. Milk which is an important part of diet, is not taken by many of the poorer section because whatever their cattle provides for, they sell it but themselves are unable to buy at the market price. Thus almost all the villagers suffer from under nourishment. Moreover vices like drinking and smoking have also added to their misery in the form of illness. Although Guajrat is a state which is declared to be a dry state, illegal liquor is easily available. In Suskal, villagers besides buying such drinks, also consume local made drinks. *Taari* is the most common one. The juice is extracted from *Taar* (Palm Tree). Smoking of *bidis* is very popular among the villagers. *Bidis* are made at home from leaves of *Asatra*, which is stuffed with *Tambakhu* (Tobacco). The villagers are aware that excessive smoking of *bidis* is responsible for the high rate of tuberculosis but this has not deterred them from abstaining from smoking. As one old woman points out that smoking keeps them "active" all day long.

The Rathwas of Suskal, defecate and urinate in the open, preferably in the fields. Bathing and washing of clothes are done in the backyard for which they get water from water sheds, hand pumps, wells etc. Due to the absence of proper drainage system, rain and waste water from houses collect and gets stagnant near the houses itself and acts as a favourite place for the breeding of mosquitoes and germs. The wells too act as good mediums for mosquitoes and germs to breed as they are uncovered and have not been cleaned for ages. This is why malaria is on the rise in Suskal. Moreover, they use the water from the wells for drinking even though they have been provided with two water sheds for this purpose. I have noticed that they do not clean or purify the water from impurities before drinking. They do not realize that drinking dirty water may lead to illnesses. It is no wonder that a large number of people suffer from dysentery, diarrhoea, jaundice and typhoid.

## Disease Causation

Disease can be caused by both natural and supernatural means. When a comparison is made between the two, it is found in tribal societies that "only a few diseases are ascribed to natural causes, the common diseases being headache, diarrhoea, cough and consumption" (Jaggi 1982).

In Suskal, the Rathwas beliefs about disease can be classified into three categories:

1. Disease caused exclusively by supernatural powers like spirits and ghosts.
2. Disease caused by magical means—Sorcery and Witchcraft.
3. Disease caused by natural means.

Disease can be said to occur by supernatural powers when a human being is attacked by a supernatural being (deity or god) or a non-human being (ghost or spirit). This idea is well laid out in the minds of the villagers in Suskal. When goddesses are not given due recognition and reverence, they show their wrath by causing disease and death among men. The Rathwas believe that *Sitala-mata* or *Devi* (Goddess *Kali*) usually causes small-pox to express her anger. The other local deity, *Tilau Mata* when provoked, afflicts a person with leprosy. In order to free oneself from such tormenting and painful experiences, the deities have to be carefully appeased. A sufferer of leprosy is taken to the *Tilau Mata Mandir* where the sick is given a bath at the pond

(*Sarovar*) which is outside the mandir. Then they offer prayers to *Tilau Mata*. The ingredients used for worship are coconut and *agarbatti*. After this, they return to the pond, and the mud of the "holy" pond is smeared all over the body of the patient. The villagers believe that the mud contains miraculous particles which cures the afflicted. These are beliefs of the present population though no such case was found. The older generation however insist that they have seen such miracles occur. In case of small-pox *Sitala Mata* is propitiated. When a child has measles it is called *Holi* while for adults it is called *Bariya Dev*. The patient is not allowed to venture out of the house. Women of the family go and offer prayers to *Sitala Mata*. The *prasad* is given to the sick, which will make the disease disappear. So that this deadly and disfiguring disease is not let loose by *Sitala Mata*, a *puja*, *Sitala Satav* is organized every year in the month of September. On this day the villagers take cold food in order to please the goddess.

The Rathwas believe that a person who dies an unnatural death becomes a ghost. This ghost may enter the body of a man and do him damage. A person who is possessed is always restless. The villagers are of the view that ghost or spirit intrusion takes place when a person passes through the forest alone at night. Thus one should not venture out after sunset. The immediate effect of spirit possession is, the victim gets hysterical and becomes unconscious. Ghosts and spirits however do not cause any disease in man but cause death and destruction.

Disease is said to be caused by magical powers when there is an intrusion of a foreign body into a human being. The Rathwas mention "evil-eye" and "witch-craft" as two agents of illnesses caused by magical powers. It is believed by the Rathwas that some individuals have the faculty to cast a spell on others by just looking at them. Evil eye can be cast voluntarily or involuntarily. As they cast the spell, the person to whom it is done, faces misfortune. The person may fall ill or more often have an accident as a consequence of this. Children are particularly susceptible to the effect of evil eye. The Rathwas call this *Nazar Lagana.* When a spell is cast on children it is called *Bafara*. When someone comments on a child's beauty and intelligence, and if the child falls sick after this, it is blamed on the evil eye. The child usually loses its appetite and vomits out whatever it consumes. The child becomes paler and weaker too. It is not just children who suffer from the evil eye, adults suffer too. The indications are severe headache and pain in the eyes among them. When a woman faces complications during delivery or when a woman is not able to give birth at the prescribed time, all these are attributed to the vices of the evil eye. Once a woman falls under the influence of the evil eye, she might not be able to conceive for many years to come. To counteract this, a woman is gifted a *Sapan*, by her brother on Diwali. It is a black thread on which a spiral shaped silver pendant rests. It is tied on her arm or worn on the neck. Children are made to wear copper rings, called *balyut* on one of their fingers of the foots. Other means of defying the evil-eye are, applying black spots with *kohl* on the corner of the forehead of children, tying black threads etc. Chanting of mantras in the name of God, also helps. They are of the opinion that the evil eye is cast because of the envious nature of humans. It is usually done by the 'have-nots' on the 'haves'.

Magic is a morally neutral term which may be used with or without social approval. It refers to the activities or craft of the magician, a person who, suitably prepared, performs rituals aimed at controlling impersonal supernatural forces held responsible for the succession of events. In these rituals, the magician manipulates material objects and substances, often having the characteristics or origins symbolically related to the objectives desired, while reciting an appropriate verbal formula (Marwick, 1970). The following definition holds true in the form of *dakan* (a witch) in Suskal too. A *Dakan* is said to possess supernatural powers by which she causes disastrous results. The Dakan, according to the description of the tribes here, is hard to recognize as she projects the appearance of an ordinary person. But the Rathwas conceives that a *dakan* in action wears white and leaves her hair loose. A *dakan* attacks a person in order to bring misery in a family. As by nature, she is an envious person and cannot bear other's happiness and prosperity. She catches her victim at night preferably at a lonely spot. She drinks his blood, takes out his heart and in its place she fixes a chicken's or a pig's heart. The victim falls into a delirium and suffers from high fever. After a few days he expires. Acute pain in the chest is also said to be the handwork of a *dakan*. The local term used for such a chest pain in "*Dakan ne mudd mar diya hai*". *Dakans* do harm to women too, specially pregnant women and newly wed ones. Hence, the Rathwas never let pregnant women to move around alone.

The causes of disease and illness are given in naturalistic terms too by these *adivasis*. Illness and disease are personal misfortunes which people may explain in various ways. Illnesses which are considered to be "natural" may be an upset in the balance of hot and cold inside the body. Excessive work leading to headache, perspiring heavily leading to fever, unclean body giving rise to boils, dryness etc. are all attributed to natural causes. For such ailments the people either opt for home remedies or visit the village "doctor". If they are not cured, they then visit the Primary Health Centre at Jabbugaon. Visit to the herbalist also cannot be excluded.

Just as the knowledge of disease and their causes are part of a person's socialization, so are its curative systems. After the discussion on disease causation, we now shift our attention to the various availabilities of therapy and cure present in Suskal. The adivasis of Suskal, exhibit the presence of a multitude of systems ranging from home-remedies, herbalistic treatment, shamanism, snake-bite healing and of course the Primary Health Centre which provides allopathic medicine. All these systems co-exist but differ in choice patterns. In Suskal medicine defines what is normal, proper and desirable. Etiological interpretations of illness, here are representations of the world as it is experienced and comprehended by the members of a society. Here too the *adivasi* Rathwas give their own meaning to the sufferings they experience and accordingly as their mental prowess allows them search for a benefiting solution.

## Curative Measures

*Home Remedies*: As mentioned earlier, enculturation enables an individual to be knowledgeable in some rudimentary cures or attain some medical knowledge. Thus, the curative and therapeutic aspects are not just limited to the specialists but can be practiced at home as initial medical treatment. This can be called 'home remedies'. It is a section of folk medicine with a limited number of drugs which are readily prepared by housewives with materials available in the kitchen or the area surrounding the household. The importance of home remedies can be readily seen when we realize that the entire Indian population depended on them for centuries without the aid of any professional western medicine or even the codified systematized ayurveda, siddha, unani or homoeopathy (Nagla, 1997). In home remedies when illness is first experienced, it is labelled and treated by the individual (this is self-care) or more often by family members and other members of the social network. Some of the things which are used for such treatments are special foods, diets, local herbs, massage etc. Mother plays an important role in determining as well as giving the remedy for the illness to a child. The Rathwas basically make use of home remedies for illness like cold, headache, earache, fever, nausea, pain in the eyes, stomach ache, cough, difficulty in urinating etc. Easily available items like milk, ginger, garlic, red chillies, mustard oil, juice of lemon, *ajwain*, cinnamon, turmeric, black-pepper corn, dates, papaya are used in varying degrees for the preparation of different home-remedies. For example, when a person has a cold, ginger and garlic paste is made to be inhaled. Along with it water is boiled and the steam too is taken in through the nose. For fever, red chillies fried in mustard oil is to be inhaled. For cough, turmeric powder is mixed with milk and to be drunk. The Rathwas make use of a home remedy to abort a child. *Kali mari* (black-pepper corn) is mixed with gur, papaya, dates and ginger. All these when boiled together is drunk by the pregnant women and the foetus gets eliminated in the womb itself.

So it is seen that as far as possible, a physical problem is first treated in the family. If the patients do not get cured within a week, he/ she can then be referred to other medical systems.

## Folk Medicine

The folk sector of the health care system comprises non-professional, non-bureaucratized 'specialists'. Folk healing can be divided into sacred and secular subsectors, indicating its roots in both religious (e.g. Shamanism) and empirical (e.g. herbalism). The folk practitioners are part-time, non-registered practitioners functioning within the context of village organization. The folk practitioners adminster simple folk medicine and remedies to clients on a regular basis. In return they may or may not receive some form of direct or indirect remuneration.

## Herbal Treatment

Herbal medicine is a part of the medicinal institution in societies where the medical importance of plants is recognized. The treatment here is obviously done through the administration of herbs on the body. A vague idea about herbs which have curative affects are known to almost every Rathwa *adivasi* in Suskal. This knowledge has been gained either from one's own family or from the village elders. But besides the individual's knowledge of herbs, a herbal specialist by the name of Maka Bhai who resides in Suskal with a wider knowledge of this treatment through herbs and this is an essential aspect of the curative system. The local treatments administered by the Vedji (herbalist) were made available to me. Here it is important for me to mention that only the local names of the various herbs have been used as I was not able to collect their botanical names. Some of the remedies provided by Vedji Maka Bhai along with the names of the herbs and diseases are given below:

| *S.No.* | *Local Name of the Herb* | *Name of the Ailment (English/Gujarati)* | *Manner of Use* |
|---|---|---|---|
| 1. | Limra | Body Ache (*Sharir Dukhao*) | Leaves to be taken and boiled in water. To be taken thrice a day. |
| 2. | Bawar | Jaundice (*Kamra*) | Flowers of Bawar (Acacia) to be crushed, and the extract to be taken with boiled water three times a day. |
| 3. | Vel | Asthma | Leaves to be crushed and taken with water. |
| 4. | Tulsi | Vomiting (*Veti*) | Juice extracted from its leaves and to be taken with water. |
| 5. | Asopalav | For child with stomach ailments (*Pet Dukhao*) | The stem is taken and put on the abdomen. The touch of the stem provides coolness and removes the heat inside the stomach. |
| 6. | Limbu | Vomiting and heat (*ulti/garmi*) | Juice to be extracted and to be taken with water and sugar. |
| 7. | Arjun | Cough (*Khasi/Dam*) | Bark to be taken and vigorously rubbed on a stone slab. The paste formed is to be applied on the neck. |
| 8. | Bhendigare | Tooth Ache (*Daat Ma Dukhao*) | The juice extracted from the seed is to be applied on the check and the tooth. |
| 9. | Kapas | Constipation | Leaves of cotton to be mixed with castor oil and smeared over the stomach. |
| 10. | Thor | Ear Ache (*Kaan ma Dukhao*) | The juice taken out and to be put inside the ear. |

*Contd.*

| *S.No.* | *Local Name of the Herb* | *Name of the Ailment (English/Gujarati)* | *Manner of Use* |
|---|---|---|---|
| 11. | Nagni | Swollen red eyes | Juice to be extracted from the bark and to be applied on the edge of the eyes. |
| 12. | Hardera | Neck Fracture (*Mauch*) | Leaves are to be boiled and the boiled leaves are to be tied in a piece of cloth and to put it on the neck. |
| 13. | Asuro | Chest pain | Leaves to be boiled with water and to be taken. |
| 14. | Koski | Scorpion Bite | Small fresh leaves to be spread over the affected area. |
| 15. | Hawhar/Shant Hawa | Numbness of joints of leg and hands | Its branch is ground and mixed with salt and boiled water. The paste thus made is applied on the affected area. |

## Shamanism

Shamanism is another sector of folk medicine. Here folk medicine bears its roots in religious and massaging system of healing. The Shaman, like the herbalist is a part-time, non-registered practitioner. He has some other occupation (in this case agriculture) as his economic mainstay. Social recognition and prestige are the main rewards. The Shaman functions in the context of local oral folk traditional and local health culture with heavy magico-religious overtones. He knows his clients and their problems personally. The folk health system has deep roots in the local culture.

In Suskal, the role of the Shaman, locally known as *Bhua*, is confined to that of a healer. The Shaman whose name is Bharat Singh Bhai, is a young man of 30 years or so. Whenever a sick is brought to him, he either makes him lie down or sit in front of the Goddess (framed pictures that he has in the room where he operates). He then starts meditating. After a while he goes into a trance. This means that the Goddess has entered his body. The Goddess through the *Bhua* asks the victim and the family about the ailment and proclaims that only after an offering of *Sawal* (Rice), *Gehu* (Wheat), *Agarbatti* (incense), flowers and coconut is made, will the victim recover. When these ingredients are put forward, the *Bhua* takes them and revolves them around the victim's body five times in a row and then takes a broom made either out of neem leaves and branches or peacock feathers and wafts it separately for three or four times over the affected area and chants mantras. Besides chanting mantras, the *Bhua* sometimes also resorts to medicine made out of herbs. The medicines are similar to what the herbalist prescribe the only difference being the *Bhua* chants mantras over the medicine while giving it to the patient. Besides the *Bhua*, there is another person in the village who treats snake bites. He is Chandu Bhai and is a follower of *Bhateji Maharaj* (God of snakes in Gujarat). Whenever a person is bit by a snake, he/she is brought to Chandu Bhai's place. Before taking out the poison he starts meditating before *Bhateji Maharaj*. After a while *Bhateji Maharaj* enters his body and Chandu Bhai goes into a trance. Then the offerings of coconut *dhoop*, flowers etc., is given. While still in trance he takes out the poison from the victim, after which he makes the paitnet chew some neem leaves. If the patient finds the taste to be bitter, then it is regarded that the poison has left the body but if the patient does not find it bitter then the poison is considered to be still inside the body. Chandu Bhai then recommends him to the allopathic doctor.

## Allopathic Treatment and the Presence of a Primary Health Centre

The Government of India has done its bit by providing for a Primary Health Centre which is situated in Jabbugaon, 6 km away from Suskal and occupies a prime place in the health care and disease management system of Suskal. An institutionalized form of the western and modern medical system, it offers free medication to people compared to other specialists who may ask the sick or his family members to spend some money on the healing ingredients. The efforts made by the health workers and the village's link with the nearest town Bodeli has made the people start believing in the goodness of the allopathic system of cure. The female health workers along with the female health supervisor visits the village twice a week. The male health worker also accompanies them. They call the people to the *Anganbadis* or the schools and medically checks them. They also provide free immunization and advice to the villagers on family planning. The health workers encourage them to go for Leproscopy. They advice pregnant women or their diet and give lessons on the proper techniques on health and hygiene. The PHC has a staff comprising of the Medical Officer, two female Health Supervisors, one Sanitary Inspector, one Auxillary Nurse Midwife, one Male Health Worker and the Leprosy Supervisor.

The doctor at the PHC does not search for the symptoms in his patients but the patient himself/herself describes the problems. Once this is done, the doctor makes a thorough check up and accordingly prescribes medicines. Besides this, minor operations like abortions, leproscopy, delivery etc., also takes place here. Even though Suskal has a high rate of T.B. patients, the PHC does not have any facility like X-Ray machines to help the T.B. patients. This makes the people go to private hospitals in the nearby towns where they have to pay a lot. Such high expenses in treatment makes them stick to their age old local healing facilities. True, allopathic medicine provides instant relief but non-availability of medicines at times, absence of provisions, distrust among villagers for orally examining women etc. makes it a safer bet to visit the herbalist or the *Bhua*.

In this portion I include a brief discussion on women and their known gynaecological problems in Suskal. Here I try to probe into the various disorders and the causes for such ailments. The causal explanations given by the women and the remedies availed have been taken note of.

Over-work and stress affect women's health and that of their families. The net effect of the cultural, social and economic, biases that women suffer from are reflected in their excessive mortality, poor health, inadequate access to health care and medical services and increasing gap between men and women in literacy (Usharao, 1993). This difference is much wider in rural/tribal societies. In such societies moreover, parents wish to marry off their daughters as soon as they attain puberty. Traditional practices regarding marriage and the status of the daughter-in-law in the household along with the practices associated with pregnancy, child birth, lactation, fertility control and health care utilization, further aggravate the health impairment of women. The situation in Suskal is no different where women work as peasants and housewives and yet are not given any respite. These women carry huge responsibilities which prevent them from spending time on their health. "Maternal and child health service in India are very poorly developed. Only 40-50 per cent of the pregnant women at present receive antenatal care, less than 15 per cent are delivered by trained birth attendants, only about 20 per cent receive tetanus toxoid and some 30 per cent are covered by the nutritional supplement programme" (Usharao, 1983).

Repeated pregnancy, short birth intervals and pregnancies occurring at the extremes of reproductive age and lack of family planning practices are responsible for unfavourable outcome in mothers and children. Many women in Suskal do not practice family planning because of high infant mortality, the social custom to have sons to foster the family tree and fear of desertation by husband and family members. The role of illegally induced abortions, in case of maternal death is well recognized in this group but difficult to prove because of the secrecy surrounding abortion as a cause of death and lack of data. As mentioned earlier these *adivasis* are married off immediately after their menarche and she enters the new household as yet another labour hand. These women work in the fields, do all the domestic chores and look after the needs of their husbands and in-laws. The heavy tasks assigned to them have a significant toll on their health. Pregnancy at an early age and lack of adequate diet, makes them weak and feeble.

In Suskal, most women are found to suffer from sterility, the reason being the frequent occurrence of white discharge after the onset of the first menstrual periods. Other than this, the women also suffer from Reproductive Tract Infection (RTI), Dysfunctional Uterine Bleeding (DUB), Pelvic Inflammatory Disease (PID), Anaemia etc. Along with these, the disorders related to menstruation like menstrual cramps (*Masik me Dukhao*), irregular menses (*animit masik*) and heavy menstrual flow (*Satar masik*) are also quite common. Though I have named these disorders, they have been in reality collected from the doctor's records at the PHC and the women themselves do not realize that they are victims of such malicious diseases. They do not understand the complications connected with such disorders and since every other women in the village have one of these disorders, they feel it is nothing to worry about. They go about their daily routine without much thought about their personal health and hygiene. Like the case of DUB, the women think of it as eating of hot and spicy food leading to bleeding for which they immediately either resort to home remedies or go to the herbalist. The state of pregnancy is not taken as something that would require complete rest throughout the gestation period. A pregnant woman carries out all her daily activities (heavy and light) without any thought of the baby inside and its care. In fact hard work during pregnancy is considered to be a sign of good health by the people of Suskal. It is only during the last week of pregnancy that a woman is confined to rest.

Here I mention some of the local remedies followed by the women for ailments about which they have no scientific understanding:

1. For white discharge which they call *Safed Pani* or *Wakhul*, roots of *Meori* are dried and made into powder which is then consumed with water.
2. For a burning feeling during urination (*Jalan*) the roots of *Khar Vindu* are ground and the juice thus extracted is applied at the area where the sensation occurs.
3. To stop bleeding from the uterus, juice of *Thikri* is extracted from the root which is taken with water.
4. For abortion (which is of course not any disorder, but done to curb unwanted children), seeds of *Deveri* are taken and the upper layer of the seeds are removed and swallowed with milk.
5. For excessive bleeding during menstruation, the bark of *Ashok* tree is boiled and the juice extracted is administered on the patient once or twice daily but not while menstruating.
6. For painful menstruation, ten grams of the root of *Ulat Kambal* is ground with two pepper corns and one betel leaf. The mixture is given with water when the pain occurs.
7. The juice of the stem of *Thikri* is given with water twice during the day to women suffering from irregular menses.

Along with these remedies, the visit to the *Bhua* and the PHC is not to be forgotten which is done when these medicines do not have any effect on the body or these medicines may be used when they are not satisfied with the *Bhua* or allopathic medicines.

**Conclusion**

In Suskal, ethnomedicine has an enduring and indispensable part in the social life of the Rathwa *adivasis*. I have made an attempt here to discuss how much the traditional means of healing has an influence over the modern (or western) medical system which is of course a late entry. I have talked about the various medical system available in the village, their integration and the changes which have taken place in the set of medical beliefs and practices as a consequence of changes occurring in the social system, as a whole. In Suskal, we see the presence of a multitude of systems ranging from home remedies, herbalistic treatment, Shamanism, Snake-Bite healing and of course the Primary Health Centre which provides allopathic medicine. All these systems co-exist but differ in choice patterns. Medicine in Suskal, defines what is normal, proper and desirable. Etiological interpretations of illness here are representations of the world as experienced and comprehended by the members of a society. In Suskal disease causation is attributed to the wrath by Goddesses, ghosts, witches and by natural means also. They are scared by the supernatural powers and hence try to remain in harmony with such powers. These they do by observing taboos and making regular offerings to the strength which symbolizes their Gods. For the adivasis of Suskal, witch craft exists because of the universal vice, jealousy. The Rathwas believe that, people are envious of one another's progress and time and again try to inflict miseries in the form of illness with the help of magical performances. On the basis of the theories of disease causation, there are a variety of therapeutic practices available. Thus accordingly the *Bhua* is present to curb off diseases which arise due to the infliction of the "evil eye" or "ghost intrusion". Similarly for ailments like cough or cold, remedies like turmeric mixed with milk is recommended. The villagers have great faith in the herbalist who is called *Vedji*. It is not only the medicines which brings the Rathwas close to the different specialists, but it is also due to the psychological effect, they have on the patients.

Besides the supernatural reasons, the life style of the Rathwas which is exhibited in the form of poor sanitary habits, lack of cleanliness and unhygienic conditions are responsible for the prevalence of disease among them. Though they are aware that the germs and dirt can cause illness, they are careless about basic things and thus do not bother about cleanliness. Moreover, they would rather attribute their discomforts and sufferings to paranormal wickedness than to their own doings.

Lack of education and acute poverty combined with a detachment with the "real" world has made the way the Rathwas are today. Though the government has done the "needful" by placing a Primary Health Centre, where the health workers, try their best to educate men and women alike on the basic concepts of hygiene, cleanliness, proper diet consisting of nutritious food, there is still a long way to go. The health workers meet the men and women at the *Aanganbadis* and schools and many a times visit their homes too. The PHC has even introduced the concept of trained mid-wives who are instructed to help women live a clean and disease free life. The mid-wives do their best to educate women on pregnancy, problems related to pregnancy, child care, family planning etc. But such attempts have highly remained unsuccessful as for example instead of understanding that dirt and germs may cause ill-health in a child, the Rathwas would rather blame it on a "evil-eye" and resort to amulets, *tabeez*, or black *kohl* applied on the forehead. The ideas about causation of disease by paranormal means have become ingrained in the minds of the Rathwas as they have been socialized to believe so. Socialization is a vital part of growing up and is thus almost impossible to shun away such deeply rooted beliefs from one's thought process. The confusions about which medical system to visit will remain with the *adivasis* as long as they do not remove the suspicions regarding western medicine or the fear of being punished by supernatural powers for their deeds. Along with these the indigenous healers, obviously consider the existence of the PHC a threat to their survival. Their wish to stay in control of the naïve *adivasis* lives makes them bad mouth the western form of medicine. The presence of herbal medicine is of course of great importance and its healing powers can never be denied but treatments provided by the *Bhua* in the form of magico-religious rituals has in reality no positive effect on the Rathwas though they would like to believe otherwise.

From the above discussion, it is seen that religious beliefs, superstitions and magic play an important role in the lives of the Rathwas of Suskal. The presence of various curative systems show the existence of medical pluralism, though in different degrees. The allopathic system of medicine is making its entry felt though at a low pace. Education is much needed in this society and which has to make an impact on erase them for a hygienic life. In the times to come, with changes in the society which may be due to economic upliftment and education, the traditional folk medicine will hopefully merge with the bio-medical system and thus provide a continuity in change.

## REFERENCES

Jaggi, O.P. (1982), *Folk Medicine,* Atma Ram and Sons. Lucknow.

Landy, David. (ed.) (1977), *Culture, Disease and Healing; Studies in Medical Anthropology,* Macmillan, New York.

Marwick, Max. (ed.) (1970), *Witchcraft and Sorcery,* Penguin Books, Great Britain.

Nagla, Madhu. (1997), *Sociology of Medical Profession,* Rawat Publications, Jaipur.

Usharao, N.J. (1983), *Women in a Developing Society,* Ashish Publishing House, Delhi.

19

# Healing Practices amongst the Gaddi Tribe of Himachal Pradesh

SONIA KAUSHAL

## Introduction

"Health is of universal interest and concern." (Forest Clements) All human societies not withstanding the scale of development have a concept of what makes a healthy living as well as conception of illness. According to Mukherjee and Nandy (1986:274), health is not only the result of interaction between an individual's hereditary contribution with his natural and cultural environment but it is largely determined by the biological and cultural adaptation and evolution of the society and the population. In fact, health and illness are two polar words. World Health Organsation (WHO) gave a utopian definition of Health as "a state of complete physical, mental and social well-being and not mere absence of disease or infirmity". Landy (1977) defined a state of health as "the condition of an organism that permits it to adapt to its environmental situation with relative minimal pain and discomfort, achieve at least some physical and psychic gratification and possess a reasonable probability of survival." While on the other hand a state of disease according to Landy "is a condition of the organism that seriously obtrudes against these adaptive requirements and causes or behavioural dysfunction". Every society has cultural objective to prove whether or not there is a case of illness and whether or not individual is healthy.

Tribes are relatively isolated and autonomous groups. They have their own cultural system and medical system is one of the important system of tribal society. The tribal social structure has its own structural and ethnic specificity and the disease that inflict upon the tribals are likewise specific to the attribute of their social structure. The knowledge of disease, their classification and etiology is a part of their cultural system and they develops methods and ways of curing the diseases.

In tribal societies, health, disease and medicine is inextricably linked to the area of social relationships and to the magico-religious world. Physical diseases, psychic disorders and even death are mostly, thought of as the result of personal hatred and as having been affected through the intervention of spirits, ghosts, gods or other forces belonging to collective belief. Only a few types of illnesses, disturbances and death are viewed as being independent of human responsibility or supernatural agency. In tribal societies, "Health is not an isolated phenomenon, but part of the magico-religious fabric of existence", and of the social, ethical, and cosmic equilibrium. "Disease is considered as a disequilibrium in the body as well as in society" (Appiah-Kubi, 1981, pp. 2,14). Such diseases are cured by magico religious healers.

In tribal societies, system of cure is not only based on magico-religious means but also on plants. Tribal people have a developed pharmacopoeia and some rudimentary knowledge of medical techniques at individual level. Both these techniques, i.e. magico-religious and herbal medicine are used to cure sick either together or separately. People have knowledge about the plants in their surroundings and also attribute cultural beliefs and practices to the plants.

Thus, medicine in tribal societies address both supernatural and empirical theories of disease. It includes various systems of medicines—herbal, supernatural, home-remedies and even surgical methods.

The social structural practices of tribals put some sort of implications towards the concept of health. It acts as a preventive medicine. Thus, many practices like avoidance of the house in which a death has occurred, distinction of hot and cold food and hiding of bodily waste for fear of their being used by witches and sorcerers, serve hygienic purposes.

As tribal communities are insulated from the impact of wider world, there is every probability that it would have its own medical system. But in the contemporary world, tribal societies giving way to the outside world and other medical systems. It may not be possible to find a community thriving on its own medical system with no impact of the western bio-medicine. There has been a wider spread of western medical system but at the same time, indigenous system still co-exist with deep rooted belief in curing and giving possible explanation behind the cause of disease and illness.

In this paper an attempt has been made to focus upon the disease causation and healing practices of Gaddi tribe of Himachal Pradesh.

## The *Gaddi*: Disease and Cure

The Gaddi is one of the tribe of Himachal Pradesh and according to 1991 census, their population is 86,511. The *Gaddi* is the generic term used for all the indigenous population who live in the Chamba and Kangra district of Himachal Pradesh. The largest bulk of the population lives in Bharmour tehsil of Chamba district and few are scattered in Kangra district. The abode of *Gaddi* is popularly known as *Gaderan*—the home of Gaddis. They follow Hinduism with special emphasis on *Shiva* and *Shakti*. The land they inhabit is also known as *Shiv-Bhumi*. The language spoken by them is *Bharmauri Gadiali* which falls under the Indo-Aryan family and its *pahari* sub-family. Their script is known as *tantrik*. Occupationally, Gaddis are agriculturists, it is the primary source of their livelihood. They are also transhumant and own large flocks of sheeps and goats, as a subsidiary occupation.

The Chamba district is situated in the alpine pastoral zone between north latitude of 32°–10' and 33°–13' and east latitude 77°–55'. The whole region is mountainous and remains under snow cover for about 5-6 months. The community occupies the inaccessible, inhospitable terrain. It is a high altitude area and remains cut off most of the time because of heavy snowfall. The area has thick and dense forest with low rainfall and low humidity.

## Common Diseases

Such a physical environment poses a severe challenge to the Gaddis and also affect their health. The common disease prevalent among them are: goiter, venereal diseases and all types of leprosy. The staple diet of the people is maize and due to this indigestion and bowel-complaints are common. Symptoms of malnutrition, especially pallegra and night blindness are common due to deficiency of vitamin B and vitamin A, respectively. Other diseases are chest diseases such as tuberculosis, pneumonia, etc. Eye infections, rheumatic infection and skin diseases, anaemia, diarrhoea, dysentery, small pox, cholera are also common.

## Supernatural Disease Causation and Treatment

The seeking of the causes of disease is an almost universal trait and the *Gaddi* believe in supernatural cause of illness. Sickness and disease amongst them is thought to be punishment inflicted by deity a form of in some cases and in others, it is seen as a result of an evil consequence. *Gaddi* have profound faith in disease caused by *dayans*, spirits, ghosts, etc. To satiate them, offerings and sacrifices are made to respective spirits and deities.

## Illness Caused by Spirits, Ghosts and their Treatment

### *Autars*

The Gaddis believe in spirits whom they seek to propitiate by sacrifices. They are known as *autars* (or ancestral spirits), which means spirits raised to the level of local deities. The spirit of a deceased person who died childless is worshipped as *autars*. It is regarded as malignant spirit causing illness but thoughtful enough to warn people in their dreams of any impending disaster.

To propitiate *autars* appearing in dreams and threating death, *jemanwala* is performed with offerings made four times at night, of *ghunganian* (four balls), nettle baths and bran bread. The sick person dons clothes which are made for the spirit, with a silver image of the dead and then worships the *autars* idol, which is always set up near any stream and a he-goat is sacrificed. In order to ward of evil eye, the children also wear similar images. *Autars* are also propitiated on *puranmasi* and the *amawas* days.

### *Kailung*

*Kailu Bir* or *kailung* is believed to be a demon causing abortion. Kailung is propitiated in the form of *darat* (or sickle). To propitiate him, the woman puts 4 copper coins along with her necklace invoking the name of the *kailung*. Two or three months after the delivery, the mother and the *purohit* worships and offer sacrifice to the demon by putting up a large stone under a *kointh* (or walnut).

### *Gunga*

*Gunga* is an equally menancing spirit but attacks only animals. It is a disease-spirit of cow and when it attacks, they fall ill. It is believed that it is a very powerful demon.

*Gunga* is propitiated by settling aside a *tawa* of bread in its name. A piece of iron is made and thus the deity is taken into the cattle shed where it is worshipped by the sacred fire, on Thursday. A he-goat is sacrificed and some drops are sprinkled on the iron. Some cakes and sweets are served to the family members, while the rest are burried. *Gunga* is worshipped every fourth year.

### *Super Natural Agencies*

Apart from abôve spirits, the Gaddis believe in super natural agencies like *Joginis* (the rock spirit), *Rakshanis, Banasats, Chungu* (the demon inhabiting on walnut tree or mulberry tree and under the *Karangarh* Shrub), Naags, Sidhas, Devis, Birs, respectively.

### *Devo Sanskars*

Gaddis are very particular about observing what they call *Devo Sanskars* (rituals connected with the spirits of the dead), lest they haunt their living relations and can cause illness and other misfortunes to them. To please them, small houses are built on the village outskirts called *bangalands*, and the spirits are supposed to live there quietly.

## Illness Caused by Magicians and their Treatment

### *Magic*

Like other tribes, the Gaddis believe in magic. It is believed by Gaddis that human beings are also instigator of disease through magic. According to them *dayans* (witches), *chellas*, black-magicinas, who has knowledge of manipulating the power and know the other objects used in causing illness. People take help of them to harm others or they use their magic to harm others. There are four types of magic:

(a) *Vashikaran*: The patient's eyes become as that of an owl's and he cannot speak.

(b) *Maran*: Poison is given to a person through magic for killing him.

(c) *Contagious*: A part of a animal is carried to acquire its characteristics or as a protection against it.

(d) *Others*: To make anybody a leper or a skeleton.

### *Witchcraft*

The *dayan,* according to Gaddis, masquerade in the disguise of women during the day. They leave their abode at night and put their broom-sticks in their place and cast the spell on their family members, so that they may not become aware of the *dayans* departure. The *dayan* rides on *garur*, lion or *mrig* and flies away and assemble in a forest, where they dance and sing throughout the night but return to their home before the people are awake.

If a *dayan* wants to kill a person, she flies to a *jot* or *dhar* and brings some herb with her. Then, she feeds the herb to the person she wants to harm and the person becomes ill. If such person is not treated in time by a *chella,* he dies of an unknown disease. The *dayans* are considered very dangerous by the community.

To counter their spell, there is a supernatural witch doctor, *gardi chella* possessing powers. He worships almost every God. He cures those patients who are afflicted by black magic or witchery. The *doli* (the patient) gather at his residence for treatment. He begins by playing *dupatara* (a stringed instrument) to the beat of a drum. Meanwhile, he throws a small shell, cowrie towards the *doli* who fall in trance and start dancing. At the end, *chella* discloses the name of the *dayan* who gave him *booti* (herb). Then, *chella* ask patient to dip their palm and feet into a bucket full of water, while his body is dusted by *mor-mutha* (peacock's feathers). As a result, some dust, hair, thread, etc. come out of the patient's body and fall in the bucket of water. This process continues for a week, till the *doli* recovers his health.

### *Mani*

Illness is also said to be brought on by burying some objects—a tuft of hair, *dhoor* (soil) of the dead or an effigy of *satisaryan* (turmeric) over which spell has been cast—in the house of enemy with the help of magician. Due to this, all the family members fall sick. To cast away this evil, a ceremony is held. The *chella* keeps a *mani* (a wooden pot) in the house. Some neighbours are collected around it and a *kangana* (red thread) is tied on the wrist of one of them and then the *mani* is put into his *kangana* tied hand. The *chella* chants the mantras and scatter the grains of rice or *mah* around. The man with *mani* starts moving and fetches the man to that place where spell was cast. This action is performed for three times. The *chella* asks the people to dig the floor, where the *mani* turned down and thus the buried articles are found and dugout.

## Magico-Religious Treatment for other Ailments

### *Stomachache*

A patient with stomachache is treated by the *chella,* who gives a thread to the patient after chanting some mantras, for wearing around neck. Purified *dhoor* is also given to the patient.

### *Fever, Backache and Snake Bite*

For fever, backache and snake bite, the *chella* waves the *bhang* plant over the patient with chanting of mantras.

### *Small Pox*

In order to recover from small pox, people pledge *manauti* to *Shitla Mata* and they offer *akhi* to the goddess after cure. The *chella* waves the *bhang* plant over the head of the patient and a *dhuni* consisting of *Harmala, satisaryan* and *mithi dhup* is offered. Prayers are also observed in her praise.

## Natural Remedial and Curative Practices

In addition to such magico-religious practices, *gaddis* also make use of their knowledge of home remedial practices and surgical treatment to cure diseases.

## The Disease and their homely Treatment

| *Name of the disease* | *Indigenous Name* | *Treatment* |
|---|---|---|
| Cough | *Khang* | The maize cob after removing the grains is reduced to ashes and administered in small doses. |
| Stomach ache | *Petepeer* | A brew of powdered *ajwain*, sump and common salt is prepared. A pinch of sugar or *bura* is added and given to the patient. |
| Fever | *Tap* | *Choti ilayachi* and *ajwain* are boiled and given to the patient. |
| Backache | *Dake peer* | The affected portion is massaged with warm mustard oil. Then a lump of salt heated in the fire is wrapped in some old clothes and the concerned part is fomented with it. |
| Snake-bite | *Kira dank* | The *lim* is tied tightly with a black woollen string above the bite. Sometimes the effected portion is also cut. |
| Anaemia | *Lizsa* | *Vaidya* or doctor is consulted. |
| Eye itching | *Chippad* | *Rasaut* is rubbed into water or milk applied inside the affected eye. |
| Dyspepsia | *Kabj* | *Summaken, trij, pesori gulab* and *khand* are mixed up and boiled. Thereafter the juice called *duchhandu* or *Kadhu* is given to the patients. |
| Diarrhoea | *Jangal* | *Belgiri* is grinded and given to the patient after mixing up the same with *khand*. |
| Dysentry | *Marore* | *Dodas* or *happu* (opium) are boiled in water and *kadhu* is prepared. Thereafter it is given to the patient. |
| Scorpion sting | *Bichchu Dank* | Iron is touched on the affected portion. |
| Small pox | *Mata Dhammi* | No medicine. Only precautions are taken. |
| Cholera | *Haija* | *Chhoti ilayachi, soya* and *podina* is mixed up with *khand* and boiled in water. Thereafter it is given to the patient. |
| V.D. | *Firang* | This disease is rare in this region. However, if anybody falls victim of this disease, he consults the doctor for treatment. |

## The Surgical Techniques of the Gaddis

| *What for?* | *Techniques* |
|---|---|
| Bleeding from a wound | *Gudar* (cotton) is burnt into fire and prepared *dhor* from it and is pasted on a wound. Thus the bleeding from a wound is stopped. |
| To cure a broken bone | The broken bones are kept in joint form and the *phun chaks* (bamboo pieces) are placed around the affected part. There after a *patti* is rolled on it. It is untied after 3rd day, then one week and so on and again tied after examining the limb. |
| To cure a wound | (1) Turmeric is applied over the wound. (2) Sometimes pepers are grinded with mustard oil and applied to effected part. |
| Eye's operation | No technique. Doctors are consulted. |
| Teeth removing | Some local dentist, if available, removes the teeth from mouth with help of a *jamura* (an instrument). |
| To operate a boil | When the boil becomes yellow, they operate it with *kard*, a type of knife. Thereafter some solution is applied to the part. |

## Conclusion

The Gaddis of Himachal Pradesh believe in disease caused by spirits, *dayans,* and deities. To propitiate them, they often sacrifice animals for the deities and spirits, and worship these deties. They also use talismans and observe certain taboos to avert the ill-effect of evil-spirits. Besides this, they put nature into use such as medicinal herbs, roots, etc. for curing purposes. The Gaddis also have good knowledge of surgical treatment. Medical facilities are also made available to them by the government which they accept and utilize with willingness but the presence of these medical facilities does not improve their health because they are very scarce and out of reach. To avail medical facilities they have to travel long distances, as the area occupied by *gaddis* is highly undulated. Doctors, nurses and other health providers are not much interested in working in such areas. Besides this, area remains covered with snow for almost 4-5 months which results into meagre transportation and communication, which directly affect the medical facilities provided to them. Thus, the Gaddis of Himachal Pradesh are left with no choice but to rely upon their own indigenous medical system. At the same time, their indigenous medical system is 'hope-generating' and the explanation of disease causation given by them falls within their world view and they look for the cultural answers and solutions of such cxplanations.

## REFERENCES

Balgir, R.S., (1995), Environmental constraints, Health and Population Trends among the Muslim Gujjars of Himachal Pradesh, India, *J. Human, Ecol*; 6(3): 191-196.

Bhasin, Veena, M.K. Bhasin and Indera P. Singh, (1991), Ecology, Culture and Development: Gaddis and Pangwals of Himachal Pradesh, *J, Hum Ecol*, 2(3):253-302.

Channa, S.M. (ed), (2002), *Encyclopedia of Religion: Health and the Super Natural Diseases and Cure in Tribal Society*, India: Cosmo Publication, Vol. 11.

Clement, Forest, (1932), *Primitive Concepts of Diseases*, University of California Publications in American Archeology and Ethnology, 32.

Gupta, S.K., V.P. Sharma and N.K. Sharda (ed), (1998), *Tribal Development—Appraisal and Alternatives*, New Delhi: Indus Publishing Company.

Jerath, Ashok, (1995), *The Splendour of Himalaya Art and Culture*, New Delhi: Indus Publishing Company.

Joshi, P.C. and Anil Mahajan (ed.) (1990), *Studies in Medical Anthropology*, New Delhi: Reliance Publishing House.

Kakar, D.N., (1977), *Folk and Modern Medicine*, New Delhi: New Asian Publication.

Kayastha, S.L. (1964), *The Himalayan Beas-Basun: A Study in Habitat, Economy and Society, Varanasi.*

Lamba, Rajni and Shalini Mehta (1995), Priorities in Indian Medicine: A Tribal Perspective, *Indian Anthropologist*; 25: (2)-12.

Landy, David (ed), (1977), *Culture, Disease and Healing: Studies is Medical Anthropology*, New York: Macmillan Press Ltd.

Mandal, Hrisikesh, Sumit Mukherjee and Archana Datta, (2002), *Anthropological Survey of India*, New Delhi: Caps Micrographics (P) Ltd.

Paul, B.D. (ed), (1995), *Health, Culture and Community*, New Delhi: Russel Sage Foundation.

Shashi, S.S., (1977), *The Gaddi Tribe of Himachal Pradesh: A Sociological Study*, New Delhi: Sterling Publication (P) Ltd.

Verma, V., (1996), *Gaddis of Dhauladhar: A transhumant tribe of the Himalaya*, New Delhi: Indus Publishing Company.

# 20

# Stress due to the Modern Work Schedule : Problems and Management—A Case among Gonds

ANIMA SHARMA

---

In the present trends of modernization the work conditions are also becoming more demanding. The competition is cut throat; hence there is emphasis upon specialization, learning skills and high goals. Unless one performs well, he could be thrown out of the race at any moment. The performance pays back or not is a debatable issue because it is directly related to one's expectations and ambitions, but in the process, the price we pay for achieving it comes as a very late realization. The higher we rise in the ladder of success, lonelier and greedier we become. It becomes a vicious cycle from which there is no escape. This often leads to several types of social, psychological and health related problems.

With the encroachment of modernization, the job conditions and job situations *vis-à-vis* socio-economic aspects are also changing in the tribal areas. They may not be at par with the urban world in terms of professionalism but they are also undergoing a great deal of change and having experiences of different kinds. On the one hand they have to leave their traditional modes of earning and on the other the new jobs have brought change in their socio-cultural life. This has affected them psychologically too. The interesting thing about stress is that it means different things to different people. We may share common physical reactions to stress-muscle tension and rapid breathing, for example, but what one person finds exciting may leave another person frightened. You may say that, in some ways, stress can be a state of mind.

## The Area and Population

The present study includes various primary and secondary sources of information. For the Primary data collection Interview method was adopted. The survey done by MIND, a Mental Health Charitable Society was taken as the standard because its validity is accepted worldwide.

A two months long social anthropological fieldwork was carried out during 2002 to collect the primary data. The sample selected for the present study comprised of 75 Gonds (tribal) working as labourers in the villages of District Narsinghpur and 75 urban people working in government and private offices in Jabalpur.

The reports appearing in various journals, newspapers and on the Internet were used for the secondary data.

## The Data Collection Tools

The Primary data was collected by using interview method. After establishing the rapport a number of questions were asked and some of the questions were reformulated and simplified on the spot for the convenience of the respondents and to get the information. The observation went on simultaneously to note down the behavioural components.

The thrust was to know if the respondent thinks that he is satisfied by whatever he is getting in his own way. Does he think that whatever he is getting is in proportion to what he deserves? Is his earning sufficient for him and his family? Is he able to spent enough time with his family and children? Can he express his ideas freely at workplace or does he work under any obligation or fear? Has joining the job brought any change in his social or personal life?

These and other related questions were explored at length.

## The Reasons of Stress

There have been a number of factors observed which may cause stress to an individual. These factors vary from person to person and from one situation to another but the universality of the stress at workplace and due to work itself cannot be denied. The often cited reasons include too much of information or may be lack of information. Too much information confuses one in the matter of selection while lack of information deprives him of several opportunities even at an arm's distance. The timed schedules sets ones nerves always at a wreaking point, which has effects (often ill-effects) on his overall mental and physical health. The stress thus caused slows the recovering process at the time of illness and the person is not able to give enough time to recover completely. Not only that the monotone at the workplace also rides on one's nerves and he finds himself in a circle from where he sees no way out or respite.

## The Danger Signs due to Stress

Stress is a slow killer, which often gets manifested when it is already too late. But, it has a trail of silent yet overt symptoms, which if diagnosed in time may prevent from a greater loss in the terminal stage. As mentioned in TOI, Sunday Magazine dated March 18, 2001; these symptoms are indeed the danger signs, which are broadly divided into three categories. These are:

- *Psychological*: Irritability, Anxiety, Defensiveness, Anger, and Feeling of helplessness, Sadness.
- *Physical*: Muscle Aches, Falling Ill Frequently, Headaches, Grinding Teeth, and Clenched Jaws.
- *Behavioural*: Impatience, Withdrawal from others, Overeating or loss of Appetite.

## Work Place Stresses Common to the Tribal as well as a City Dweller

In spite of the fact that a tribal may not be working in a very technically sophisticated and much advanced work environment, the stress conditions affecting his personal and professional life are more or less the same. The degree of intensity with which they realize it may be different but its presence cannot be waived off completely. Various studies have shown that the types of stresses include: Anxiety, Depression, and Insomnia; Job Problems and Job Pressures; Marital or Relationship Problems; Family Problems and Financial Worries; Self Worth Problems; Burnout and Personal Health Problems; Communication Problems at Work or at Home; Anger Management and Hopelessness or Helplessness.

These types are common for all the working human beings in every part of the globe. So we can say that "Mental Health Problems Are Common At Work Place..."

## The Data Collection

Mind, the mental health charity, conducted a survey. Its results are given below:

Mind questioned 1,500 people and found that 61 per cent of people believed work stress was the main cause of mental problems from depression to severe illness. Loneliness was thought to be a common factor by 59 per cent of people, followed by bereavement (55%), traumatic events (52%), and the demands of modern life (50%) and relationship problems (50%).

The Primary data shows that: 66 per cent urban and 45 per cent tribals blamed work stress as the main cause of mental problems, 55 per cent urbanites complained of loneliness being the reason, but among the tribals this concept was not found relevant. For bereavement and traumatic events were quite comparable that is 52 per cent and 53 per cent among both. Similarly, 52 per cent urbanites and 35 per cent tribals found modern ways of life responsible for these diseases. 46 per cent urban and 28 per cent tribals identified relationship problems.

### *Findings*

It can be concluded that:

- The high-pressure environment of the modern work place is fuelling widespread problems with mental health.
- More people blame stress at work for problems with mental health than any other cause.
- People believe job problems are more likely to cause mental illness than marriage breakdown, bereavement or loneliness. However, among tribals the network of social relationships is such that loneliness is not the identifying characteristics.
- Similarly in Indian social set up bereavement and traumatic

events are found to leave similar effects on the psyche of the people irrespective of their place of residence.

### *Few Specific Stresses Identified during the Interviews*

This survey data showed that there are several common stressors for the tribal and city dwellers. Yet there are few stressors specific for each group.

For city dwellers, working in the stringent network of professionalism the most common problems causing stress came out to be time pressure and deadlines and kid's education.

For tribals this list of problems is little longer including, cultural uprootment and change in life style, exploitation due to ignorance, lack of information and guidelines and lack of proper training for skilled or unskilled labour.

### *Few Stresses Where both are Working Together*

At the common workplaces for both the groups few more factors emerge out which cause disparity in goals and achievements between them and become the cause of stress for the weaker group, here the tribal. The conceptual literature on stress suggests that tribal people are prone to the same stressors as experienced by city dwellers. Yet, they are also confronted with potentially unique stressors such as discrimination, stereotyping, social isolation, and work/home conflicts. They face segregation at the work place due to socio-cultural and ethnic reasons and also barriers to career progress because of the same reasons. These also push them into the vicious cycle of stress.

### *Few Suggestions to Learn How to Avoid the Stress of Work*

Though stress management is a highly technical field and lie within the domain of the Clinical Psychologists. They use various sensitive techniques to make people able to come out of this cycle and to learn the ways in which they can combat with their conditions in a healthy way without getting affected or victimized by it. Still, without challenging or interfering with their area yet drawing inference from their experiences here are few suggestions for the stress management,

- Tap into renewed vigour and productivity.

- Time management skills come from the process. Good time management is critical, but normal time management techniques add to your workload instead of relieving it. Poor time management skills is a symptom NOT a cause of problems
- Learning how to work with information in an organized manner increases your productivity and stress is eliminated. But, steps should be carved out to work with too much information.
- By learning to work effectively you increase your value in the world, significant amounts of self-induced stress is eliminated. You feel better, and achieve more.
- Work-related stress could be reduced by learning to recognize stress.

## Exercises to Manage Stress

It is always beneficial to follow a healthy routine and begin your day with few physical exercises, which keep you active and agile throughout the day. There are few more exercises which could be done at any time and place according to the convenience. The following exercises are designed to help change a stressful frame of mind into a calm, peaceful one:

A. Meditation
B. Daydream Away
C. A Stress-Less Frame Of Mind

## Some More Attempts to Reduce Stress

The need of stress management would be half met of those are carried out at personal level only. There should be advocacy to reduce the basic reasons, which cause individual stress. If the reasons of stresses are cured at its origin then it would be great attempt to check it from becoming an epidemic. At work place if equity is promoted, pay conditions are made justified, occupational segregation is not observed, the rigidity of performance evaluation system is reduced, equal opportunities are provided then much of the load of stress would be eliminated from the lives of the people. These are but few basic requirements, which need immediate and appropriate attention of the state and the people.

In the concluding remark I would like to add briefly that the stress is an inseparable part of the lives of the individuals. Some amount of stress is necessary to keep the ongoingness and productivity of the system. But, it assumes a threatening position when it starts riding on one's nerves to an extent that not only his performance gets affected but his discretion and decision making also gets affected. Then it needs serious consideration and societal intervention to combat with the situation. In today's fast paced, dog-eat-dog corporate life, high stress levels can assume alarming proportions. This makes it imperative that companies approach this problem in a healthy manner and organize stress management programmes to boost morale and increase productivity. Such programmes are common in West and implementing it here would only help develop positive lifestyle changes.

21

# Bon Medicine among Monpas in Western Arunachal Pradesh

ATSUKO IBATA

## Introduction

Not only practitioners of biomedicine, it is commonplace in this side of the 'modern world' to assume biomedicine as essentially and exclusively 'true' in theory and practice, their 'science' which professes the cellular, biochemical basis of pathology. Hence anything that is said or done by a professional practitioner of contemporary orthodox medicine is assigned to 'scientific' culture of 'biomedicine ' that culture is seen indeed a dominant and all encompassing (Atkinson 1995:28). Thus traditional unorthodox medicine is assigned here to be 'scientific' to secure a room in the 'modern' culture.

In recent years, however, anthropologists of medicine have attempted to characterize contemporary medicine as a cultural system (Atkinson 1995:21). Thus for the most recent anthropological studies, biomedicine is itself an ethnomedicine. It is 'the pre-eminent professional ethnomedicine of Western cultures' (Gaines and Hahn, 1985:18,n.1) , although anthropologists began by defining the scope of their interest as ethnomedicine and originally excluded biomedicine from that categorization ( Atkinson 1995;21).

As Gains and Hahn articulates (1985;3), anthropological and medical critics have been struck by the reductionism which excludes alternatives and which asserts biological universalism and individualism which ignore, if not deny, basic anthropological understandings which see cultural and social forces as wellspring of human behavior, including healing and suffering (Gains and Hahn,1985;3). Arnold (1988:18) also delineates in same manner in relation to medicine in European colonies, 'seeing it as rational, scientific and universalistic, western medicine defined itself in opposition to the presumed irrationality and superstition of indigenous medicine. The customs and beliefs of the people were treated as obstacles to overcome, obscurantism to be brushed aside by the new scientific age' (Collins 1999: 182-183).

Therefore to have a garb of 'scientific' seems to be the only left solution for the 'obstacles' in this perspective to avoid being labeled as 'uncivilized'. This force of knowledge colonization and the rhetoric of biomedical supremacy may be persuasive because it forms part of larger discourse which has dominated Western thinking since the birth of the industrial era (Gordon 1988)—a discourse which assures by means of accurate observation and rational deduction human beings can attain an objective knowledge of the nature of reality that will enable us to predict and control nature (Lupton 1994:87).

Modern medicine appeals to the dominant social institutions and imagery of 'science' is a source of legitimacy, probity and integrity. Important to the legitimating of science, in contrast to religious and other systems of knowledge, its procedure are regarded as objective and value free. The conduct of objectivity, as sociologist Will Wright (1992:23) has explained, gives science a 'desperate privilege', so that in Western societies, knowledge is virtually equated with the achievements of science.

While other systems are constructed as other by being treated (by social scientists, biomedical practitioner) as 'folk' 'ethno' 'alternative' 'unorthodox' 'quack' and so on, The anthropologist of medicine reverses the polarity. For now it is the conventional and dominant system of medicine that is treated as other (Atkinson 1995:28). Inevitably, the world can not be reduced into sole line of thought or enlightened mode of Western value system in this plural multicolored world. The coercive degradation of another knowledge by making it 'Other' cannot be granted uncritically by those who touched the world of the knowledge of which purview is more than the modern framework.

As the application of this trend of decentralisation, this paper illustrates Bon Medicine not as complemented to the biomedicine, but as one distinguished system of knowledge on its own right. In other words, paper does not attempt to examine through biomedical standard, but to describe the thickness of the causality and efficacy beyond scientific proof through the logic of Bon world view. For being inside the logic and frame of the science can not help involving oneself with reproduction of same prosaic discourse.

This principle of symmetry in this context insists that it is necessary—as a methodological imperative—to apply the same anthropological analyses to domain of knowledge that are conventionally regarded as 'orthodox' as to the 'rejected', the 'failed' or the heterodox (Atkinson,1995:45). In the field of medical knowledge, therefore, it is the task of the anthropologist to pay equally serious attention to the practices of orthodox cosmopolitan medicine as to the non-orthodox or non-Western.

Against that background of methodological precept, therefore, there is no difficulty in recognizing that all knowledge-including scientific and medical—is socially produced.

Of course, says Kenwood (1999:180), no social constructionist denies the existence of true organic problems and diseases (e.g. epilepsy, Alzheimer's). It would be ludicrous not to acknowledge the existence of organic diseases that require ' treatment' at both the biological and the social levels. However, she warns, mislocation is more likely to occur from lack of clarity about the term 'social'. The danger is in assuming that the interesting sociological issues- of cultural variation, of belief, practical reasoning—are to be found only in the interaction of the patient's biography and the practioner's expert knowledge-. This bias therefore parallels the classic anthropological preoccupation with illness behavior.

The anthropological literature tell us far too little about how medical knowledge and practice are produced and reproduced, how it is shared and transmitted, how it is legitimated in practice. The principal of symmetry requires that we acknowledge how knowledge is made, legitimated, shared and transmitted within socially organized contexts. Since health and its promotion may be seen to be universally valued end, it is widely recognized that medicine serves sectional interests (Atkinson 1995;34) like between religious group such as Bon and Buddhism.

**Background**

***Process of Bon***

Bon is a name of religion which used to be widely followed in pre-

Buddhist Tibetan cultural sphere. Buddhism reached in Tibet in the seventh century and became state religion in the year of 762 A.D. Since then, though, once there was severe persecution at the initial stage in eighth century, the configuration of life, culture and discourse in the world of Tibetan culture has been centering Buddhism value system. Although Bon elements have been underpinning of their version of Buddhism which colors originality of it.

To our interest, some of the pockets of this cultural sphere fall in the land where a 'tribe' of India settles. It covers Ladakh, Kinnor district of Himachal Pradesh, and Tawang and West Kameng District of Arunachal Pradesh, the vicinal area of Tibet. Although people living there are linguistically and historically distinct from mainland Tibetan, the spatial continuity exposed people into profound influence of Tibetan Buddhism culture. The inter-exchange of people and goods with ambient culture has configured the multicolored medical knowledge and healing practice on its own right in each different geographical and cultural context.

In present day the modality of the Bon differs between these two kinds of communities. Although both are exiled from main Tibet in different historical phases, the former Bon, which is practiced among indigenous communities in India, is a healing tradition, dealings with the ailments of the locals through ritual performances The Monpas of Tawang and West Kameng district of Arunachal Pradesh take part in the fabric, and this is the community, which this paper focuses on. They has been less exposed not only to Buddhist influence, to any other outer force due to geographical location, thus Bon among them remains in the art of healing.

Besides these autochthonous communities, India also embraces the very community of Tibet fled from main Tibet after the Chinese uprising in 1959. Among them, Bon forms institutionalized religion still followed by the people now reduced to minority in Tibet. To the Tibetans in general, Bon is identical to this form of legitimate 'Yungdrung (Nine Swastika) Bon' which officially recognized as one of the five tradition by Tibetan government in the year of 1988, hence highly in Buddhist garb.

The term 'Bon' has variant meaning and depends on the interpretation in historical sources and understanding of the interpreter, one of them means to invoke, being related to 'bod pa'(to invoke or to invite in Tibetan), another one means "seed". In Zhang Zhung term, it is identified with 'gyer 'means to chant ( Bansal 1994 ). Zhang Zhung was a kingdom where Bon religion originates and flourished before it was conquered and incorporated by Tibet in 7th century. According to Namkhai Norbu, it is identical with ancient word 'bzla', to recite mantras or magic formulae (sNgag ) (Namkhai 1980).

On the other hand, Ekval says, it is not certain that the word 'Bon' referred to one unified religion, for there is some evidence which suggests the possibility that the early religion of Tibet was not a unified system (Ekval 1964), it was rather belief system of population which seek the service for riddance of ills and misfortune of everyday life, also in the court for kings and country's well-being. Later on, this form of belief acquired 'unified' shape in the course of encounter with ' international' 'organized' foreign religion, i.e. Buddhism.

Following the term 'bonpo' represents this crucial difference between these two forms of Bon. In Tibetan term, Bonpo is follower of Bon religion (Bon =Bon religion, po=of people), however bonpo in these community of pre-Buddhism Bon denotes medicine man or faith healer, more precisely, it often referred to 'pujari', priest or ritual conductor in Hindi. In the area covered by Tibetan Buddhism, bonpo commonly is used (though there is slight alteration such as onpo in Ladakhi, mun in Lepcha), and it does not mean the follower of Bon religion, hence their creed is Buddhism in basic.

They are succeeding the popular tradition of healing art of pre-Buddhism Bon till present day, as it remains in the designation. Or it may be actually continuation of Bon as aristocratic priests in Yarlung Dynasty, as Sammuel emphasises the bon priest in the earlier 'court religion' of Zhang Zhung, which were merely one kind of various court priests at this time (Sammuel 1993). Whether this hypothesis is veracious or not, it profoundly comprises the vestiges of pre-Buddhism knowledge and practice. To them, pre-Buddhism Bon is contemporary living experience, not the past relics confined within the texts and historiographies.

However, this form of continuation is not tangible to the authority of 'official' Bon viz. 'Yung Drung Bon', of which headquarter locates in the Tashi Men-ri monastery in Sirmour District of Himachal Pradesh. To the supremacy of this version of tradition, 'unorganized' pre-Buddhism belief and practice in those periphery is not their 'sophisticated' Bon , in fact the existence of this mode of Bon itself is not much known to them. Rinpoches, who are the source of knowledge of Yung Drung Bon does not accept the 'older worship' as the part of 'modern' Bon teachings' (Crossette 1995:77).

However, according to the oral history of Tashi bonpo in Zung village of Lumla circle, Tawan district of Arunachal Pradesh, they are the descendants of the exile who were expelled at the time of Buddhist persecution during eighth century. Moreover, his writen texts in Tibetan script which he succeeded from his forefather do tell the name of 'Tonpa Shenrab ' as the source of their knowledge for healing rituals. (Tonpa Shenrab Miwo is the name of the founder of Bon religion, who occupies equivalent status as Buddha).

Bon at that time was mainly associated with the cult of the divine king included the belief that he was endowed with both magical power and a special magnificence (Lopez 1997). Bon dominated the community in general and its leaders in particular, above all the king. In this sense it is said in some chronicles that the Bon looked after the life (tsho) of the king or aid his ministers with the word and deed, or that they keep in view the defense of the country's borders (Tucci 1980: 232).

According to Karmey, this worship of sacred king and his appendage started between 6th and 7th century, which closely connected to the divinity of a special tutelary god of the king, the "body spirit"(sku bla) who protected the king's power, encompassing everything from his body to his political authority to the order of universe. This tutelary god was mostly mountain gods (Karmay 1975 ), these kings did not leave earthy remains when they died, but ascendant bodily by means of 'Mu', luminous rope to heaven. This belief in the divine nature of the king and their gods, especially the gods of mountain, originally formed the nucleus of their belief system (Bansal 1994).

One of the primary responsibilities of the royal priests and ministers, who were Bon from Zhang Zhing kingdom, then seems to have been the maintenance of the king's health, for if the king become ill or if the body spirit was determined other to be displeased ,the safety of the kingdom an even of the universe was in jeopardy, and epidemics and droughts were interpreted as signs of this displeasure. Then Boŋ were summoned and performed a range of sacredotal functions in service of the divine king, such as officiating at coronation ceremonies and rites of allegiance to the king ( Lopez 1997).

### *Process of the Monpas*

The Monpas are one of the Scheduled Tribe in India living in western Arunachal Pradesh. When we look at broader perspective of space and time, the word Mon appears to have a chequered history, and was not confined to a single group of people defined by a definite geographical boundary. Monpa is a broad term in fact, given to various groups living in parts of Arunachal Pradesh, Bhutan and the south of Tibet, but also some groups of Eastern Tibet. According to Stein, even in the earliest text, mention is made of Mon people in the east, along the Sino-Tibetan border. In the west, the name is given to other low-caste communities in Ladakh, and lastly it is applied to Sikkim and Bhutan. In western Himalaya, Handa (2001) reports, the Mons or the Monpas are known to the Tibetan as the Molan, that is 'the dweller of the valley beyond the Himalayan frontiers' who inhabit in the Lahul and Zanskar areas, to suggest their non-Tibetan origin, Alexander Cunningham is of the opinion that the ancient sub-Himalayan people were the Mons. The Kashmiri historical work the Rajatarangiri of Jonaraja mentions the bs Kal Mon as the original non-Tibetan inhabitants of Gu gc. It would appear that as the prehistoric Tibetans moved south and west across the plateau they encountered people of various tribes who came to be known generally as Mon (Tucci:1949:6).

The main habitat of the Monpas in India locates in the district of Tawang and West Kameng which is in western side of Arunachal Pradesh. It is separated on the North by province of Khams or Khamsyul of Tibet along the 700 mile long crest of the eastern Himalayas, from the tri-junction of Bhutan, Tibet and India to the tri-junction of India, Tibet and Burma; on the West by Bhutan; and on the South by Assam (Bose 1997).

The term Monpa covers three distinct groups who may be conveniently divided into Northen, Central, and Southern. Taking each by turn, the Northen Monpa are mainly concentrated along the broad valley of the Tawang Chu north including a pastoral group at Mago. They can also be divided into Major distinguishing features between these groups are the dialects. Tawang area broadly falls into three popular divisions, mainly Cha-chum,Thakpa and Pangchen. Central Monpa lives south of thc Se la in the region of Dirang and Southern Monpa is in the further south in Kalaktang area both of which fall into district of West Kameng.

Historically Monpas inhabits eastern lower jungle are labeled by the 'civilized 'and 'cultured' Buddhist Tibetans as savage and outsiders living in thick forest an untamed environment of which they posses a great knowledge, traditionally subsisting not as farmers but rather hunter-gatherers. Their milieu and way of life does not appeal to

Tibetans since 'savage' nature does not represent an ideal state to the Tibetans mind. It may even be said that part of the aspiration of Tibetan religious ideology is to eliminate wilderness by subjugating it. We often see this schema that promotes to control nature in the name of civilization, that is, science. And once fierce and uncultivated nature, and that of Bon deities, is included within the sphere of Buddhism and re-presented Buddhism language, nature and supernatural is tamed.

The process to reach present Buddhist Monpa has been parallel to the process of Tibetanization of original inhabitants of the land which had distinctive characteristic which simply cannot subsumed into homogenous sphere of Tibetan Buddhist culture. As the impact of Buddhism was less and low comparative to the main Tibet due to geographical and political distance, this land of Monyul have sustained more liberal in terms of 'un-tamed' life and interaction, which could be, cradle of Bon faith.

## Bon Medicine among the Monpas

### *Cosmology and Etiology*

The world of pre-Buddhism Bon is configurated by the interplay between the microcosm and the macrocosm, with multifarious divine manifestations and all appearances were suffused with religious significance for the people's life (Tucci 1980:177). The entire existence of the Monpas, their knowledge and practice, cognition and construction is suffused and colored by the experience of the spiritual. In ancient time, the sphere of nature and man was integrated whole. Theg lha (celestial spirits), srin (terrestrial spirits) and klu (subterranean spirits) and humans were not separated, and could exchange conversation, and stones, trees and earth all spoke the language of humans (Belleza 2001:36). In those days, cosmos was not stratified, everyone resides in the same horizon, and human could commune with nature and that of spirit directly.

In Monyul, this tight bond between human and nature is not yet to be relics, human still can commune through the bonpo's age long inherited art of healing, and also through the Menpa's (Medicine man) dream. It is a gift from the abode to ease the suffering of the people.

When menpa is asleep, Phu (Mountain spirit) goes to the menpa's dream, and when menpa wakes up, it returns to its body again. Menpa in Dirang village says, the night before patient comes to him, he sees the dream visited by Phu of Medicine. When he wakes up, there is medicine under the pillow. Or, Phu informs treatment for the coming patient on tomorrow, and instructs the place and time that he can get necessary healing material such as herbs. It is only through dream he can cure, otherwise he is just one of the member of the village. Not only to the side of physician, in the Sarali village of Nafra circle, patient also see the divine dream which foretells the own coming disorder, which often is the capture by don, evil spirit, and dream in red is a sign of illness.

This interrelatedness of the macrocosmos is homologous to the microcosm, the relationship of 'Lu-Lha-Yong'. Lu is aquatic spirit resides and rules the underworld, Lha is generic term of the gods dwells sky, but in this context it indicates the guardian spirit on the head of individual accompanying the whole life. Yong is soul in Dirang Monpa word.

This trinity is so intently united, something bad happen to Lu or Lha, Yong falls ill in response to the offence. For the Lha who resides the top of the head, the body of the host is a shrine. Therefore when watery area where Lu lives gets polluted, or when Lha defiled by the host's visiting to polluted place, for example the house just after delivery, Yong fall into the state of grip, defilement.

Usually it manifested swelling some part of body and eye, bad throat. But the ailment can be cured when the Lu or Lha is purified ritually or through retrieval of cleanliness. In the rite, the smoke of juniper reaches to realm of gods and spirits, and the rage appeased by the fragrance of the juniper.

This relation expressed by another formula: Lhadhan-Medhan-Ludhan Sum (Lha, Human, Lu, Three) (dhan is suffix for plural). Since all three kinds of being are living together under one roof, if Me, human conducts simultaneously reflects to other two, and human receives the return of what s/he did.

The hallmark of the Bon supernatural geography overlaps the holistic phenomenology of illness, and the structure of the triad cosmos corresponds to the spiritual arrangement of the therapeutic intervention and expertise of specialists. And the earthly experience of the illness is projected to the cosmological happenings (Tucci 1980). In the Monpa tradition, cosmos was triad, not the six realms of Buddhism. The world of supernatural forces is divided into three planes of existence: the sky, intermediate or atmospheric space, and the earth and underworld, respectively dominated by the Lha, the Nyan and Lu (Namkhai 1995).

The sky and the subterranean world each have several storey, usually nine above and nine below. This application of number nine is specifically Bonpo concept, they storey are reached by a 'sky door' and an 'earth door' the former being the hole in the roof for the light and smoke, the latter the hearth (Stein 1962).

To delineate pre-Buddhism Bon etiology, briefly I sketche illness causation of don following to the triad cosmology. In the realm of sky, Lha resides to watch out the human deeds and morals. Any mistreat of the things and waste of the food and resources leads to sickness which attributed to the disrespect to them. For example, Chu lha, god of water feels offended when pairs of socks are washed in water (meant for public usage), or if someone spits or urinates there. He punishes the defilers by causing pain or sore to their feet, mouths or genitals. At the banks of the rivers and ponds, the two-meter filthy stretch of water should be left untouched before using it for consumption.

Nyan, the spirits of the trees and rocks are easily annoyed and send sickness and death by way of retaliation. Nyan is also offended by the chopping down of any trees that may be held sacred locally, by the digging up of the sacred ground, by the smell of burnt food, and by the beams of torches or lamp cast on the tops of hills or mountains consecrated to him (Mukherji 1995:150). There are certain places, one have to conduct rite to ask for permission to cut trees. In same fashion, there is rite to unearth stones to prevent from illness by those deeds.

Sadag are spirits of the grounds of any locality to which on many occasions offerings are brought. In general terms, they can become irritated when one 'wounds' soil, their domain, through work, excavation, or building. The grounds, which held the hearth should be dug out and thrown into water, in default make Sadag annoyed and punish the owners or defilers with the disease (Mukehrji 1995:174).

Among Monpa in Dirang circle, Sadag is called 'Lou'.The stone with lou has to be kept clean always. It has synchronic linkage with villagers, for when some one put the fire on the lou, the offender or his/her family members would get burn in his body. It is not healed by applying the medicine, but by a performance of rite.

The land that has been inherited since forefather days, has a lou in particular stone of the land. If the lou is not kept clean, any members of family are subject to fall ill. Bonpo can detect which stones is a lou by pouring goat's milk. If the stone is lou, it gives bad smell, and it absorbs milk as if it drinks. If it is offended by any means even without intention, unknowingly, it causes swelling in the body. In Chug village, one child had swelling at his leg, and it was not getting better against medication. When his parents consulted with bonpo who diagnosed it is due to the stone thrown to the ground, which provoked lou. When it is removed from the ground, he was cured.

In Monpa villages, if villagers do not treat Lu proper way. In other words, if the place like Lu dwells such as stream or spring was polluted by washing socks or dishes, then not only the offender, sometimes entire family fall the ill-state such as sick or fail of crops. In Monpa villages, Lu lives in the dry area. It is much more powerful and readily enraged.

From ancient time to the present day, the sacred mountains are 'god of the country' or 'masters of the place'. They are regarded both as 'pillars of the sky' and 'pegs of the earth'. The summit of any of the sacred mountains was a place of contact between heaven and earth, the two being linked by a sky ladder (Bansal 1994). This concept of connection between heaven and earth is nucleus of the Bon faith, and the mountain was, and is until the present day, the midpoint of two spaces. (Tucci 1980).

This worship of mountain is strongly observed among the Monpas and it is also the core concept of bonpo practice of healing. The mountains where the ancestor descended or on which he lived acquire special sacredness, and cosmogonic or theogonic accounts or complex philosophical attempts at interpretation become attached to them. Because of their sacred nature such mountains become in a sense the soul of the country, they assure its perpetuity, and protection for the men living at their feet.

In Monpa word, the spirit of the sacred mountain is called 'Phu'. It occupies the most important seat in the Monpa pantheon. The 'father' Phu protects and watches out villager's deeds and thoughts, and governs all aspect of everyday life. This is the deity bonpos contact for their service of healing. It is Phu who instructs the treatment, for he is also a cause of the illness. Particular Phu causes particular illness, which can be healed only through that Phu. Task of bonpo is to detect that enraged Phu by divination and to contact that Phu for propitiation by performing rites. Not all the mountain is worshiped as Phu. The chosen grandiose mountain is venerated at the same time feared by all the communities at his feet. Phu manifests everywhere, in every place, in every object or happening. It is thought that most of the illness in Monpa community is his influence by depriving of the soul or possessing into soul by them. The river in the Phu's mountain is symbolised as his blood where the spirits Lu, Tsang Dut and Rimong resides. If river is polluted by human, naturally, it leads that offender to sick. So does by pollution to all nature where those spirits resides such as water, stone, tree, even hearth.

In the Monpa context, most important and involved into people's life is Phu, the mountain spirit. As we have seen above, each locality has their own Phu in the mountains surrounds the village. It is said that Phu resides on the mountains top. It is believed among Lish villagers that if a helicopter flies over a mountain where the 'Phu' stay, the helicopter will fall or meet with an accident. Phu is the soul of the village, core of the Monpa's everyday life. It protects, watches, and governs the every aspect of living at their feet. Yet, like other deities, the nature of the Phu is also ambivalent and this is a main cause of the peoples illness, too. Each Phu has unique character according to the village context. In the case of Lish villages, there are three Phus. Each Phu affect the man its own way. If any of the Phu possesses a man, the rite has to be performed to that particular Phu which possessed the man. Although the source is peculiar to the Phu, the attack manifests in common symptom. The main symptom of these possession is madness. It also causes the body pain and shivering.

Thus, illness does not merely have a physical origin. One has to distinguish the primary cause (rgyu), which consist of a disturbance of the equilibrium of the three "humours" and contributory cause (rkyen), which is to be sought or in an impurity, a shadow, a defilement (grib) (Tucci 1980:173). The malefic power, which represented as 'Don', evil spirits is often provoked by these contributory causes.

The impurity or shadow can be of various kinds; it can originate in a sinful action, and also arise through associating with men who emanate a dangerous sacredness, as for example with smiths and armourers. (Tucci 1980:173).

Grib is generated by defilement such as at the time of delivery, death, and menstruation. During this period one has to abstain contact with religious settings. It is also caused from eating various impure foods. Thus food offered by a widow or a murderer brings about a dangerous condition, or burnt food, which offend the phug lha also cause defilement, as does the pouring on the hearth of liquids or substances producing evil smells or smoke, which anger the god of the hearth. An example of this violation of taboo can be observed among religious specialist particularly, as bonpo in Salari village said, when bonpo defiles his body by eating prohibited food such as onion, garlic, and meat, he falls into the grip. This provokes the Phu, which leads bonpos get sick. If one falls into grip, the bla also got affect and exposed to the vulnerable condition.

For people of Tibetan culture, radiation covers every time, everywhere. Anytime it may turn negative as 'don'. All sacred nature is continually beset by a whole variety of don, who were presumed to be directly responsible for the ailments and misfortunes. According to the lama in Rama camp village in Dirang circle, there are three hundred thirty kinds of don.

Don is the condition, which breaks out as a result of above contributory cause of dregsi (uncleanness) mi gtsang (impurity) or, more generally, grip. Then the malevolent radiation intrudes into corporeal interiors and brings about in a human a particular state of weakness. That is the moment illness haunts people. On the other hand, it also haunts in the condition of low vital life-forces by other means such as soul loss.

Poisoning is one of major cause of the not just illness, usually it leads to death. Poisoning is committed by : 1) hand (la doh) 2) eyes (me doh) 3) food (rhe doh). Death by poisoning is a part of black magic, also specializes in powers, which can kill outright, without any physical contact with the person. In Tawang, sickness is often attributed to ritual poisoning. But once a person has been poisoned through witchcraft and black magic he can only be cured by the services of another black magic priest. It is also common in Lumla and Zimithang and is practiced mostly by female who are occasionally known and identified. At other times, even ordinary person practices poisoning as a matter of ritual.

The poisoning in Dakpanang is it the widely acknowledged that poison is not necessarily administered to an enemy. According to the Nanda's (1982) report, it is a matter of ritual or even habit. The ladies who believed to poison the people also do it regularly as their macabre profession. As tools should not be allowed to rust, so must a sincere witch sharpen her craft and remain in practice by continuing to poison people at regular intervals. The main motive behind the administration of poison is luck—a desire to obtain the luck and good fortune of the other person ( Nanda 1982). At that time all the government officer from main India were duly warned that they should eat and drink with these people at their own risk and peril. A Circle Officer of Zimithang would not even allow the villagers to watch him while eating, for fear they would poison him through their eyes. In Tamang in Nepal, which also has bon tradition, it is believed that witches gain control over spirit by promising them food in the form of human sacrifice by poisoning.

The withdrawal of the bla from the body and the consequent danger can be the work of dons, which we observed above, because the person is psychologically weak and has no resistance to don. It also is believed for threatening death of the man for whose benefit the ritual is to be performed. The la is especially susceptible during dreams and can be carried off by dons, who particularly covert the life force of children.

### *Doctor as Modulator*

As the answer or receptor to these ailments in this setting, bonbo takes up the role of modulator between nature and supernatural, and that is role of this form of 'doctor. To be a bonpo, one has to bear the responsibility of becoming 'public goods', in the sense that he has to be prepared for the house call of the villagers. A bonpo in Lish village said, 'Like a doctor, if anyone falls sick in the night, early morning or noon or whatever time it may be, and if the bonpos help is sought, and he is obliged to do so. (Interview from Lish bonpo on 27.11.02). Thus villagers seek the assistance of bonpo to protect them from the malignant activities of spirit as well as to secure their own health, and service of bonpo is done through the assistance of 'Phu', as a mouthpiece for Phu and to control other subsidiary spirits (Belleza 2001:78).

When people fall sick, the first resort is be diagnosed and prescribed through Bon lama's oracle and the divination to take next action. This 'health seeking behavior' is common to the Tamangs in Nepal, the community which is also 'bonpo', is active. Peter reports, "Just as western laymen rely on doctors to diagnose the cause of illness, so the Tamang laymen leave it to the bompo "(Peters 1998: 72). In a similar bon tradition of Sherpa Yolmo who Desjarlais (1994) met, "bonbo can cure outer illness, but not inner engines. If the inside is broken, the healers cannot cure us, so we go to the hospital." The outer illnesses to which patients of bonpo refer often involve feelings of malaise due to personal distress and social conflict.

For the Bon medicine, these somatic sensibilities borne of the communal exchange of everyday life is the most adept field for healing (Desjarlais 1994). But these entire adept does not give full play without patient faith. One can do at certain level if the bonpo's spirituality or purity of the mind and body to contact to Phu is high enough. For bonpo's ability to divine the particulars of an illness rests entirely on his relationship with the supernaturals. A bonpo in Dirang village says, without prayer, medicine does not work, a bonpo says, and the work of poison is due to power of evil spirit (don), and the work of medicine is due to god (lha). It's not the bonpo who breaks epistemic barriers but rather the gods whom he has the talent for hosting within his body. Through the medium of bonpo's voice, Phu reveals information about the world, knowledge that humans are otherwise incapable of obtaining access to (Desjarlais1994). The spokesman for this transaction, a bonpo learns much of what he knows through his relationship with a Phu who teaches and empowers him. The ritual is the forum of this communication, bonpo reaches the Phu who diagnose, and also cures, for the particular Phu is also the cause of the ailment.

However, the purview of the Bonpos among Monpa do not delimit only 'somatic sensibilities', people consult bonpo first for all the kind of illness. In the case of the natural cause, they recommend bed rest or change in diet. In the case of bone fracture bonpo makes fire by iron load and recite the mantras. Then locally available first-aid, such as bandage and herbal paste is applied. They do not perform rites for patients suffering from natural causes. Bonpo in Dirang village said, all rite was done after the diagnosis of the cause such as palpation, palm and pulse reading. On the basis of this examination, bonpo detects if it is due to don or poison or possession or physical cause. If the result tells that it is the intrusion of don, then bonpo goes for divination to fix the ritual to that particular don. For different kind of illness, treatment is also done through different gods. What is physically caused is cured physically, and what is spiritually caused must be spiritually cured (Govt. of India. 1996:231). However, what is caused physically also ultimately, it was the work of divine providence in the larger cosmological framework. The task of bonpo is to guide most suitable and reasonable way to retrieve normal state of the patient under guidance of divine, the beyond of human intellect.

Bonpo knows the purview of his art. For the case of natural illness with no involvement of witchcraft or dons, he sends the patient to the hospital. For bonpo intuitively knew what he could treat successfully, and what he could not. He frequently acknowledged that doctors are superior at treating cholera and preventing rabies. If it is beyond his control, the death of the patient gives a bad name to him.

There are some illnesses (like related to blood) that can be cured by medicines, but the patients those who are harmed by don cannot be cured by medicine. The patient Dejarlais (1994:228) met says, "The doctors in a hospital didn't touch even my pains, but after performing the ceremony, all the pain and nightmares left when bonbo beat me." The ritual healing is not merely exercises in the treatment disturbing emotional states and interpersonal relations, it gives some effect physically by dealing with those sphere of the ailments. To bonpo, patient's aches, pains, weakness, blindness appears as the development of the family conflict, quarrel with neighbor, frustration due to unemployment all these events and relation afflicts patient and it seems that this anxiety laden social situation may have been responsible for the physical symptoms.

The greatest success of bon medicine among the Monpas is with illness especially acute, sudden at the onset, yet not incapacitating. According to Bonpo of Salari village, this kind of illness is mostly attack by 'bad air', or don in the form of headache, body ache, eye problem or mental problem. They can distinguish whether the cause is spiritual or physical spiritual by seeing facial expression, shadow, etc. If the illness is ritually or spiritually caused, then it must be treated ritually or spiritually. Bonpo in Salari tells that without the rite, mad person would remain as such.

At first bonpo palpates the patient at his hands, feet, his forehead and his heart. He then diagnoses the cause such as the kind of intruding spirit and accordingly he prescribes the rite. No rites are performed without thorough examination. If a rite is performed thorough checking, it is detrimental to the recovery of the patient.

Nanda (1982) reports her observation on Bon during her tenure of D.C, which is sole written information about then practice of the Bonpo in Tawang area. Bonpo in Hoogla village reads the pulse as well as palm with prayer for clear reading; it should be done in the morning, preferably on an empty stomach and not at night. Bonpo in Hoogla she encounter could predict events of coming future through divination (Nanda 1982).

In the case of bonpo in Dirang village, firstly he palpates the palms the name and the age of the patient is identified to consult either of brother Phu whose name is 'Dimpu' and ' Bangle' through divination by wheat in water. The divination starts from the recitation of mantras. The mantra bonpos recite consists of special term of Bon. It was common to the rite of bonpos in Dirang circle, the rite itself is conducted to contact particular Phu who is tormenting the patient, but bonpo have to recite the names of all Phu in the area. If he misses the names, it touches the wrath of forgotten Phu. After this, he throws some seeds of wheat in water in the bowl. From there he prescribes the treatment, it would be either ritual or other solution. As like the bonpos in Salari village, the common tool for calling Phu is Dorje bell.

According to Peter (1998:119) bonpo of Tamang also reads the pulse to diagnose the attack by don or not. For treatment, bonpo blew a mantra at patient's head. This consisted of repeating the magical formula designed to dispatch the don and intermittently slowing on the afflicted area. Bonpo believes that the magical formula he whispers has the effect of a command: i.e., the recitation guarantees the god's obedience (Peter 1998:123).

A bonpo in Zung village of Lumra circle also examines the planet position through his inherited astrological texts. He examines whether the patient's birth star and the planets are in order and whether the favorable and adverse elements connected with his birth star have come into conflict. He then recommends a date on which the rite should take place.

According to Tucci's classification, the relevant rituals and magical formulae of pre-Buddhism knowledge have two principal objectives in view; in the first place prosperity, well-being, good fortune (bde legs) in the most material sense, as well as long life (tshe ring), health (nad med), riches (longs spyod), victory over enemies etc., and then the driving out (bzlog) and elimination of all which stands in the way of this legs, such as poverty, illness and early death (Tucci 1980:155). The activity of bonpo thus has an infinitely wide field open before it; in case of drought he can invoke rain, he can banish hail or conjure up inflict vengeance, he can call a halt to epidemics among men and public. In this immense area of ritual techniques for the furtherance of good and defense from evil and the traditional heritage of Monyul can be clearly distinguished.

Hence bonpos ritual for objective of health is not merely exercises in the treatment of physical/biological illness and diseased organ, but attempts at re-organizing the environmental disunity and imbalance. At the time of communal ceremony such as Phla Festival, the domain of bonpo and the scale of re-organization expanded from individual level to the public level.

In everyday life, when one faced with unfortunate events, which approached realization, he/she has available service to improve by option of the numerous types of rites. Broadly, rites are consists of purification (sel) by aromatic plants water or blood, driving out of adverse forces through powerful exorcistic actions (to), and rituals of ransoming (glud). The bla, the soul, can for example be ransomed from danger as in cases of unconsciousness (Tucci 1980:175) by soul loss or possession by dons.

A bonpo in Sarali village says, for different illness there are different rites, as like for doctors there are different medicine for different illness. The kind of rites selected thus, according to the kind of 'dons'. By performing the appropriate ritual actions, for example through an ablution, every stain left by bad actions is cleansed, and the don lose their power over the man so purified. In describing the don it should also be mentioned that they appear in three groups, outer, inner and secret (phyi, nang, sgang).

To exorcise native forces, the cause of poison viz. grip which weaken positive forces is to be removed. It is done through purifying by fumigation (sang) of juniper and sprinkling of lustrating water called Tsen. The juniper tree is a sacred tree of Bonpos.

There are a variety of rites for reconciliation with don to repair harm dones by them (Namkhai 1995:131). The first task was to evoke the beginning of the world, kind of illnesses. Since the world took form, since it became a mode of being (srid), man has intervened to create the necessary ordering and to give an appropriate form to the habits of his/her life. This process, however, has brought a new situation into existence, which often disturbs or injures those powers that hitherto called particular domains their own. The building of a house, the erecting of a tent on a particular spot, building a bridge over a river, digging in the earth, each of these are intrusions into the domains of other powers which require expiation through appropriate rituals (Tucci 1980:142) to reconcile with natural.

According to Tucci, the bonpo sources account for these rituals or narrate the origins of particular customs in the appropriate contexts. In other words this event was the origin of the custom. The treat of these subjects and their narratives not only provide an explanation for the origin of the custom concerned, but also contain the assurance that no harmful effect can arise from it, and that its repetition will evoke once more the primal moment when after an offence had been committed against the divine and demonic powers the sure means to remedy it was found. In short, the recital expiates the offence, which has taken place and provides protection against its consequences (Tucci 1980:154).

The mdos, yas, lud are devices to extricate one from the threatening dangers of hostile powers. These powers can be of bodily and material or immaterial and invisible nature.

It is called curative image (ngar lud). The image of the person afflicted by illness or misfortune, the accompanying shapes of tsamba dough, the little tsamba figures of man and animals all around the main figure these are all transformed in a magical fashion into real things beings able to satisfy the demand of don. Tsamba are used to symbolize gifts for the gods. In the preBuddhism context, animals such as horse, sheep, dog were sacrificed communication between the deities and the man to maintain the relationship as the medium of "intercessional prayer".

A bonpo in Salari performs the rite with the white hen and after that the hen is released into the jungle, in initial phase of rite. If the confrontation takes place without success, then recourse is done finally by means of magical compulsion if it doesn't work one had to commit real sacrifice of animal such as white hen or black sheep.

Interestingly, after visiting of fourteenth Dalai Lama in Dirang for Kala chackra initiation, a number of Bonpo have given up the sacrifice by hearing his speech.

Bonpo can heal the poisoned patient, too. In the protracted rite, he detects the cause such as bewitchment and its persecutor and venue. Through meditation in front of the patient, and ritual sips from a cup of chang and recitation of mantras, bonpo approached patient and lowering his head, placed his mouth against patient navel. Slowly he sucked the navel and then lifting his head turned and spat into an empty cup, which he had placed nearby. Bonpo repeated this ritual thrice, sucking a curious liquid out of the navel till the cup was almost half-full. Then he lifted the cup, examined the contents and declared. "The poison had been administered to you through a red chillie but now it is out of your system." Needless to say, the patient improved and was soon backing to normal health (Nanda 1982).

If a person falls sick due to soul loss, there are rites designed to bring the la back into the body, known as " calling the la"(bla'bod). Magical procedures also enable the soul of an enemy to be called by force. For this rite, family summons a bonpo, he divinates how the spirit was lost, where it has wandered, and how best to receive it .He then ritually searches for and attempts to call the lost life-force back into the body of his patient (Dejarlais 1994:13).

In this connection of the cosmological arrangement, there is clear territorial distinction between Buddhist lama and bonpo in the religious performance for healing. The domain of lama is sickness caused by 'Lha' the gods resides highest part of cosmological hierarchy. Thus, lamas do not deal with Phu, by saying that is too low for them. The strata of Lha are also extended the seat for the Buddhist gods and saints. In Monpa context, the class of Lha and Sange (Buddha) is almost identical.

The difference reflects also to the therapeutic effect. People say in Monpa villages, the rite of bonpo is more 'quick' and 'cost effective' than that of Buddhist lama. The healing rite takes brief time hence cheaper, but needs more repetition. Because in the case of bonpo, it is bargain between Phu and bonpo over the recovery of the clientele. Bonpo demands strongly the return at the cost of the offering of Torma (dough made of flour), cloth, ornament, sometimes sacrifice. According to one villagers description, it is like 'corruption type' bribing the Phu or don to release or leave from the patient soul. But it can also express as 'reciprocal', in the relationship one negotiated in equal basis. On the other hand, lama takes one day fully. It is time taking because lamas go step by step with patience and compassion by reading lengthy texts to implore and convince the spirit to make patient free. According to Nyingma pa village lama (Buddhist), therefore the result is 'permanent', no repeater. But according to bonpo, villagers come more to bonpo. Some says bonpo is more effective. According to bonpo in Dirang village, after consulting lama, if it is no recovery, patients come to bonpo.

## Conclusion

The most focal point of this so-called faith healing lies on the subject of the healing. It comes from the nature or supernature; it is never of the healer himself. He is a just medium who serve the seats by its purity and pristine of the self and body. Illness is caused by may be some infection or imbalance of the humor, but all that is administrated by supernatural. Therefore only supernatural can cure and heal the source of illness, through the medium such as bonpo, but it not the deeds of bonpo himself.

In this system of thought less tends to aggregate a certain view which construct the discourse to specialize particular individual or group and less intentional manipulation for proliferation of own belief exists. It does not impose the own philosophy or framework of doctrine, rigorously remains as the third person that is mere medium. It remains a farmer as same as other lay person, it does not accumulate special attitude to distinguish medical professionals. The power is not attribute to the particular individual as bonpo, but to the Phu, the almighty power that governs every sphere of the life and word. It is not the bonpo who cures and ails, but it is Phu who does everything. For them, what bonpo announce through divination is not by him, but Phu, and more important relation is with Phu, and bonpo's transparency as medium. In the Monpa context, bonpos are aware their knowledge came from Shenrab, but he does not share the position of absolute supremacy like Buddha in Buddhism, or Shenrab in post Buddhism Bon. The worship of sacred mountain is the core of Bon in preBuddhism version, and the mountain is very pervasive all the main controller of the all power whether it cause illness or heal illness.

On the other hand, so-called 'world (or International religion) religion such as Buddhism are founded by one individual and every virtue and merit is attributed and accumulated to that particular human, irrespective of contents of the teaching. That is utilized for the enlargement of the organization by legitimizing it. In this process, the power and legitimacy has to be augmented by subjugating other way of seeing, i.e., knowledge, and it is become the absolute truth to the member of organization, and other knowledge was transmuted dominant version which subservient to the 'truth'. Thus, the knowledge is structured of the composition of hierarchy. However, this movement is not one-sided and top down. It is realized because of the involvement of the subservient into the logic of dominant discourse. Unknowingly in uncritical manner, one conspires the strength and cogency of the discourse. In this structure there is no victim and no explorer. Everybody is the confederate by ignorance of the position of the self.

Through this paper researcher intended to rethink the extant notion of popular medicine not by evaluation through modern medicine framework to promote allopathy, but by placing same line as the expertise which is already existing always and playing a role in its own right. From the viewpoint of different culture, it looks the very 'construction', but for them it is a reality hence the 'bonpo' rite works out and they get relief.

This everyday life of religion system is same to all cognitive structure of knowledge also from the other cultures point of view; it may be seen as fabrication. But in the same way, the common sense knowledge we take its authenticity for granted is based on strong faith. As Burger ascertains these common-sense-knowledge intrinsically has religious structure. In this 'plausibility structure', one of the realities is justified to take for granted by people commonly convinced, as a result it confines the all speculative question. The essence of the plausible everyday life is, in fact, consist of a kind of agreement.

If we wish to make sense of perdurability of non-biomedical knowledge and techniques to some in these places, we need to understand how they thought it rationalized more adequately than its competitors, the frailties of our concrete existence in the world. Human beings act rationally in the sense that their actions are purposive rather than expressive. Even through human action can appear irrational or senseless to an outside observer, according to this perspective, individuals always have reason for acting the way they do. Moreover, these reasons are always contemporary in that they are grounded within structures of meaning which mediate between the environment and the individual's experience of it. In other words, human action is rational from within the structures of meaning individuals use in order to realize their interests as they perceive them. (Wiling 1999:46).

They, like ourselves, held that some beliefs and practice were sensible and others foolish. Destructive disease were particularly terrifying deformations of human existence, and the belief, that we have won or are in the process of winning some degree of apparently rational mastery over them counts for a great deal among us. And this system of reasoning is true to all knowledge modality. By analyzing the very nature of popular medicine and religion thought, it provides a context for understanding not only present medical system but also the possible structures of forms, which have yet to be invented.

## REFERENCES

Atkinson Paul, (1995) *Medical Talk and Medical Work*, Sage Publication.

Arnold, David, (1988) "*Introduction: Disease, Medicine and Empire*" in David Arnold ed. Imperial Medicine and Indigenous Societies, Manchester University Press, Manchester.

Barbara, (1995) *So Close to Heaven*, Alfred. A, Knopf, New York.

Bansal B.L, (1994) *Bon: Its Encounter with Buddhism in Tibet*, Eastern Book Linkers, Delhi.

Berger P.L and Lackmann T., (1966) *The Social Construction of Reality*, Penguin, London.

Belleza vincent John, (2001) *Antiquities of Northern Tibet*, Adroit Publishers, Delhi.

Bose M.L., (1997) *History of Arunachal Pradesh*, Concept Publishing Company, Delhi.

Cunningham, A., (1997) "*Religion*" in Sharma, S.K & Sharma, Usha ed., Religious Heritage of Tibet, Encyclopedia of Tibet, Series-4, Anmol Publications Pvt Ltd, New Delhi.

Collin Samson, (1999 ) *Health Studies*, Blackwell Publishers, New York Crossette.

Dejarlais, R. Robert, (1994) *Body and Emotion*, Motilal Banarsidass Publishers Private limited, Delhi.

Ekval, B. Robert, (1964) *Religious Observances in Tibet*, The University of Chicago Press, Illinoi.

Gains A.D and Hahn R.A, (1985) '*Among the physicians: Encounter, exchange and transformation*' in in R.A. Hahn and A.D. Gains (eds) Physicians of Western Medicine: anthropological Approach to Theory and Practice. Dordrecht: Reidel. pp. 3-22.

Govt. of Arunachal Pradesh, (1996) District Gazetteer of Tawang and West Kameng District, Directorate of Research, Itanagar.

Gordon, D.R, (1988) "*Tenacious assumptions in modern medicine*", in M. Lock and D.R Gordon (eds), Biomedicine Examined, Dordrecht: Kluwer Academic.

Kenwood, Christine, (1997) *Social constructionism: Implications for psychotherapeutic practice*, in Cromby Jhon, Nightingale J. David. eds., Social Constructionist Psychology, Open University Press, Buckingham.

Karmey S.G., (1975) *A General Introduction to the History and Doctrine of the Bon*, Memoirs of the Research Department of the Toyo Bunko. No. 33, Tokyo.

Lopez, S. Jr., (1997) *Religion of Tibet in Practice*, Munshiram Manohrlal Publisheres Pvt. Ltd., Delhi.

Handa, O.C., (2001) *Buddhist Western Himalaya*, Indus Publication House.

Lupton, Deborah, (1994) *Medicine as Culture: Illness, Disease and the Body in Western Societies*, Sage, London.

Norbu Namkhai, (1980) *Bon and Bonbos*, Tibetan Review, December, Delhi

Norbu Namkhai, (1997) *Drung,Deu and Bon*, Library of Tibetan Works and Archives, Dharamsala.

Mukherji Priyadarsi, (1995) *Chinese and Tibetan Societies Through Folk Literature*, Lancers Book, Delhi.

Peters, Larry, (1998) *Tamang Shamans*, Nirala, Kathmandu.

Sammuel G., (1993) *Civilised Shamans Buddhism in Tibetan Societies*, Smithonian Institution, Washington and London.

Stein, S.A., (1962) *Tibetan Civilization*, Faber and Faber, London.

Tucci Giuseppe, (1980) *The Religions of Tibet*, tra. by Samuel Geoffrey, Allied Publishers Private Limited, Delhi.

Wright, Will (1992) *Wild Knowledge: Science, Language and Social Life in a Fragile Environment*, University of Minnesota Press.

# PART IV

# TRIBAL MEDICINES

# 22

# Technology Road Map for Herbals as Renewable Bioresource and Tribal Health Care

A.K. SRIVASTAVA

## Introduction

Natural products have always fascinated human cultures since centuries. For several thousand years, the plants and herbs are being used in traditional systems of medicine in India and China. Today, Ayurveda co-exists with modern systems of medicine, and is widely used and practiced. India is bestowed with a wealth of medicinal and aromatic plants, majority of which are being traditionally used as most popular systems of tribal healers for generations. Medicinal plants have their existence in almost every part of the country and the globe, under a well defined, value added biodiversity group. These herbs are the symbolic representatives covering diverse disease scenario in the healthcare sector with the tribal and rural communities. These herbs, therefore, form the most active ingredient in the formulations of pharmaceutical drugs. India is a repository of over 45,000 different plant species out of which around 15,000 are medicinal plants. The Indian systems of medicine have identified 1,500 medicinal plants, out of which around 500 species are used in preparation of drugs. Millions of rural households use medicinal plants in a self-help mode. Around two million practitioners of the Indian systems of medicine in the oral and codified streams use over 7,500 species of plants for preservative, primitive and curative applications. As per latest record in the Indian scenario about 860 botanicals are in greater demand with high market value, and annual domestic turnover has been to a tune of

Rs. 4,000 crores with the export potential of around Rs.400 crores/ year. In order to revitalize the bioresources in their ecological niche and to get out of the alarming situation associated with declining healthcare resources, awareness for the bio-resource conservation and utilization has to be given priority. About 4635 ethnic communities have been using the herbal resources for human and veterinary health care covering a wider range of biogeographical regions from Ladakh in the Trans Himalayas to the southern coastal tip of Kanya Kumari and from the deserts of Rajasthan and Kutch to the hills of the north east and majority of them to say around 1800 have been fully documented for their concerned regulatory properties, actions and drug formulations in the healthcare activity sector but at the moment no exhaustive and reliable inventory for the herbals representing the ethnic communities in different Eco-systems are available.

## Biogeographical Background of Medicinal Plants and their Uses in Healthcare

Medicinal plants are distributed across all biogeographic regions, diverse habitat and landscape. Tropical areas on the whole have greater predominance of the medicinal plants, which cover around 70 per cent of the total of India's herbals. These are spread across the Western and Eastern Ghats, the Vindhyas, Chota Nagpur plateau, Aravalis, the Terai region in the foothills of Himalayas and the North East. Less than 30 per cent of the medicinal plants occupy the geographical areas in the temperate alpine region and higher altitudes. The thermo-medicinal diversity has been the unique distinct features of bioresources in the dense tribal inhabited forests. Tribal specially have vast knowledge about the medicinal characteristics of the plant species in and around the dense forest in the adjoining areas. The tribal in general move around the known ecological niches in the forest and they collect resources, which form the vital component for their food security and healthcare.

The art of herbal uses and medication is almost as ancient as human history itself and has remained everlasting practice with fluctuating demand and supply. There is enormous number of evidences confirming the wide scale use of herbals in Medicare, which dates back to the ancient period known to human history. The system of herbal medicine known as Ayurveda has been followed in India from time immemorial. The germplasm for this science which is now receiving worldwide attention can be traced to the most ancient of Sanskrit texts known as the *Vedas*. In the *Rig Veda* the Aswini twins were described as divine physicians who used herbs and medicinal plants as a source for medicare, curing diseases to the extent that those could even ward off death. In the legendary account of their marvels, it is reflected that during that period it was possible to some extent to restore youth to the old, rejuvenate the debilitated body and invigorate the aged *Kal*. Such old heritage and the popularity of herbs and medicinal plants are gradually loosing its sanctity and it has now remained mostly the treasure of health vitality with the tribal in different part of the state. Many valuable, rare medicinal and aromatic plants have been reported from various parts of the country and those are the treasure for the present and future generations as a source of medicare, regulating the control of lethal diseases and also a good source of promising tonic in healthcare. The knowledge of herbals have mostly grown and remained as treasure in the real perspective with tribal who occupy only 8 per cent and the next users of the herbals in their native origin are the rural population which occupy 70 per cent of the total population. There are many exciting examples where the herbals once domesticated in the tribal and rural sectors now have become the most sought for the herbs in modern medicine. Plants have provided modern medicine with more diverse and important drugs than any other natural resources (Farns worth and Morris, 1976). The daring examples of tribal treasure—the opium poppy (*Papaver somniferum*) is now being widely used for the production of morphine and codeine, two well-known opoid analgesic drugs. The alkaloid is extracted from the dried sap obtained by lancing the unripe seedpods of opium poppy or by solvent extraction of poppy straw (Casey and Parfitt, 1986). This drug in India and many other countries is of greater choice for the control of acute and chronic pain of malignant origin such as cancer (Gorlay *et al.*, 1986). Another important medicinal plant, *cinchona ledgeriana*, the bark of this plant is being used from the ancient time by the tribals for the treatment of cardiovascular suffocation is being widely used for the extraction of the alkaloid quinidine and put to wide use in medicare as a cardiac depressant or antiarrhythmic (Rosketh and Storstrein, 1963; Stern, 1971).

There are many such important plant treasure and knowledge with tribals in their own ecological niche which have great potential and future in modern healthcare sector. If one visualizes the total scenario, in the present context, tribal communities are becoming displaced, acculturated and impoverished and the consequences are the dilution in their strategy concerned with healing knowledge, disappearance of their traditions, along with culture with the wide scale deforestation and moving in of new drugs and modern medicines. In India, wider range of medicinal plants of high value has been extracted from the wild to meet the increasing demand of raw material for domestic consumption and export. This has resulted in the depletion of natural habitats at a very fast pace. Another more alarming situation has arisen which accounts for the use of unscientific methods of extraction and adulteration in the modern system of medicine and this has accentuated this complex problem to a greater extent (Shastry and Chatterjee 2000). Tribal know-how therefore has to be tied up at an initial stage, developing a knowledge base to get the authenticated herbal extraction. The ancient heritage of one of the rural community of the central Himalayas known to be "Raji Van-Raut" (king of forests) from two districts of Uttaranchal (Champawat and Pithoragarh) as one of the important tribal pocket like few others, majority of them (60-65%) use herbal medicines for the treatment of their common ailments. There are almost 50 important very common species which are used even raw as specified part of the plant, dried powder, but interestingly their response in curing the ailments are very positive and competitively more effective than the allopathic medicines and remarkably with no side effect. Bhotia-tribals of Garhwal Himalayas also have their major dependency on the herbal medicare. These tribals carry tremendous informations about the natural wealth—the herbals, more than herbal practitioners do.

## Modernization of Herbal uses in the Historical Perspective

In the past, medicinal plants were harvested from the forests where they were in abundance and the consumption was also very less. Now, the situation has been reversed due to deforestation and increasing demand for herbals, inviting a major disaster which is going to risk the existence of entire herbal resources and biodiversity in their ecological niche, that points to an unethical commercial exploitation of the wild species for marketing. This kind of "feeding frenzy" is beginning to take its toll and throwing the majority of medicinal plants as scarce and endangered. Under these circumstances, it has become necessary to cultivate medicinal plants to have sustainable supply of herbals to provide highest quality of herbals to consumers and also to protect the endangered species as well as the environment. The building up of such pressures on the herbals, due to high demand from the pharmaceutical companies and the poor revitalizationary practices for their sustainable growth and development in the natural habitat, many of the species are threatened under extinction. The Medicinal Plant Conservation Centre (MPCC) at Pune has made a beginning of medicinal plant conservatory and some of the local Non-Governmental Organizations (NGOs) under support from United Nations Development Programme (UNDP) has made possible to maintain the population in their natural habitat. Perhaps what appears to be mos important is to facilitate the tribal communities to participate effectivel in conserving their botanical heritage while reaping the benefit o income generation simultaneously with the improved access to th plants needed for healthcare. This is mainly because of their inheren potential to give a soft handling of the herbals in their respectiv heritage. In the year 1987, women groups working in healthcare uni from all over India identified themselves to enter into the venture t develop a ready reckoner about herbs and their healthcare recipes fro nine states of India. This effort made it possible to generate some ver useful information related to 600 remedies corresponding to 300 plan and the collection so made were preserved for the future knowledg based research making their uses most effective. These women grou while working in eight states got the clinical test of these herbs ar recorded their remedy measures which were experimented by heal workers in rural areas and slums.

## Action Plan

With the widespread growing resurgence throughout the wor' developing knowledge based data bank on herbals and their uses medicare, the lost interest and seriousness in their conservation a cultivation has to be regained back. The shift in the socio-econor and cultural changes for the upliftment of local tribals and changing dimensions in health care measures warrant to redisco the old traditional knowledge based herbal medicare to fight out chronic upsurge of tribals which presently have mostly domestic the forest area with their activities as a source of their liveliho Herbals are the richest bioresource for the generation of a str entrepreneurship in the area. The beneficiaries are mostly the fo officials as they are the biggest client to get the knowledge learning about the value of medicinal plant resources along with the communities. The best part of it, the awareness about the medicinal plants has grown several folds in the tribal community as well as the forest officials. This has given a better stand to the threatened species for their conservation and also rejuvenation. There has been a tremendous change in the tribal communities and the entrepreneurs in the area of marketing authentic and genuine herbals as planting materials for nurseries for their sustainable use. Eventually cultivation of medicinal plants could meet the increasing industrial and pharmaceutical demand and forests could become a source for planting materials rather than decamping the forests from the medicinal plants, which are at the verge of extinction.

Educating the community about the practical application of herbals as a highly value added bioresource with medicinal properties has benefited the large community. The entrepreneurs in this sector have been motivating community to protect natural resource and undertake the cultivation of medicinal plants. Majority of interested entrepreneurs including tribals at large who were the innocent participants in this programme have now grown up with their wisdom and skill and are being benefited largely from an exciting venture, new income generation and employment opportunities. Globally the growing importance of herbals in healthcare, protective fencing of the herbal niches in the forest, specially the tribal belt are being implemented and knowledge exchange group for their conservation practices, cultivation and agro-cultural practices, post harvest processing and packaging for transport are picking up fast. Local people and tribals will have an access to the set up for the upsurging of their knowledge and skill and on the same to enhance livelihood and entrepreneurship. In close association with NGOs and State Forest Departments, lot of input is being added for quality raising of nurseries and herbal production to meet the everlasting demand of cultivated medicinal plants. Global support for popularizing the herbals in healthcare practices, MPCC has ventured in a bigway to make the herbal development programme backed by strong scientific research, community development and education with sustainable income generation and revitalization of traditional medicinal practices. Initiative in this direction has already been undertaken in a bigway. Bangalore forms a part of the wider plant conservation network covering around five states in India and over 54 conservation sites which has a basic back up from the Foundation for Revitalization of Local Health Traditions (FRLHT). The tribals more tuned to therapeutic uses of herbals are now being encouraged for their participation in the conservation of their botanical heritage.

Given the fact about the widespread traditional use of medicinal plants by the rural poor and women folk, it is important that the plans for the conservation and sustainable use of these resources are gender sensitive, promote equity and social justice. With the change in herbal habitat scenario due to over exploitation and also shifting priorities, there has been great upsurge in cultural diversity. The erosion of local and mainstream cultures related to biodiversity has a great impact on the biosphere which has remitted subsequently in the loss of biodiversity itself as both cultural diversity and biodiversity go hand in hand. The latest development in the conservation of medicinal plants, global consciousness has developed for the check and balance of their erosion and resurgence for the long term sustainability of herbal in their ecological niche to meet their increasing demand as medicine for health care. A special attention has to be given to conserve the natural flora—the herbals in and around the tribal belt and involving them in the authentication of the herbs and their medicinal uses with knowledge based back ground information in the historical perspective. This continuous effort has made it possible to conserve around, species of medicinal plants across sites in the network. The enthusiastic scientists group in Maharashtra have undertaken a serious exercise in this sector doing the botanical inventory exercise and launching a collaborative project for mapping the scattered bioresources and this has laid the foundation for further conservation work. This has to be given priority as an essential component in the healthcare sector.

## REFERENCES


Anonymous (2002), *Medicinal Plants Scenario in India*, Technical Report No.1—Ministry of Environment and Forests, Published by Medplan Conservatory Society, Bangalore pp. 1-21.

Casey, A.F. and Parfitt, R.T. (1986), *Opioid Analgesics, Chemistry and Receptors*, New York: Plenum Press, pp. 9-10.

Farnsworth, N.R. and Morris, R.W. (1976), Higher plants the sleeping giants for drug development, *Am.J. Pharm*, 148, 46-52.

Gorlay, G.K., Cherry, D.A. and Cousins, M.J. (1986), A Comparative study of the efficacy and pharmaco kinetics of oral methadone and morphine in the treatment of severe pain in patients with cancer, *Pain* 25, 297-312.

Rosketh, R. and Storstrein, O. (1963), Quinidine therapy of chromic auricular fibrillation, *Arch. Intern Med.* 111, 184-189

Shastry, A.R.K. and Chatterjee, S. (2002), *Setting biodiversity conservation priorities for India* (eds. Singh, S. *et al.*) WWF-India Vol. II pp. 467-473

Stern, S. (1971), Treatment and prevention of cardiac arrhythmias with propranolol and quinidine, *Br. Heart J.* 33, 523-525.

# 23

# Plant Use among the Tribals of Jharkhand

DOLLY FLORENCE MURMU

## Introduction

It was in the month of September when I had an opportunity to visit a Munda village for a small research study. During my visit, I realised that the villagers pay a great importance to the trees and plants in their surrounding, they consider trees as an auspicious for their deity to reside. Some consider them as mother, a second home for their ancestors spirits, which bestow them the blessing they need.

The tribal concept of viewing the plants convey lots of meaning. They do not look at it as a mere object but have a great sense of belongingness to the plants. In this paper I would like to focus the use of medicinal plants among the tribes of Jharkhand. The medicinal properties of plants are known to the general people also but there exist medicine man, like Pahan, Bhagat, Ojha, Jaributi Ranin etc. who with great care prepare medicines for the treatment of various diseases, like cholera, fever, amoebic dysentery, scabies, anaemia, diabetes, and female diseases like barrenness, undesirable fertility, etc. During my investigation, I saw pahan grounding some medicine on a stone slab, in front of the small worshipping place. After my enquiry he said that, the medicine is for his daughter who is suffering from stomach cramp due to menstruation. It was an amazing sight, within 15 minutes of intake of raw medicine his daughter got relief from pain. But the fact remains that it is the medicine man who prepares the medicine in front of the worshipping place believing that, the magic property of the medicine will have a great effect if he seeks blessing from his deity.

Therefore in present context we find that, it is not the medicine which is valued by the tribals but it is the medicine men who are given much more importance because the people think that, the magical properties of the medicine will be effective only when it is prepared by the medicine man at an auspicious time.

## Origin

Regarding the origin of the large number of medicines practically nothing is known. The tribals must have hit upon some herbs in some or the other way and found them efficacious and this way they have been guided by experience. But as far as the literature is concerned, their uses are not so far recorded and especially the particular medicinal property which the tribals attribute to the plants is not known.

Therefore I am trying to make an attempt to document few plants with its medicinal properties, along with therapeutic preparation and remedies with hope that this could help us to understand the effectiveness of the treatment and secondly, the government should help tribal people finding out a way for profit sharing by aiding them with adequate facilities in other words a small farm houses should be encouraged so that the tribal wealth should be cultivated on the commercial ground, and people should also be ensured the profitable marketing by opening co-operative markets.

## Present Status of Medicinal Plants and Human System

Plants remedies are harmless provided they are selected carefully and taken under medical guidance. Curative effects of the medicinal plants were known to the people long before scientific explanation were advanced. They soon came to separate edible species from the poisonous ones and gradually learned how to select the most useful parts of such plants. This wealth of acquired knowledge was passed on verbally and still it is continuing among the tribals. Slowly and gradually the facts are distorting and all kinds of imaginery power are attributed to the certain plants.

In the present context, scientific research has greatly clarified the study of plants, medicinal plant now have accepted botanical name. Attempts have been made to analyze them chemically and distinguish at least some of the many components and active principles. Such analysis have recently been utilised in the production of similar compounds by synthetic means. These are not only more convenient to take but are also easier to store. Experiments have shown, however, that from a curative point of view, substances extracted from medicinal plants and the equivalent substances produced synthetically behave differently. There is a variation in the absorption capacity and the natural product has a milder effect on the system than the man made one. Other tests have shown that synthetic drugs afford a faster rate of recovery, but that plant substances have a much more positive and lasting effect.

## How Medicinal Plants Work?

Since ancient times, orthodox pharmaceuticals medicines were the only solution to sustain life and counter infections. Despite of the dramatic advances and advantages of conventional medicine, or biomedicine it has been established that herbal medicine has offered a great solution to cure diseases such as tuberculosis and malaria. Today, herbal remedies are coming back into prominence because the efficacy of conventional medicines such as antibiotic which one had near–universal effectiveness against serious infections is on the wane. Over the years, infectious organisms have developed resistance to synthesized drugs and the herb qinghao (*Artemisia awanua*) and its active consistent artemism for example, are now being used to treat malaria in areas of the world, where the protozoa causing the infection no longer respond to conventional treatment.

Herbal medicine offers conventional treatments, providing safe well-tolerated remedies for chronic illness. It is experiencing a dramatic renaissance in western countries, partly because no effective conventional treatment as yet exists for many chronic illnesses such as asthma, arthritis and irritable bowel syndrome. In addition, concern over the side effects of biomedicine is encouraging people to look for more gentle forms of treatments. It is estimated that 10–20 per cent of hospital patients in the west are there due to the side effect of conventional medical treatment. This is one of the major reason that tribals use herbal medicine to combat not only acute disease but also chronic diseases.

Herbal medicines should be used wisely. Most commonly used herbs are extremely safe to use. But some plants can produce side effects and like all medicines, herbal remedies must be treated with respect. It is necessary to take or use certain plants only under the guidance of a well trained practitioner, to avoid adverse consequences. It has been observed that Ephedra (*Ephedra sinica*) can be extremely toxic at the wrong dosage, and comfrey (*Symphtum officinale*), a very popular herb in the past, is thought to cause severe or even fatal liver damage in rare circumstances. Therefore herbal medicine should be used correctly, however, the chances of developing a serious side effect are remote.

**Value of Whole Plants**

Biomedicines are literally God/Goddess gift, rather developed in laboratory. Though it is difficult to understand the action of individual active constituents of the herbal medicine. In fact biomedicine is ultimately about the use and actions of whole plants. Therefore it is essential to identify the key parts of the plants. The whole herb is worth more than the sum of its parts and scientific research is increasingly showing that the active constituents of many herbs, for example those in ginkgo (*Ginkgo biloba*) interact in complex ways to produce the therapeutic effect of the remedy as whole. Plants contain hundreds, if not thousands of different constituent chemicals that interact in complex ways. Frequently we simply do not know in detail how a particular herb works even though its medicinal benefit is well established. The pharmacological approach to understanding how whole herbs work is like working in jigsaw where some of the pieces have been provided. Furthermore, although it is very useful to know that a plant contain certain active constituents, such information can be misleading on its own. For example, tea (*Camellia sinensis*) and coffee (*Coffea arabica*) contain approximately the same levels of caffiene. Tea however contains a much greater quantity of tannins which give tea its sour astringent taste.

These constituents reduce the amount of nutrients and drugs that are absorbed from the intestines into the blood stream and consequently less caffiene is absorbed. As a result, and true to most people's experiences, tea is less stimulating than coffee. This example reveals a couple of fundamental truths about herbal medicine. Firstly, the experience of the herbal practitioner and of the patient often provide the most reliable guide to the medicinal effects of individual herbs. Secondly, the value of a medicinal herb cannot be reduced simply to a list of its active constituents.

Similarly we have to find out what other ways in which the tribals attribute value to the plants and only then we can realise the actual value the plant hold in the eyes of tribals.

## Herbal Market

Man has been exploiting nature for various reasons from time immemorial. Out of 25 million species of plants worldwide, only 20,000 have so far been listed as being of known medicinal value and only 5,000 have been studied in detail. According to WHO, about 25 per cent prescribed human medicines are derived from plants with medicinal value, containing specific pharmacological activity, which depend on traditional system of medicine for primary health care need. India accounts for 17,500 species of higher plants, over 2,000 documented species having medicinal value around 1,100 species used in different systems of medicine. Out of these 600–700 species are used much in the country and 150 species with commercial usage, 95 per cent of the plants are obtained from wild sources and not cultivated.

The world herbal market according to a report published by U.K. based consultancy McAlpine Thorpe and Warrier, stands at $ 14.2 billions or Rs. 51,210 crore (*Business India*, November 17–30, 1997). This presents a big opportunity since India's share is currently only Rs. 280 crores against China's figure Rs. 18,000 crores.

## Conclusion

So far pharmacological experiments or clinical tests have been done on a very small number of medicinal herbs. Hence it may be emphasized here that, if we have to exploit, the exploitation should be effective harnessing of medicinal plants resources available in tribal areas, and secondly, the modern scientific test on these medicinal herbs should be intensified.

The use of tribal medicine, particularly the herbs have been studied by many including botanist and some have also pointed out the importance to document them and use them after adequate experiments. Beside this, there is a need to understand how tribal people perceive these plants? In what way they categorise the medicinal properties of the plants? How emotionally they are related to the plants? What role a plant plays in the life of tribes? Do they look at medicinal plants as God or Deity? Do they consider that the plants has a magic property? How tribals are bound in their cultural construct can only be understood, if we make an effort to know what type of meaning is being conveyed by the plants. It was found by Dr. S.P. Singh and Dr. V.L. Singh that, contraceptive plants were used by the tribals of U.P. They were experimentally evaluated, for the purpose and positive results were observed. It has been suggested that these plants may be utilized in the preparation of an indigenous contraceptive pill. Such valuable plants need to be preserved carefully.

The Government should help the tribal population to take important measure for the conservation of forest, for the cultivation of medicinal plants. Medicinal wealth of tribal be experimentally benefited. We ensure the effective harness in other words, farm-houses should be opened, where medicinal species of plants should be cultivated on the commercial ground. Marketing should also receive aid from government. It should be co-operative kind so that all the benefit should go to the tribals. It should be checked that no middleman (*Thekedar*) receives the benefit from the tribal wealth.

**Documentation of Medicinal Plants used among the Tribals of Jharkhand**

| Sl. No. | Botanical Name & Family | Vernacular | Tribe | Part used | Therapeutic preparation | Remedies |
|---|---|---|---|---|---|---|
| 1. | *Holarrhena antidysenteric* (Apocynaceae) | Karchi | Santhal, Munda Oroan, Ho | Tree | The bark of the stem and root, preferably of the young plant and the seeds are well known as remedies. | Amoebic dysentry |
| 2. | *Zingiber Officinalis* (Scitamineae) | Ada | Santhal, Munda Oroan, Ho | Tuber | Zingh pieces are boiled in water and solution is taken for the treatment. Zinger paste is made along with honey and taken for cold, cough and respiratory problems. | Toxia, indigestion, respiratory trouble, cough, cold |
| 3. | *Swerita Chirayita* (Roxb. ex Flem.) *Karsten* (Gentianaceae) | Chiraita | Santhal | Leaves | The whole plant is extremely bitter. It is used in the form of infusion. (Half an ounce of the bruished plant infused in one pint of hot water for 20–30 min. and the solution is administered to the patient. | Liver and spleen trouble and as tonic |
| 4. | *Saraca Indica* (Leguminoceae) | Ashok dari | Santhal, Munda Oroan, Ho | Leaves | The bark is strongly astringent, as it contain tannin. A decoction of the bark in milk is generally prescribed. The dose is 1 ounce 3 times a day commenced from the 4th day of the monthly period, and continued daily till the bleeding ceases. | Uterine trouble internal bleeding dysentery |
| 5. | *Andrographis penicculata* (Acanthaceae) | Kalmagh dari Adihara dari | Santhal, Munda Oroan, Ho | Leaves | The whole plant is intensely bitter and yields its properties readily to water or spirits The root has stomachache, tonic and alternative properties. | Liver and spleen & trouble diarrhoea for children etc. |

(*Contd.*)

(*Contd.*)

| Sl. No. | Botanical Name & Family | Vernacular | Tribe | Part used | Therapeutic preparation | Remedies |
|---|---|---|---|---|---|---|
| 6. | *Sidacordifolla* (Malanaceae) | Berola | Santhal, Munda Oraon, Ho | Whole plant | The roots of all these species are regarded as cooling, astringent and toxic, given in infusion in nervous diseases.<br>The powder of root bark is given with milk for the various diseases. | Heart trouble, Neuralgia, sciatica, paralysis |
| 7. | *Adhatoda Vasica* (Acanthaceae) | Baikash | Santhal, Munda Oraon, Ho | Whole plant | The root, bark, leaves and flowers are all used medicinally, mostly in the form of powder, or infusion of the root and extract of leaves in cough, asthma. | Respiratory trouble, worms |
| 8. | *Withania Somnifera* (Solanaceae) | Aswagandha | Santhal, Munda Oraon, Ho | Roots | The roots are grinded to make paste and patient is administered internally. | Seminal weakness Rheumatism Ricket |
| 9. | *Rauwolfia serpentina* (Apocynaceae) | Chandra | Santhai, Munda Oraon, Ho | Roots | The roots are known as an antidote to poison and to the bites of poisonous reptiles and stings of insects.<br>The roots are also administered for various diseases. | Madness, High blood pressure, Tension |
| 10. | *Butea monosperma* (Lam) Taub. (Fabaceae) | Murhu dari | Santhal, Munda Oraon, Ho | Seeds | The seed paste are administered with butter milk against worms. | Worms |
| 11. | *Terminalia Chebula* (Combretacea) | Aaunla dari | Santhal, Munda Oraon, Ho | Fruits | The ripe fruits are used for the constipation powdered amla with sufficient ghee is used for ulcer. | Bowel trouble, Ulcer, high blood pressure |

| Sl. No | Botanical Name & Family | Vernacular | Tribe | Part use | Therapeutic preparation | Remedies |
|---|---|---|---|---|---|---|
| 1. | *Acalypha indica* (L) (Eupyorbiaceae) | Khokali | Munda | Leaf | Leaf juice is prescribed to the patient. | Diabetes |
| 2. | *Aegle marmelos corr.* (Rutaceae) | Luwa dari sinjudari | Santal Munda | Leaf | Leaf oil is administered to the patient. | Diabetes |
| 3. | *Argyria Nervosa* (Burmf.) Boj. (Convolvulaceae) | Marangarin | Santal Munda | Leaf | Paste of leaf is used in diabetes. | Diabetes |
| 4. | *Asparagus racemossus wild.* (Liliaceae) | Mahadijat Kaisago Huring Atikir | Santal Munda Oraon | Roots | Boiled roots are administered to the patient. | Diabetes |
| 5. | *Azadirachta indica* A. Juss (Meliaceae) | Nimdari | Santal Munda Oraon | Leaves | Paste of leaves with black pepper is used in diabetes. | Diabetes |
| 6. | *Bambusa bambos Druce.* (Poaceae) | Bansdari | Munda Santal | Young leaf | Paste of young leaf is used. | Diabetes |
| 7. | *Butea monosperma* (Lamk) Taub. (Leguminosae) | Palas baha | Munda Oraon Santal | Leaves and fruits | Leaves and fruits are used. Its antidiabetic property is well known. | Diabetes |
| 8. | *Cissampelos pareiral.* (Menispermaceane) | Huring Pitusing | Santal Munda Oraon | Root | Root extract is used to control excessive urine discharge. | Diabetes |
| 10. | *Coccina grandis* (L) Viogt (Cucurbitaceae) | Kendari Tilkakriba | Santal Munda | Roots, leaves fruits | Roots, leaves and mucilage from the fruit is used. | Diabetes |
| 11. | *Ficus bengalensis* L. (Moraceae) | Bardari | Santal | Bark | Bark is used for diabetes. | Diabetes |
| 12. | *Momordica charantia* L (Cucurbitaceae) | Korla | Santal Munda Oraon | Fruit | Fruits are used. | Diabetes |

| Sl. No | Botanical Name & Family | Verna-cular | Tribe | Part use | Therapeutic preparation | Remedy |
|---|---|---|---|---|---|---|
| 1. | *Plumbago Zeylanica* (Plumbaginaceae) | Chitaor | Oroan | Root | The roots are grinded and rubbed over the effected parts. | Goitre |
| 2. | *Trigonellafoenum graecum* L. (Fabaceae) | Methi | Oroan | Seeds | Seeds of methi are soaked in water for 8–10 hours after that it is filtered and the solution obtained is taken to cure diabetes. | Diabetes mellitus |
| 3. | *Lawsonia inermis* L. (Lythraceae) | Mendi | Oraon | Seeds | The seeds of mendi are used as medicine for weakness. | Anaemia |
| 4. | *Bombax malabericum.* (Malvaceae) | Samri | Oraon | Leaves | The leaves of semal are boiled and is taken with sugar in case of anaemia. | Anaemia |
| 5. | *Shorea robusta* Gaertn.f. (Depteracarpaceae) | Salgom dari | Oraon | Gum of tree | The gum of sal tree is powdered, mixed with fresh curd and then drunk. | Diarrhoea |
| 6. | *Euphorbia hirta* (Euphorbiaceae) | Dudhia | Oraon | Root | The root of dudhia is powdered and is taken with water in bowel complaints. | Amoebic dysentry |
| 7. | *Eugemia jambolana* (Mytaceae) | Sow dari | Oraon | Bark | The juice of the bark of jumun is taken to cure dysentery. | Amoebic dysentry |
| 8. | *Sida carpinifolia* (Malvaceae) | Bariari | Oraon | Leaves | The leaves are powdered and mixed with Talmishri is taken in the form of paste to cure jaundice. | Jaundice |
| 9. | *Cucumis Satinus* L. (Cucurbitaceae) | Khera | Oraon | Seeds | The seeds of an old cucumber are grinded and given to patient suffering from cholera. | Cholera |
| 10. | *Bombax malabaricum* (Malvaceae) | Samri or Sambar | Oraon | Bank and Root | The bark and root of this plant are powdered with water and sugar and then filtered. The mixture so obtained is used to cure retention of urine. | Genito urinary disease |
| 11. | *Jatropha curcas* L. (Euphorbiaceae) | Baghrandi | Oraon | Latex | Baghrandi latex is used to fix loose teeth and to check bleeding. | Gum problem |

## REFERENCES


Chaudhuri, Buddhadeb, (1986), *Tribal Health: Socio cultural dimension*, Inter-India Publication.

Das, Sarita, Das, S.K., Pandey, S.N., (2003), Ethnomedicinal information from Orissa state, India A Review, *Journal of Human Ecology*; Vol. 14, pp. 165-227.

Ghosh, Abhik (1996), Oraon World views and concepts of Health and Medicine, *Man in India*, 1966, Vol. 76, No. 1, pp. 67-80.

Green, Halgh Trisha (1987), Drug prescription and self-medication in India, An exploratory survey, *Social Science and Medicine*, Vol. 25, No 3, pp. 307-18.

Michael, F. Brown (1987), Towards a Human Ecology: Medicinal Ethnobotany and search for dynamic model of plant use, *Review in Anthropology*, Vol. 14, Number 2.

Pandey, B.N., Das, P.K.L., Jha, A.K. and R.N. Tripathi, (1995), Association of Blood Groups with diseases and uses of medicinal plants among the Oraon, *Man in India*, 1995, 75, (3), pp. 307-11.

Schroder, Ekkehand (1978), Ethno medicine and Medical Anthropology, *Review in Anthropology*.

Sen, Sharma Priyadarshan, (1988), Ethnobotanical investigation in the Indian Purans, The Vayu Purana, *Man in India*; 1988.

Silvakalinga, Tudor; (1991), Ayurveda, Malaria and the Indigenous Herbal Tradition in Sri Lanka, *Social Science and Medicine* 1991, Vol. 33, No. 2, pp. 153-60.

Srivastava, Ratish, (1979), Future of Tribes in Bihar Anthropological perspective, *Man in India*.

Swarankar R.C. (1995), *Indian Tribes: Health Ecology & Social structure* Printwell Publication.

# 24

# Science in Society: The Case of Tribal Medicine

BUDDHADEB CHAUDHURI

## Introduction

The prevailing health and medical system, the western system, has unfortunately failed to meet the need of the world's majority. The failure of the Alma Ata Declaration in fulfilling its objectives of achieving Health for all by the year 2000 gives more urgency for looking for an alternative. In most countries a very frightening policy change is being manoeuvered by agencies like the World Bank and IMF (International Monetary Fund) to give less and less emphasis to the social and welfare sectors and higher emphasis to the economic and infrastructure sectors. As such the financial allocation for health is going down in most Asian countries. The implications of such a trend in countries where health insurance is unaffordable to the majority is unimaginable. Based on current trends in health care financing and the failure of the Alma Ata Declaration to take a grip of the situation there is an imperative need for evolving an Alternative. In this whole changing situation, the condition of the poor, particularly the indigenous people has become more critical and difficult. Generally, when we talk or think about science, we refer to the western or industrial society. In the context of scientific development, we prefer to discuss more about the so called modern scientific innovations assuming that science is only there in those societies and quite often implying that scientific rigour or interest is absent in other societies. The role of science is to help mankind to meet the various demands exploiting the natural resources in the best possible way without adversely affecting the environment. People have developed their own science and technologies based on the demands of the concerned societies, but quite often these are ignored. What I want to impress here is that we need to look at indigenous science and technology particularly when an exiting body of knowledge is available: perhaps it is better to develop it instead of replacing it in the name of scientific development and modernization. Besides, the traditional knowledge and wisdom have important implications in the contest of globalization process. The traditional tribal medicine and treatment in India have been examined in this context.

## Tribal Demography

The different tribal communities in India do not represent a homogenous group. There is considerable variation in the context of economy, life style, behaviour and practices. Similarly, considerable variations are also there in the context of demographic features. Thus, population of communities varies from around 20 as in the case of the Andamanese to over 40 lakhs as in the case of the Gonds. Thus in one context, the survival of the community may be the most crucial factor while in another context economic development may be more important. If we examine the growth rate of tribal population it is obvious that the growth rate of the total tribal population is quite high and in fact it is higher than the all India average. But this does not really reflect the true situation as considerable variation is there so far the growth rate of the different tribal communities is concerned. In fact, it would be wrong to categorise the tribals as homogenous group, as there are tribal groups where, (1) the population is decreasing, (2) the population is stagnant, (3) the population is increasing, and (4) the population is increasing very fast. In case of some communities, there is a definite decline, threatening the survival of the community. In this context, the study of socio-cultural habits and health practices becomes imperative. The decline might not be only because of a lower rate of fertility but also owing to high mortality and problems in the existing health practices. The decline may be related to their food habits or certain types of food that the tribals consume which may adversely affect the fertility of the concerned population. Again, it may be worthwhile to examine what is the minimum viable population of a group. In other words, it may be examined, whether the size of the population is, in anyway, related to decline, if so, what is the size. Unfortunately, till today we do not have many studies to answer some of these crucial questions.

## Health and Culture

Every culture, irrespective of its simplicity and complexity, has its own beliefs and practices concerning diseases. No culture works in a meaningless fashion in its treatment of diseases. Every culture evolves its own system of medicine in order to treat diseases in its own way. This treatment of disease varies from group to group.

*The belief in the supernatural:* The belief in the interference of supernatural agency is particularly strong in the case of their main economic pursuits and in the context of health and disease. The different economic activities are associated with rituals. Similarly, different deities and spirits are connected with various types of diseases. Most of their socio-cultural activities revolve around gods and spirits. They identify the supernatural powers with a group of powerful forces and deities which control and influence the happenings in the community. Thus, they have specific gods for their health and disease, for calamities, for the cattle and so on. All these deities have their own respective departments and areas of influence, effect and control, as well as nature of action. A number of tribal communities of West Bengal like Santals, Mundas and Oraons have a village deity who is the general protecting goddess of the villagers. But a number of specific deities are also there like Sitala and Manasa, who are connected with different diseases. Thus, when there is an epidemic like small pox or cholera, she is always propitiated. Manasa is the controlling deity of the snakes and naturally her blessings are sought against snake bites or in case of an incident involving them. Dessauli among the Hos is a deity who protects the villagers form evil spirits, diseases and epidemics. Among the Oraons, there is spirit—Pat or Pat Raja Raja who protects the village from sickness or other misfortune.

The tribals have such a strong faith in these deities that figures are often drawn on the walls or in the case of the Malers, to represent a god or goddess, and his or her presence protects the family members. The deities of epidemics are temporarily kept in the house to deal with illness.

It is important to understand and identify the cause of illness as the nature of treatment is intimately connected with it. The present author has noted this link in his study of the Mundas (1967; 1979); Valunjkar and Chaturvedi (1967) too have noted this relationship. Religious performances occupy a prominent place in the treatment of disease, like small-pox and plague which are associated with supernatural causes. Lewis (1958) too has noted that the advantage in learning about the indigenous beliefs and practices of the community is the insight that one can get regarding the world view of the people as concepts of disease causation are part of a society's total world view, which is also reflected in other spheres such as agriculture, politics and interpersonal relations. Elwin (1955) enumerates various gods associated with different diseases in the Saora pantheon. There are gods associated with children's disease, cough, cold, blindness, madness, disease of pregnant woman, of animals and so. Propitiating these gods directly or through shamans can cure most of these diseases. The association between gods and disease is so intimate that 'in many cases, the only thing a Saora can say about a god is to name a disease he gives'.

## Health, Medicine and Community

Health and treatment reflect the social solidarity of a community. In a tribal community, for example, illness and the consequent treatment is not always an individual or familial affair, but the decision about the nature of treatment is taken at the community level. In the rural areas, in case of some specific diseases, not only the diseased person or his/her family, but the total village community is affected. All the other families in the village are expected to observe certain taboos or norms and food habits. The non-observance of such practices often calls for action by the village council. One cannot deny the impact of this psychological support in the context of treatment and cure. In some societies, illness may be an individual affair, and the patient may be looked after by the administration (state), while in tribal societies it is a familial or sometimes community affair where necessary action and care is taken by the community as a whole.

Among the tribals, there are a group of specialists—the priests and/or magicians or medicinemen whose services are sought after, depending on the cause of the illness. Among the Hos, there is the Deuri or religious headman and Deonwa or the spirit doctor. The Deuri worships the deities and when epidemics or diseases are there in the village, he offers a sacrifice at the sacred place. He is entrusted with the benevolent deities. The malevolent spirits are controlled by the Deonwa, often through magical performances. Among the Mundas and the Oraons the religious headman is Pahan who propitiates the village deities on behalf of the entire village to word off disease and misfortune. Again, among some tribal groups, there is one person who officiates as priest and magician. The Bhils have Badava, who is the priest and performs the role of a medium, diviner, worshipper and healer. The Korwas beat an ailing person with iron chains and insert a burning wick into nose to cure him. When a Kuttia child of Orissa has its first serious illness it is generally decided that it is time for its naming ceremony to be performed. The medicineman is called in for magical performances. Among the Kuttias the village priest is the magician. Tharu women of the Himalayas are pioneers in the magical arts. Dube (1970) has noted the strong belief of the tribals of invisible powers which help in controlling an epidemic and curing an ailing person. Buch (1964) has noted two types of medicinemen: Janka, who works through divination and Barwa who works by calling to his aid a superhuman force.

The dependence on and confidence in traditional medicinemen or magicians and shamans are again often responsible for the non-acceptance of modern medicine. The traditional approach establishes faith and assurance in the patients, while modern medicine lacks this. As the shamans, traditional medicine-men and magicians share the common cultural beliefs and practices of the patients, naturally they have more faith in them. Carstairs (1955), a medical psychiatrist and anthropologist, pointed out that the difference between the points of view of the physician and the village folk with regard to theories of etiology, techniques of curing and conceptions of roles of the physician, resulted in misunderstandings between himself, a physician and his clients. Marriott (1955) has shown how the contrasts and conflicts between the roles assumed by the indigenous and the western medical practitioners resulted in obstacles to the acceptability of western medicine.

In most of the tribal communities, there are number of folklores related to health. Certain practices are suggested to avoid illness or diseases, while some are prescribed to have better health. These should not be ignored as mere folk-beliefs, but need careful attention. There are different folklores to avoid illness, during illness, regarding food and so on. Documentation of such folklores available in different socio-cultural system may be very rewarding and may provide the model for appropriate health and sanitary practices in a given eco-system.

**Health, Food Habits and Nutrition**

It has been noted by many that tribals living in remote areas have a better health status and more balanced food than those living in less remote areas (Chaudhuri, 1986; Chaudhuri *et al.*, 1989). In two projects related to tribal health, it has been noted that the various roots and tubers available in the forest or small animals they can hunt supply a more balanced nutritional status to the tribals (Chaudhuri *et al.*, 1989). Again, in many cases, it has been noted that certain diseases may be common in certain areas but they remain controlled because of certain food habits based on vegetation available locally or certain practices which have been generated through tradition. There is no doubt that any disturbance in the eco-system is likely to affect the balance and adversely affect the concerned population.

Another survey has shown that contrary to the general expectation, the shifting cultivating tribes like the Padam, Riang were having better nutritional status than those of the settled agricultural tribes like the Santal and the Ho. Again, in the context of deforestation, the hunting and gathering tribes were having lower nutritional status. It is quite significant that death rates are consistently lower than the national average in some of the tribal predominant states. Roy Burman (1990) has noted that physical well-being of the tribals is inextricably linked up with the forest ecology. In fact rapid disappearance of forest, commercialisation of minor forest produce, replacement of food crops by cash crops and tendency towards monoculture forestry and lastly, privatisation of communal lands may affect the health and nutrition and physical well-being of the tribal population.

***Crucial Issues and Myths***

A number of myths have been systematically created against the non-western system in general and indigenous system in particular. This system is based on a wide range of biological resources using thousands of plant species, hundred of animal species and animal parts and various minerals and metal sources. Unfortunately, over the years traditional knowledge and skills have been neglected and a prejudice has been engineered and encouraged by powerful nations and multinationals in order to subjugate non-western cultures. In order to evolve a proper health policy in the developing countries particularly for the indigenous people and the poor, a number of issues are to be examined.

1. Often it is said that health is the exclusive domain of medical science. By restricting it in this way, the socio-economic, cultural and environmental issues are often ignored.
2. Following the above logic, more and more expenditure on sophisticated research is promoted. It is not my intention to discourage research but when the resources are limited, it is to be seen how best possible way the resources can be utilized and whether it should provide more expensive sophisticated facilities to a few or minimum less expensive facilities to a larger population. Perhaps there is a need to make a balance between the two.
3. Quite often it is said that the rural people, particularly the tribals are all superstitious. Thus if a tribal worship a deity for cure, automatically it is assumed that they are superstitious and would not accept the so-called modern health practices, but when that the same thing is done in the cities of India it becomes tradition and when it is done in the Churches of Europe, it is levelled as convention. The question of rationality cannot be judged or examined in isolation, without examining the eco-system, health facilities available and economic condition. Again, the mere presence of a health centre does not necessarily mean that people would depend on it, if proper and adequate facilities are not available or if the people are not convinced about its efficiency. In fact, bulk of the social scientists, who have studied health culture of the rural population in India have been over enthusiastic in discussing superstitious health beliefs and practices but they have not paid adequate attention to the force which have been instrumental in causing decay and degeneration of their health culture.
4. The advocacy of traditional method of treatment does not mean that something counter to development is suggested. The point is that there may be many positive aspects in a traditional system, which should be encouraged and propagated. In fact, the need is to provide all the alternatives and not to depend on only one system.

5. The argument often put forward in favour of the introduction of the modern system (and of the replacement of the traditional) is that tribal and similar traditional approaches do not have an answer to many diseases. This is an undeniable fact but does not necessarily reflect a limitation of the traditional system. Apart from the fact of the non-availability of many herbs, one should add that many of these diseases were formerly unknown. Naturally, the question of any traditional system having a remedy for them does not arise. In fact, for the same reason, modern medicine also does not have remedies for many diseases.

***Strategy***

1. Documentation of traditional knowledge in health and medicine is urgently necessary. Most of the research and publications available in this field is purely academic in nature. Society in general is schooled into thinking that adopting traditional health skill and culture is inferior as compared to modern medicine. This attitude has contributed to the further degeneration of this knowledge. Documentation is also urgently needed because the traditional knowledge is mostly an oral tradition and hence documentation is necessary before they are forgotten. Loss of this rich and diverse eco-system based knowledge systems and skills will be no ordinary loss.
2. Legal and policy issues involving protection of traditional knowledge also needs to be examined. A legislative framework is required whereby the knowledge is kept with the people and recognition, financial or otherwise, is accorded to the individual or community by commercial firms who have to use their knowledge.
3. The changing forest policies and the changing development scenario in Asian countries have adversely affected the strength of the biological resources used in traditional medicine as much of these resources are being depleted through deforestation. The mono-plant afforestation programmes where emphasis is given on commercial plants has not helped the people much. There is a need to promote conservation measures for saving medicinal plants on various eco-systems and habitat.

4. A number of studies have pointed out the nature of health hazards in the context of unplanned/uncontrolled use of insecticides and pesticides. It has been noted how they have killed the small fishes in the paddy field and thus the poorer families, who generally consumed this protein were deprived of it. This is also true in case of many tribal areas. Thus the whole development strategy needs critical analysis as it may adversely affect the environment and consequently the health status of the people, particularly the tribals.
5. Multinational drug companies, medical lobby and the western media have played a major role in disrupting and negating the indigenous knowledge systems while on the other hand exploited this traditional knowledge and resource base to develop new drugs. Current efforts at research in ethnic pharmacology have often proved to be counter-productive to the development or advancement of local cultures as the objective is not to strengthen the traditional knowledge and resource base but to get information for multinational drug companies. It is well known that drug multinationals have been robbing traditional knowledge for their own interests.
6. There is a need to perpetuate and revive the traditional/indigenous system, which is close to the people, non-commercial in nature and curative in approach. It this context, it may be necessary, for—
   (a) identification of factors responsible for erosion of indigenous health care system and formulation of action programmes to countermand it,
   (b) formulation of appropriate methodology to institute traditional health care system in rural/tribal areas, and
   (c) identification of methodology for more intensive and integrated documentation, research and development.

## Traditional Knowledge and Wisdom: Limitations and Scope

A number of studies were made in different villages to examine the traditional knowledge and wisdom related treatment. Besides the studied villages, an attempt was made to ascertain the traditional knowledge present among the tribal communities in this region, covering the tribal dominated areas of West Bengal, Bihar and Orissa. It may be added here that by virtue of close association with some activist groups who are working in the area specifically on health and treatment, a large number of traditional herbal medicines used by them were identified.

Disease and treatment particularly in the tribal societies cannot be properly understood in isolation. Health and treatment are very much connected with the environment particularly the forest ecology. The traditional health care system and treatment are based on their deep observation and understanding of nature derived through their observation of other animals in nature. Though we have limited ethno botanical studies with reference to the tribals, but all of them have indicated deep knowledge of the tribal people regarding the medical value of different plants, which they regularly use for cure and treatment. It may be added here that many of the tribal groups use different parts of the plants not only for treatment, but even for population control. This knowledge can be fruitfully utilized in a wider context. Again, many tribal groups plant certain varieties against insects. Instead of going for insecticide, these shrubs can be planted since they would not adversely affect the environment and may be more helpful to preserve the ecological balance.

Even though we have only a few ethno botanical studies with particular reference to the tribals, ethno zoology, which seeks to know the medicinal application of animals and aims to study the interrelationship between man and animal in this context, is still less developed. In fact, there are hardly a few studies in this field worth mentioning and, incidentally, the first ethno zoological study conducted by the Zoological Survey of India (Joseph, 1989) was in M.P. having the largest tribal population in India covering about 23 per cent of the total population of the state. Out of 58 Scheduled Tribes, the study covered 39 communities and the utility of the animals in food, medicine, family-planning, age stabilization, mechanical and industrial uses, fuel, fertilizer, religious purpose, witchcraft, harmful animals and for other uses (total 28 uses) was studied. The study indicated about 894 medicinal applications of various animals of which the maximum number of applications as that of mammals (433), followed by birds (136), reptiles (107), mollusc (64), insects (44), crabs (39), fishes (35) and other animals. A review of literature clearly indicates our meagre knowledge of traditional animal-medicine, even though medicinal application of animals may be common among most of the tribal communities.

A knowledge and documentation of traditional tribal medicine are also urgently necessary. It is important for the modern system to begin with the base existing in the tribal society and build on it, rather than replace it. In order to achieve this, information about tribal medicinal practices should be documented before they are forgotten. A study of indigenous method of treatment may help to identify new methods of treatment of various diseases with certain modifications. In fact, a number of ethno botanical studies have helped to identify a number of medicinal plants used by the tribals to treat different types of diseases. Many of them may be very useful to treat diseases and it is urgently necessary to document them and try them after proper scientific experiment. This has been observed in the few studies that have been made on tribal medicine, especially in terms of efficiency, which is very encouraging. This, however, needs to be further substantiated by sustained research. It may be said that the achievement of tribal medicine is quite revealing. However, to utilize the research findings for further development and application for benefiting the vast majority of the rural poor, particularly the tribals who are living in areas which have very little or no so called modern medical facilities, needs an integrated and multi-disciplinary research and follow-up dissemination efforts.

Documentation should be made and at the same time one has to be aware of the risks involved and the use the commercial interest can put to it. Hence, it should be done with certain reservations. Cases are not lacking, when after the publication of research reports on traditional medicinal plants used by the tribals, many such plants were collected in bulk by outside big industries for commercial use for profit. As a result, they are no more available to the traditional medicine men to whom they are so essential for treatment. As a result, the tribals are deprived of their traditional system without the modern system becoming accessible to them.

The relation of forests with nutrition may be mentioned. It has been noted by many that the tribals living in remote areas have a better health status and more balanced food than those living in less remote areas. The various roots and tubers available in the forest or small animals they can hunt supply a balanced nutrition to them. There is no doubt that deforestation is likely to affect the nutritional status of the tribals as most of the roots and tubers are not available. Again, in many cases, it has been noted that certain diseases may be common in certain areas but they are controlled because of certain food habits based on vegetation available locally, or certain practices which have been generated through tradition. There is no doubt that any disturbance in the eco-system is likely to affect the balance and same diseases may spread very quickly. The mode of utilization of available natural resources often determines the long-term impact on health. A number of scholars have pointed out the nature of health hazards in the context of unplanned/uncontrolled use of insecticides and pesticides for agricultural development. It has also been observed how this may affect the nutritional status of people, particularly the tribals. The use of insecticides and pesticides has killed the small fishes in the paddy field and thus the poorer families, who generally consumed this protein, were deprived of it. This is also true in case of many tribal areas. Thus the whole development strategy needs critical analysis as it may adversely affect the environment and consequently the health status of the people, particularly the tribals.

Forest happens to be the main source of getting medicinal plants and animals. Naturally the different Forest Acts restricting the use and exploitation of forest resources are adversely affecting the health and treatment in tribal societies. Thus, though apparently there does not exist any relation between the forest and health of an individual, in reality, the Forest Acts, deforestation and certain types of afforestation programmes may adversely affect the health of the tribals. In some of our studies on the health care system in the tribal areas, we observed how the tribal medicine men were facing difficulties in getting medical plants. Most of the traditional medicine men who came from the three states of Bihar, Orissa and West Bengal, while discussing the problems they faced in practicing their profession, all clearly pointed out the difficulties they were facing in gathering medicinal plants mainly from the forest. The success of their approach has to be analysed in this context, even if their treatment is not successful in one context.

The relation of treatment and nutrition with forest among the rural population, particularly among the tribal communities is quite obvious. The traditional herbal treatment is rather a people's knowledge and an oral tradition. In many cases, many persons in the concerned community have the knowledge and in some cases, a few selected persons, the traditional medicine men are more knowledgeable. But in any case, people depend on nature, particularly on forest for these medicinal plants. Thus deforestation and commercial afforestation of mono-plant forest (?) may seriously affect the availability of these medicinal plants. Even the nutrition may be similarly affected as access to forest resources can affect treatment and nutrition. Thus some of the major problems the tribal communities are facing in general and the traditional medicine men in particular in this context are as follows:

1. Deforestation and non-availability of medicinal plants and animals.
2. Commercial afforestation and more emphasis on commercially important plants—consequently non-availability of herbs.
3. Forest Laws and Acts restricting the use and exploitation of forest resources.
4. Non-availability of medicinal plants because of commercial interest in many areas.

The observations made in this paper are based on the findings of research studies sponsored by ICSSR, ICMR, Asian Community Health Action Network and some action programmes sponsored by CAPART conducted along with some activist groups in West Bengal, Jharkand and Orissa. A number of workshops were also organised to have interaction of tribal medicine-men, researchers, doctors and planners in different parts of Chotanagpur region.

## REFERENCES

Banerjee, D. (1986), *Social Science and Health Service Development in India,* Lok Paksh, New Delhi

Carstairs, G.M. (1955), 'Medicine and Faith in Rural Rajasthan' in B.D. Paul (ed). *Health Culture and Community,* Russel Sage Foundation, New York.

Chaudhuri, Buddhadeb (1967), Magic Vs. Medicine in a Tribal Village, '*Adibasi*'9.3-9

—— (1979), Cultural Dimensions of Health: A study on West Bengal Villages'; 1st International Congress on Traditional Asian Medicine, Canberra, Australia

——(1985), *Concept and Treatment of Disease Among the Tribals of India,* ICSSR Review Study.

——(1986), *Tribal Health: Socio-Cultural Dimensions,* Inter India Publications, New Delhi.

——(1986), Social and Cultural Aspects of Health, *Journal of Social and Economic Studies* (n.s.) 379-388.

——(1989), 'Social Science, Health and Culture: The Tribal Situation', *Social Action.* 39(3): 243-253.

Chaudhuri, Buddhadeb, (1990), The Case of Tribal Medicine, in '*The Philosophy of Science*', Ed. J.V. Narlikar and others, Indian Institute of Advanced Study, Shimla.

——(1990), *Cultural and Environmental Dimensions on Health*, Inter-India Publications, New Delhi.

——(1993), Health, Culture and Environment: The Tribal Situation in India, in *Continuity and Change in Tribal Society*, Ed. Mrinal Miri, Indian Institute of Advanced Study, Shimla.

——(2003) *Forest, Health and Development: The Tribal Situation*, Inter-India Publication, New Delhi.

Chaudhuri, Buddhadeb, D. Dasgupta and K.K. Chatterjee (eds.) (1989), *Tribal Medicine*, Regional Research and Study Centre, Midnapore.

Elwin,V., *The Religion of an India Tribe*. Oxford University Press, London.

Lewis, Oscar (1958), *Village Life in Northern India*, Random House, New York.

Jain, S.K. (1968), *Medicinal Plants,* National Book Trust, New Delhi.

Joseph, A.N.T. (1992), Ethnozoology of Reptiles in Relation to Health care among Tribals in Madhya Pradesh, in *National Development and Tribal Deprivation*, Ed. Walter Fernandes, Indian social Institute, New Delhi.

Marriott Mckim (1955), Western Medicine in a Village of Northern India, in *Health, Culture and Community,* B.D. Paul (Ed.) Russel Sage, New York.

Roy Burman, B.K. (1990), Development Hazards to Health in Tribal India. in *Cultural and Environmental Dimensions on Health*, Ed. Buddhadeb Chaudhuri. Inter-India Publications, New Delhi.

# 25

# Ethnomedicine and Tribal Health: An Illustrative Appraisal

R.K. KAR

Disease and ill-health has been one of the fundamental concern of man since his emergence on the earth. Every known society has developed its own responses and methods for coping up with diseases and ailments; and eventually a body of its own medical system. "Medicine has been practised one way or another since man became a cultural animal. There even is some evidence that a first-aid technique derives from our primate ancestors..... baboons" (Clune, 1976:5)*

Ethnomedicine, a sub-division of medical anthropology refers to "those beliefs and practices relating to disease which are the products of indigenous cultural development; and are not explicitly derived from the conceptual framework of modern medicine" (Hughes, 1968 : 99). Etymologically speaking, the term refers to the medicines that are traditionally associated with specific ethnic groups. Thus, it can also be conceived of as *Folk medicine, Traditional medicine* or *Indigenous medicine* etc. (Mibang and Choudhuri, 2003 : 1).

It may relevantly be noted here that beginning with their earliest field research around some 100 years ago, anthropologists, in a routined way have gathered data on the medical beliefs of the peoples, they studied, in the same way and for the same purpose that they have gathered on all other aspects of culture to have as complete an ethnographic record as possible.

* Cited in Khan and Ali, 1992 : 11.

It was the noted British Physician/Anthropologist W.H.R. Rivers (1924) who first developed the idea that indigenous medical systems are social institutions to be studied in the same way as social institutions in general; and that indigenous medical practices are rational actions when viewed in the light of prevailing causation beliefs.

Incidentally, neither Rivers nor Clements (1932) nor any of their contemporaries, engaged in collecting data on primitive medical systems had any idea that they were doing "medical anthropological" research, and they seemed to have been unconcerned with the possible significance of their findings to the health of the people they studied. Consequently, we cannot say that medical anthropology has developed out of early research on primitive medicine. Rather, it is the other way around. Anthropologists, working in the health fields today have, in fact, recaptured and given a formal name—*ethnomedicine* to the study of traditional non-western medicine, and made it a part of their speciality.

As medical anthropology has developed, especially in the broad areas of international public health and transcultural psychiatry, the practical as well as the theoretical importance of knowledge about non-western medical systems has become apparent. This recognition has sparked renewed interest in ethno-medical research, elevating it to major importance in medical anthropology.

## II

As a matter of fact, the entire field of Traditional knowledge has attracted considerable attention in the recent past. An increasing number of global institutions (e.g., UNESCO and WIPO) are now concerned with defending, promoting and using Traditional knowledge more widely. The relationship between intellectual property and Traditional knowledge is receiving increased attention in many policy fora and debates, ranging from food and agriculture, environment, health, human rights and cultural policy to trade and economic development. In recognition of its relevance and importance, National Institute of Science Communication (NISCOM), New Delhi has recently (2002) launched the publication, *Indian Journal of Traditional Knowledge*, dealing exclusively with indigenous knowledge system. Considering the resurgence of interest in ethnobotany as a source of new pharmaceuticals, the first issue of the journal has been devoted to deal exclusively with some studies in this field.

India, as a matter of fact, is considered as one of the greatest store houses of traditional knowledge. She is blessed with a very rich and diverse heritage. Since time immemorial, the country has harboured and nurtured a variety of knowledge systems.

Along with traditional knowledge systems, India is also gifted with an immense wealth of rich bio-diversity that accounts for around 8 per cent of the world's total biodiversity. According to an estimate there are about 45,000 species of wild plants in India; and out of this around 7,500 species are in medical use in indigenous health practices (Vedavathy, 2002 : 25). The tribals who by and large, depend on forest wealth are the real custodians who safeguard the medicinal plants.

## III

The subject of ethnomedicine, in fact, focuses on the nature of illness as it is conceived by the natives; their own methods; criteria of classification of diseases; the causes and cures; types of therapists and healers who seek to alleviate illness, and their skills and social roles; preventive measures; the relation between medicine and religion; cultural aspects of medicine and also ethnopsychiatry (Hughes, 1968 and Foster, 1978). The primary concern of ethnomedicine is thus with the description of notions, people have about health and illness and about the behaviour they undertake in search of cures.

Rubbel (1977 : 120) explains the concept of illness as syndroms from which members of a particular group claim to suffer and for which their culture provides aetiology, diagnosis, preventive measures and regimes of healing. Studies of the relationship between health and harmony in the beliefs of the Navaha (Adair, Denschle and McDermott, 1957); and of the moral implications attributed to illness of several cultures (Fabrega, 1972), for example, provide ample demonstrations of the socio-cultural bearing on the notions of health and illness.

Data collected through the ethnomedical approach contribute not only to the understanding of medical systems in their cultural contents, but also lend insight into the understanding of the interface between the indigenous and western medical systems that effect socio-cultural change. The anthropologically oriented medical knowledge would be of immense use as an input to benefit disease control programmes and international health planning. Many of the disease control programmes have been introduced into areas where indigenous systems are yet strong, there have been great resistances (Khan and Ali, 1992 : 14).

An in-depth study of folk-medicine also helps to find out the forces of integration and resistance with regard to the implementation of certain modern medical programmes. Once we come to understand the cultural forces that hinder the successful implementation of the programmes, it will not be difficult to work out and modify the framework of the programmes according to the suitability of the culture or community for which they are meant.

Also by going into an in-depth understanding of indigenous materia media and pharmacopoeia of various traditional cultures, it is possible in ethnomedical studies to discover the medicinal value of plants and animals which are so far unknown or least known to the modern world.

The pharmacopoeia of folk medicines is copious and includes such proven drugs as quinine, opium, drossera, thuja and curare etc. Sometimes, the same species of plant is used for a host of purposes. Thus, for example, almost all parts of the Mahua (*Madhuca longifolia*) plant are used by the tribals of Madhya Pradesh in various ailments and diseases: the root paste is given to treat stomach ulcer; it is applied on scorpion sting; the bark decoction is gargled in case of gum swelling; the decoction with that of *Ficus recemosa* is used for leucorrhoea; the bark is astringent and tonic; its decoction is given in diabetes and rheumatic diseases; the flowers are given in bronchitis and cough; the flower paste is applied to take out the pierced thorn; the fruit paste is applied in toothace; the seed oil is massaged over the chest in the treatment of pneumonia; and the seed cake is used in snake bite—few drops of its decoction are put in the nostrils which results into vomitting and relief (Sikarwar, 2002 : 90).

Therapy in ethnomedicine includes both magico-religious and mechanical and chemical procedures. Indigenous medical systems show an impressive array of practices that demonstrate empirical therapeutic knowledge including trephinination, bonesetting, obstetrics including caesarian section, laparotomy, uvulectomy, comparative anatomy, autopsy, cantery, inoculation, baths, poultices, inhalations, laxatives, enemas, ointments and cupping (Acker Knecht, 1942; Simmons, 1955; Langhlin, 1963; Huard, 1969) etc.

While dwelling little bit more on the issue, particularly in the context of tribal communities, it may be noted that the practice of ethnomedicine in the form of magical cures has usually an explicit social implication reflecting socially cohesive results. Typically, the curative session involves not only the patient and the healer, but also the patient's family, clan members and other neighbours. The curative rituals serve, in various ways, as an occasion for re-integration of the group around common social values. "Especially in societies lacking strong centralised socio-political institution, the occurrence and imminence of disease with the belief that it represents punishment for aberrant, dissocial impulse or action can be functionally important in maintaining group cohesion and restraining disruptive tendencies" (Sills, 1972 : 91).

## IV

Because of a culturally and geographically diverse landscape, the North-east region of India exhibits a rich array of ethno-medical practices. But these have not been documented from several areas. Some piece-meal studies however, have been reported in a number of professional journals and edited books (e.g., Chaudhiri, 1986, 1990; Mibang and Choudhuri, 2003).

North-east India, popularly known as *Sat Bhoni* (seven sisters), comprises the states of Assam, Arunachal Pradesh, Manipur, Meghalaya, Mizoram, Nagaland and Tripura. According to 2001 census, the total population of the region is around 38.5 million, distributed over an area of 2.6 lakh sq.km. For administrative purpose, of late, Sikkim has also been included in North-east India (Population—5,40,493 according to 2001 census).

The region is considered as a cultural corridor between India and South-east Asia, and has a tremendous strategical importance, not only because of its geography, but also because of its history, demography and culture.

The region provides shelter to numerous peoples of various ethnic affiliations having different social structures, cultural heritages and cultural linkages across the international borders. There is a rich assembly of tribal cultures and communities in this rugged expanse of the eastern Himalayas. There are more than 140 major tribal groups in North-east India, having quite a good number of sub-tribes. In other words, around one-third of the total number of listed tribes for the whole of India are to be found in this region. The percentages of tribal population in different states range from 11 (Assam) to 94 (Mizoram). The average percentage of tribal population in the region is 22 (Kar, 2001).

Though the traditional outlook, customs, rituals, beliefs, habits and concepts of aetiology, as well as diagnosis and treatment of diseases are changing fast under the impact of an ongoing modernisation process, a number of studies, carried out in the recent past among various tribal groups of North-east India (e.g., among the Bodo Kacharis—Guha, 1986 a and b; Idu Mishmis—Dutta Choudhuri and Ghosh, 1984; Kaman Mishmis – Barua, 1984; Koch Rajbanshis—Guha, 1990; Pnars – Bhatt, 1986; Singphos – Dutta Choudhury, 1985; and the Noctes—Kar, 1993; Kar and Gogoi 1993, 1994) reveal that in most of the tribal and rural societies traditional health behaviours not only dominate over the modern ones, but also very often hinder the acceptance of the latter. Most of the people live in isolated high rugged terrain with a low level of technology and subsistence economy. As a result, they are much more dependent on nature. The healing system is thus intimately connected with the cosmos, emic perceptions of different natural phenomena and belief in spirits.

In most of the tribes (Plains and hills) *health* and *disease* are considered to be polar opposites. Disease refers to *a departure from the state of health*, and health is the *absence of disease*. As an illustration, the following pages have been devoted to have a fairly detailed discussion on the practice of ethonomedicine among the Mishings, an important plains tribe in Assam.

## V

The Mishings or the plains Miris are one of the major plains tribes in Assam. They are spread over five districts of the state, namely, Dhemaji, Lakhimpur, Sibsagar, Golaghat and Darrang; and a small portion of the plains of Arunachal Pradesh. In Assam, though their land spreads over five districts, their habitations are concentrated along the river courses of the Brahmaputra, Simen, Burisuti, Tongani, Chiadhol, Subansiri, Boginodi, Dikrong and the river island of Majuli. In the south their habitation is concentrated along the banks of Dibru lower part of Dihing, Disang, Dikhow and Dhansiri rivers. Waddel (1901) observes, "They are exceptionally sturdy and well developed physically although so many of them live in most malarial parts in Assam". According to 2001 census, the total Mishing population in Assam is around 4 lakhs.

The data for the follow-up discussion have been generated from a good number of Mishing villages in Sibsagar district by following standard anthropological methods and techniques. *Good health* according to the people, by and large, refers to having (i) no disease,

(ii) strong and tall body, (iii) good and white teeth, (iv) ability to carry out day-to-day work happily, (v) ability to laugh loudly, (vi) ability to plough one *bigha* (14,400 sq.ft.) of land in two days and (vii) ability to walk through a distance of at least 2 km at a stretch. In case of a woman, the additional parameters are to have (i) long and black hair and (ii) potentiality to give birth to 5-6 children. *Morbidity* episodes for one calender year reveal that the people suffer from around 58 different identifiable types of diseases/ailments. The frequently incident ones however, include asthama, boils, conjunctivitis, cough, diarrhoea, dysentery, fever, gastritis, measles, chicken pox, rheumatism, ringworm, scabis and stomachache. The data further reveal that the people very frequently become the victims of skin diseases as well as other communicable diseases. They also suffer from the ailments caused due to deficiency of minerals and vitamins (viz., night blindedness, rheumatism, vertigo, headache etc.). Many of the morbidity and mortality episodes are, however, assigned to the wrath of supernatural forces.

In the traditional medicare system, the Mishings resort to both *supernatural* (Magico-religious) as well as *natural* (Herbal or Material) means. There are at least 10 medicinemen (*Dolung-bej*) in the micro-field who are generally specialized either in one or more diseases. Some of them have been found to practise both supernatural and natural means of treatment. The diseases that are believed to be inflicted by some malevolent spirits include sudden pain in the stomach (*Alokoni*), miscarriage and infertility of females (*Delumoti*) etc. It is also believed that there are some unidentified spirits whose wrath can cause even madness in a person. The diseases that are believed to be caused by natural factors (viz. cough, cold, pneumonia, tonsilitis, influenza, diarrhoea and infection of worms etc.) are generally treated by some herbal/material medicines. As revealed by the data generated from the field, it seems, the repository of the Mishings under discussion contains; besides the animal, material and mineral items, some 40 different herbs and herbal products for the treatment of around 20 different diseases/ailments. The people very often use more than one medicine for the treatment of an ailment. The medicine varies according to the symptoms as well as secondary effects. Again, depending on the availability, sometimes alternative plants are used for a particular disease. Similarly, some plants are used for more than one diseases. The people categorise the diseases into 2 categories; (i) related to the body (Physiological), and (ii) related to mind and divine powers

(Psychosomatic). The bodily ailments are treated by using herbal medicines coupled with animal parts/products, material items and minerals etc., whereas the other ones are treated through magico-religious means.

Diseasewise uses of different medicines, as have been observed in the field are as follows:

**Asthma (Nga-nam)**

The leaf of a wild shrub locally known as ahom-phul (a kind of wild flower) and blackpepper are boiled in water; and a cup of the extract is taken twice or thrice a day for atleast one week or so for complete amelioration.

The alternative treatment, particularly for the adults is done by the smokes of dried thorn apple (Dature, *Datura stramonium*) seeds. It may be puffed or inhaled to get relief from the acute sufferings.

**Bile Juice Disorder (Pitta)**

It is diagnosed on the basis of the symptoms like stomachache, loss of appetite and mild fever. The medicine is prepared from a particular variety of turmeric (*kula halodhi*), ginger (*moran ada*), clove flower (*loung*) and bay leaf (*tejpat*). These are pounded into a paste from which pills are made. One or two pills are administered early in the morning in empty stomach and in the evening. The course needs to be continued for one week or so.

**Anyuk gakhir piram nam**

When a lactating mother does not have sufficient breast milk, she is provided with a medicinal food. The food is prepared from papaya (*amita*), red gram (*premen dali*), Jaiphal (*a medicinal nut*), turmeric (*halodhi*) and salt. This is taken 2 or 3 times a day for about a week. It has also been reported that addition of a little bit of stool of rhinoceros (*gorh*) in the food makes it more effective.

**Conjunctivitis (Lingidong)**

In order to get relief from conjunctivitis, the patient should press chopped potato (*alu*) on the eyes at regular intervals. During winter, they also use dew drops (*neor*) on the eyes in the morning. Eyes are also washed with cold water twice or thrice a day. All these measures may be taken independently or simultaneously; and it takes about a week for complete recovery.

**Cough (Sagre)**

A paste made out of ginger, a kind of turmeric (*kula halodi*) and honey is taken to get relief from the disease. In case of babies, honey is extensively used for the purpose.

**Diarrhoea (Aki gidung)**

The wild herbs locally known as *drun-bon* and *manimuni* (Indian Panny wort, *Centilla asiatica*) are taken as vegetables to get relief from diarrhoea. Intake of lemon juice is also believed to bring relief from the disease.

**Displacement of Intestine (Nari)**

The ailments like stomachache, indigestion, vomiting and diarrhoea, etc., associated with mild fever are sometimes diagnosed as the result of **nari**. The people believe that during heavy day-to-day works, the digestive canal may sometimes be accidentally displaced with the manifestation of these symptoms.

The medicine for the purpose is prepared from the bark of gooseberry (*amloki*), myroballum (*hilika*) and mango (*kedi*) trees, and leaves of a shrub locally known as *mithapul*. All these ingredients are boiled in water; and a cup of the diluted juice is orally administered twice a day until recovery.

Alternatively, they use the bark of a tree locally known as *semang*, leaf of a wild shrub (*tasing tayeng*), roots of a wild plant (*tangom*) and young shoots of guava (*madhuriam*) for the purpose. All these items are pounded together and pills are prepared for oral administration. One pill is taken twice a day until recovery.

**Dysentery (Apud gidung)**

The medicine for dysentery is prepared from a few locally available plants, viz., leaf and root of a shrub known as *yogirane*, a herb (*drunbon*) and bark of goose berry (*amloki*) tree and mango tree etc. A substance known as mosabor (latex of wild tree), bitter in taste is an important and very useful ingredient for the purpose. Alternatively, the young shoots of china rose (*joba*) and guava (*madhuriam*) are also used as a medicine for dysentery. The ingredients are ground to make paste from which pills are prepared for oral administration to the patient.

**Fever (Sagre)**

If the ailment is associated with fever, the first precaution they take is to avoid intake of solid food. In common fever, water, boiled with coriander seeds (*dhania*) is taken for two or three times a day for one or two days. Two or three glasses of the juice is said to provide relief from any fever of general kind.

In fever with cold (*yebung giying*), a kind of soup known as *jal* is taken. It is prepared with either a fowl or a wild sour fruit called *champa*, adding therein ginger, black pepper, onion, garlic and salt etc. All the ingredients are added in proper quantities and the mixture is boiled in water a get the soup.

The minors are given an alternative treatment with a wild root known as *yeero*. The root is akin to ginger and turmeric and has a unique smell resembling that of garlic. The juice is extracted by pounding the root and squeezing it. It is applied on the forehead and neck of the ailing minor. Sometimes, small pieces of the root are pierced at the centre and made into a garland by inserting a thread through those. The patient is to wear the garland around the neck. This is however, done in addition to the external use of the juice on the forehead.

**Headache (Mittupkinam)**

A paste prepared from the the bud of banana (*papuh*) and young shoots of bottle gourd (*giri lau*) is used as a topical application on the forehead in order to get rid of acute headache. Sometimes, a paste of the spongy portion of ash gourd (*kumurang*) is also used for the purpose.

**Liver Disorder (Kolpang nike)**

Pain in the upper portion of the stomach along with digestive complaints is considered to be the symptoms of liver disorder. The wild herbs used as medicinal vegetables for the purpose are locally known as *manimuni* and *drunbon*. Continuous use of the same, once a day, for a week or so, is reported to yield positive results.

## Lumber Pain (Eging kinam)

A paste is prepared from lemon seeds and ash gourd. A little mustard oil is mixed with the paste which is then slightly warmed. It is then topically used on the affected part.

## Menstrual Disorder (Mahekia bemar)

The medicine for the purpose is prepared by using a number of ingredients, viz., *kula halodhi*, roots of two wild trees locally known as *modar* and *bual*, garlic (*panaru*) and the bile glands of *rohu fish* (*Laio rohita*). All these items are pounded and boiled in water. The extract is taken in empty stomach for a week or so.

## Obstetrical Disorder (Prokota)

Birth of a child is an important event in their life. They generally do not go to hospital for delivery. Usually the old women from within the village assist in child birth.

An ailment associated with child birth is treated with herbal/ material medicine. A few items like *mosabor*, melted salt (*kala nimakh*), black pepper and turmeric are mixed together and pounded to a paste. Pills are then prepared from it and are administered orally to the patient twice a day for a week or so.

## Paralysis

The fresh and raw blood of fox is rubbed on the affected part of the body to cure paralysis. Oral administration of the same, in addition to the external application, is believed to expedite the amelioration process.

## Pneumonia

Medicine for this disease is prepared from the leaf of a wild herb (*tangloti*) and a wild fruit (*letaguti*) alongwith myrobalam (*hilika*), all boiled in water. The extract is orally administered to the patient two times a day for three or four days.

Alternatively, the ingredients are the root of a wild plant locally known as *miricot*, fruit of another wild plant (*letaguti*) and black pepper. These are pounded to a paste to make some pills out of it. One or two pills are administered to the patient orally twice a day, consecutively for three or four days. This can be administered to the minors too. In such cases, however, the pill is soaked in luke warm water and then administered along with water.

### Rib Pain (Narengia)

Infection of the rib-bones with mild fever, weakness and pain is treated by a medicine prepared from the fruits of a particular variety of emblic (*amora*) tree and a few spices, viz., black pepper, turmeric and salt. Pills prepared by pounding the ingredients are administred to the patient. Depending on the degree of suffering, one to three pills are taken a day for a week or so.

### Stomachache and Indigestion (Apid rocknam)

*Drunban* is taken as a vegetable to get relief from the ailment. The people also taken lemon juice for the purpose. *Kula haladhi* in the form of a paste is also taken to get relief from stomachache.

### Wound (Tarruk)

In the wounds, resulting out of cutting with some sharp weapon or so, the scraps of young bamboo bark (*dibaln chunch*) are applied to stop bleeding. A wild leaf locally known as *bag bon* is also useful for wounds. The leaves are squeezed and the juice is applied over the wound. It is also applied by making a paste to stop bleeding as well as to provide relief from pain. Paste of a wild herb (*tangom*) is also used on the wound with scratch or cut.

Besides, the people do use a good number of other plants and other items, either as food or as medicine as both preventive and promotive health measures. In addition, they have a number of other 'do's and 'donot's in their traditional health behaviour (cf. Singh, 2000).

## VI

According to a study carried out by the United Nations Development Programme, "eighty per cent of the world's population depend on indigenous knowledge to meet their medicinal needs ......" (Down to Earth, 1996 January, p.3)*. In the context of health, disease and traditional medical treatment, Agarwal (1996 : 53) laments, "it is a matter of great concern that India lacks a health policy worth the name. Nearly a billion people have no assured access to health care and the benefits of modern science ...... Besides traditional diseases, new diseases are cropping up due to changing lifestyles and deteriorating environmental conditions."

He continues, "...The challenge before us today is: how do we develop low cost medicine to deal with our health problem? The two major ways to reduce costs are preventive health programmes and traditional curative care ...". Traditional (ethno) medicine, as a matter of fact, can play a very important role in providing low cost service.

The modern medicare services are not only very expensive, but also have their alarming adverse side effects. In search of a real alternative we need to remember that the mother of all indigenous medicines is the tribal medicine practiced by the communities living in close harmony with the ecosystem. There is thus an urgent need for documentation of not only the herbal medicines but also the tribal health practices in totality. There is also an urgent need to translate all the available traditional knowledge as per international standards and safeguard the patenting rights of the stake holders. It should, however, be remembered that if the documentation is to be of value in modern drug discovery programme, it has to be done in relatively more details with respect to the information like symptoms, methods of indigenous preparation, doses, sources of information, modes of administration and the final outcome of the treatment.**

---

* Cited in Mibang and Choudhuri (2003 : 5).

** The author is thankful to Dr. Yash Kumar Singh for his being instrumental in generating the major chunk of the primary data incorporated in the paper.

## REFERENCES

Ackerknecht, H. (1942), Problems of primitive medicine. *Bulletin of History of Medicine*. 11 : 503-21.

Adair, John, Kurt Denschle and McDermott (1957), Some problems of the physicians on the Navaho reservation. *Human Organisation*. 16 : 19-23.

Agarwal, Anil (1996), To be healthy, wealthy and wise. *Down to Earth*, June 15.

Barua, S. (1984), A study on indigenous health practices among the Kaman Mishmis of Lohit district of Arunachal Pradesh. *Human Science*. 33 : 332-44.

Bhatt, K.H. 1986. "Concept of health and disease among the Pnars of Meghalaya", in *Tribal health*. Edited by B. Chaudhuri. New Delhi: Inter-India Publications, pp. 259-74.

Chaudhuri, B. (Ed.) (1986), *Tribal health: Socio-economic dimensions*. New Delhi: Inter-India Publications.

——(Ed.) (1990), *Cultural and Environmental Dimensions of Health*, New Delhi: Inter-India Publications.

Clements, F.E. (1932), Primitive concepts of disease. University of California publications in *American Archaeology and Ethnology*, 32 : 185-252.

Dutta Choudhuri, S.S. (1985), Herbal medicine and its implication in family planning: A study based upon the Singpho of Arunachal Pradesh. *Human Science*, 34 : 75-7.

Datta Choudhury, S.S. and G.C. Ghosh (1984), Indigenous health practices among the Idu Mishimis of Arunachal Pradesh. *Human Science*, 33-24-34.

Fabrega, Horacio. Jr. (1972), "Medical anthropology", in *Binneial Review of Anthropology*. Edited by B.J. Siegel. Stanford, California: Stanford University Press.

Foster, George and Barbara Gallatin Anderson (1978), *Medical anthropology*. New York: Wiley.

Guha. A. (1986 a), "Folk medicine of the Boro Kacharis—A plains tribe of Assam", in *Tribal health: Socio-cultural dimensions*. Edited by B. Chaudhuri. New Delhi: Inter-India Publications, pp. 191-200.

——(1986 b), Herbs in the disease treatment by Boro Kachari—A plains tribe of Assam. *Jr. Indian Anthropological Society*, 21 : 219-30.

——(1990), "Health care among two rural populations of Assam: A comparative study", in *Cultural and Environmental Dimensions of Health*. Edited by B. Chaudhuri, New Delhi: Inter-India publications, pp. 207-48.

Huard, Pierre (1969), "Western medicine and Afro-Asian ethnic medicine", in *Medicine and Culture*. Edited by F.N.L. Poynter. London: Welcome Institute of the History of Medicine, pp. 211-37.

Hughes, Charles, C. (1968), "Ethnomedicine", in *International Encyclopaedia of the Social Sciences*. 10 : 87-93. New York: Free Press/Macmillan.

Kar, R.K. (1993), Reproductive health behaviour of the Nocte women in Arunachal Pradesh. *Social Change*. Dec., 1993 (Published in 1995), 23 (No.4) : 40-52.

——(2001), Anthropological appraisal of a migrant population in Assam, N.E. India. *Presidential address, Anthropology and Archaeology section*, 88th session of ISC. New Delhi, 3-7 January.

Kar, R.K. and Juri Gogoi (1993), Health status of the Noctes of Arunachal Pradesh. *Social Change*. 23 : 164-71.

Kar, R.K. and Juri Gogoi (1994), Morbidity in an Arunachal Pradesh tribe: Some field notes from a Nocte village. *Resarun*, 18 : 133-142.

Khan, C.G. and Md. Arif Ali (1992), Relevance of ethnomedicine. *Man and Life*, 18 : 11-20.

Laughlin, W. (1963), "Primitive theory of medicine: Empirical knowledge", in *Man's image in medicine and anthropology*. Edited by Iago Gladson. New York: International University Press, pp. 116-40.

Mibang, Tamo and S.K. Choudhuri (2003), *Ethnomedicines of the Tribes of Arunachal Pradesh*. Delhi: Himalayan Publisher.

Rivers, W.H.R (1924), *Medicine, Magic and Religion*. New York: Har Court Brace.

Rubel, J. Arthur (1977), "The epidemiology of folk illness: Susto in hispanic America", in *Culture, Disease and Healing*. Edited by David Landy. New York : McMillan Publishing Corporation Inc.

Sikarwar, R.L.S. (2002), Mahua [Madhuca longifolia (koen) Macbride]—A paradise tree for the tribals of Madhya Pradesh. *Indian Jr. of Traditional Knowledge*. 1 : 87-92.

Sills, D.S. (1972), *International Encyclopaedia of Social Sciences*, Vol. 9 & 10, New York: Free Press.

Simmons, O.C. (1955), Popular and modern medicine in Mestizo communities of coastal Peru and Chile. *Jr. of American Folklore*, 68 : 57-71.

Singh, Yash K. (2000), *Health Culture Among the Misings: A Case Study in Upper Assam*, An unpublished Ph.D., thesis submitted to Dibrugarh University, Dibrugarh, Assam.

Vedavathy, S. (2002), Tribal medicine—the real alternative. *Indian Jr. of Traditional Knowledge*, 1 (No.1) : 25-31.

Waddel, L.A. (1975), *The Tribes of Brahmaputra Valley*, Delhi: Sanskaran Prakashak (First published in 1890).

26

# Ethnomedicine among the Jenu Kuruba of Karnataka

B.R. VIJAYENDRA and H.K. BHAT

## Introduction

The Jenu Kuruba is a Scheduled Tribe community inhabiting the southern districts of Karnataka. The Ministry of Home Affairs, Government of India, identified the community as a primitive tribal group in 1977, as the members of this community subsist mainly on hunting and gathering economic activities. According to the census of 1981, the population of Jenu Kuruba was 34,747 out of which 17,867 were males and 16,880 were females. They are distributed mainly in H.D. Kote, Hunsur and Periyapatna, taluks of Mysore district, Gundlupet taluk of Chamarajanagara district and in Virajpet, Somavarpet and Madikeri taluks of Kodagu district. The Jenu Kuruba settlements (*haadis*) are concentrated in and around forest areas. About 5000 people are still living inside the Rajiv Gandhi National Park. They speak Jenu nudi, a dialect of Kannada. They also use standard Kannada when they communicate with others.

Nagarahole game sanctuary, the traditional habitat of Jenu Kurubas, was declared as a national park on 1st April, 1983 (and later renamed as Rajiv Gandhi National Park in 1992). The park comes under the control of Forest Department, Government of Karnataka and as per the rules of Wild Life sanctuary; no human beings are permitted to reside inside the park. However, about 1000 tribal families (most of them being Jenu Kurubas) are still residing in the National Park. Since 1999 tribal families are being shifted to rehabilitation centres just outside the National Park. The first batch of 50 families volunteered to shift in 1995 to Nagapura rehabilitation centre. At present, there are 250 families in the centre, majority of them are Jenu Kurubas.

## The Location of the Present Study

The present study was conducted in a modern Jenu Kuruba settlement known as Basavige (pseudo name), situated 24 km away from Hunsur, the taluk headquarters. The place is 72 km away from Mysore, the district headquarters. 66 Jenu Kuruba families live in this new settlement, which was established about 20 years ago. The total population is 331 (171 males and 160 females). The literacy rate is about 50 per cent. However, all the literates had only a few years of school education.

The settlement is about 1 km away from the road, which connects the place to the taluk and district head quarters. The settlement is outside the National Park. Out of 66 houses, 65 are having tiled roofs and the remaining one house is having thatched roof. Lakshmana Ṭheertha river (a tributary of Cauveri) is flowing about ½ a km away from the settlement. The river is the main source of water for drinking, washing, cooking, bathing etc. The settlement is also having five bore wells with handpumps, out of which only one was in working condition during the fieldwork. The village is electrified and 25 houses have electrical connections. One *ashram* school is situated in the settlement. One Primary Health Unit is situated about 3 km away from the settlement.

## Ethnomedicine: An Overview

Anthropologists have been involved in the study of ethnomedical systems since the last quarter of 19th century. Tylor, Saligman and Frazer have described healing, shamanism, witchcraft, magic etc. and related them to the concept of illness in preliterate societies. In the early part of the 20th century Rivers, Ackernecht and Clements have provided elaborate descriptions and analyses of ethnomedical systems. Leslie and Dunn have discussed the ethnomedical systems in comparative perspective in the second half of 20th Century and encouraged scholars to undertake ethnomedical studies in different continents. Earlier studies of Ethnomedicine focused more on mentalistic aspects of illness and virtually neglected the biological components as pointed out by Horacio Fabrega (1974:40). Hence, the ethnomedical studies did not have much impact on cosmopolitan medicine. A major contribution of the mentalistic perspective was to broadening the horizon of Western Psychiatric categories.

The term Ethnomedicine is generally applied to the study of traditional medical systems of the non-western societies (Foster and Anderson 1978:51). Later, the meaning of the term was broadened to include all medical systems, including biomedicine, viewed within the framework of their respective cultures (Lock and Scheper Hughes, 1990: 47-72, Rhodes, 1990:159-173). Fabrega has also applied the term more broadly and includes all "Culturally oriented studies of illness" under Ethnomedicine (1974:39-43).

### *Ethnomedicine among the Jenu Kuruba*

In this study an attempt is made to give a broad outline of the traditional health beliefs and practices of a tribal community. Concepts of health and illness, classification of illness and etiological concepts, diagnostic practices, healers and healing techniques are discussed below.

#### *Concept of Health and Illness*

The Jenu Kurubas prefer to be lean and medium or short-statured and such persons are considered strong and healthy. This type of body built enables them to work hard and run faster to avoid the attacks of wild animals. Such persons are also considered to be more intelligent.

Jenu Kurubas do not have elaborate knowledge about internal structure of the body. They believe that food is going to the liver and there it is transformed into blood. Red blood is considered as the sign of healthy body, usually a characteristic feature of young people. It is said that as the person grows old, red blood turns to blackish red and the quantity of blood decreases thereby indicating lesser strength and decreased health status. Since the Jenu Kurubas traditional habitat is forest, this environment seems to have influenced certain health beliefs of the people. Sitting in front of the fire, especially during the rainy and winter seasons is a common sight in the Jenu Kuruba settlement. They believe that this practice, although desirable for present comfort, increases the thickness of blood and decreases the fastness of the body. An individual's good health and activity is also linked to the thickness of blood. Youngsters are believed to have thin blood, which flows fast in the body and makes the individual healthy and active. Aged people possess thick and blackish-red blood, which makes them less healthy and active.

Jenu Kurubas, whose traditional occupation is honey collection and hunting in the wild forest, believe in greater body movement. They do not sit idle even for a moment in one place. They think that body movement is required for proper blood circulation, which in turn promotes good health. Circulation of blood is believed to stop while one is at sleep. Weakness and illnesses are attributed to decrease in the quantity of blood.

Jenu Kurubas consider that honey, a variety of yams and green leafy vegetables available in the forest are healthy food items. Of late, ragi (a millet) is also considered as a good food item. Worship of several deities in the forest is also considered necessary to keep one's health in good condition. Another common cause for ill health is considered to be sorcery. Jenu Kurubas are very suspicious in nature due to the strong belief in sorcery. They hesitate to eat food in the houses of their neighbours and even kinsmen. In any case of illness sorcery may be suspected.

The belief in the hot-cold dichotomy of foodstuffs and other items of nature is also quite common among the Jenu Kurubas. They also believe in the balance of three elements in the body, viz. air (*vayu*), bile (*paithale*) and phlegm (*thonte*). Based on the predominant element in the body, human beings are classified into three categories, viz., hot-bodied (*kavina sharila*), cold-bodied (*sheetha sharila*) and neutral-bodied (*sama sharila*). Hot-bodied persons are believed to be lean and strong with faster blood circulation. Such persons are required to curtail the consumption of hot food items during the summer in order to keep the body heat at the required level. People prefer hot-body rather than cold-body because of the fact that the former can work hard without tiring whereas the latter gets easily tired after work. The second best body type is 'neither hot nor cold' as these elements are in balance.

### *Classification of Illness*

The illnesses identified by Jenu Kuruba may be classified into four categories on the basis of etiological factors, viz., body linked illnesses (*sharilada kayile*), deity-linked-illness (*daivada kayile*), spirit-linked-illnesses (*galiyetu*) and sorcery-linked-illnesses (*matada kayile*).

The causative factors of the body-linked-illnesses are defective diet, bad water, worm infestation and other environmental conditions. Naturalistic causative factors are mainly linked to diet and the qualities of various food items. Food items are classified into hot, cold, *vayu* (air), *paithale* (bile) and *thonte* (phlegm). Consumption of food items are made on the basis of their qualities in terms of above mentioned categories. Persons also inherit these qualities since birth and proper matching of these qualities are made before consumption. This is a clear case of interaction between the 'little' and 'great' health traditions in the Indian subcontinent. Ayurvedic concepts and practices have been in constant contact with the local cultural traditions in the historical period.

Illnesses linked to this causative factor may be roughly translated as stomachache, cough, cold, headache, giddiness, dysentery, body itching, fever, eczema, scabies etc.

Several illnesses are linked to the pantheon of Jenu Kuruba. The female deity Mari is worshipped every year by all the residents by sacrificing fowls. Failure to perform this ceremony is believed to cause measles, chicken pox and small pox. If a person suddenly falls sick or a sick person does not respond to other types of treatment it is suspected that the cause of the illness is a deity, family deities are also worshipped at the family level. The authors have recorded 12 family deities in Basavige settlement.

Another common causative factor of illness is spirits of the dead. The spirits of any dead person residing in the habitation area may cause illness to a person of the opposite sex who passes through that area, especially in the evening or at night. Any physical symptom or illness is generally attributed to a spirit if it does not respond to other forms of therapy. If the spirit is that of an ancestor or ancestress, they are addressed by using kin terms such as grandfather or grandmother. The last but important cause of illness is sorcery (*mata*). Sorcerers among the Jenu Kuruba employ different techniques to cause illness to the victims. Some of the common techniques are as follows:

1. The sorcerer puts spell-cast thorns and glass pieces inside a lemon and calls the name of the victim. The lemon is then buried on the path of the victim. If the victim passes through the path he will suffer from acute pain, swelling of a body part and ultimately looses that body part. This type of sorcery is known as *datu* (i.e. crossing).
2. There is another type of sorcery known as *Chillu Hodeyuvudu*. The sorcerer inserts certain objects such as seeds, frogs or ants into the body of the victim. The victim experiences the

movement of the object inside his body. The victim becomes restless and cannot perform his daily activities and can't even sleep at night.

3. Poisoning (*maddu hakuvudu*) is another form of sorcery. A poisonous substance is put into coffee, tea or some liquid food and is offered to the victim. The victim becomes weak and looses appetite. The victim's stomach may swell and work efficiency may reduce. He develops vomiting sensation while seeing the food or drink through which the poison was administered.
4. The another method, the sorcerer buries a spell-cast hen's head covered in a coconut shell in a pit dug near the victim's house. Due to the ill effects of this sorcery the entire family suffers from sickness.
5. The sorcerer sometimes may cast the spell on a plant in the name of a victim. This spell cast plant is supposed to dry and die within a specified period. In a similar way, the victim is also believed to suffer from weakness and die coinciding with the death of the plant. Sorcerers may also cast evil spells on any part or object which once belonged to or in contact with victim such as spittle, urine, faeces, hair, foot dust, menstrual clothes, clothes used during the delivery of a child etc. Jenu Kurubas avoid urinating, defecating or spitting in the presence of other people in order to avoid the evil effects or sorcery.
6. The belief in evil eye is also strong among Jenu Kurubas. Some individuals in the society are identified as having this quality.

### *Diagnosis of Illness*

There are mainly five types of diagnostic procedures among the Jenu Kuruba, viz., *bunde kareyuvudu* (calling their deity by the diviner), *allu shastra* (cowrie shell method), *kayile guruthu* (diagnosis based on physical signs and symptoms), *peede kadeyuvudu* (spirit exorcism) and *kenpu neeru* (red water method).

Divining is considered as the perfect method of diagnosis of most of the illnesses. A diviner does this. There are six diviners in Basavige. All of them are part-time specialists. The patient and his family members visit the house of the diviner with coconut, incense sticks, millet, areca nut, betel leaves, banana etc. These materials are used by the diviner to worship the tutelary deity, who guides the diviner in the diagnostic session. The diviner chants a verse known as *bundepada* and possesses the deity. At this time, the patient and his family members pose several questions regarding the identity and cause of the illness and the appropriate method of treatment to be followed. There is no fixed payment in cash for the services of the diviner.

In the second method of diagnosis, the expert (*allu panditha*) throws a few cowrie shells on the mat and looking at the number and position of the shells (dorsal or ventral) decides the cause of illness. The diviner actually thinks about a particular cause and then throws the cowrie shells. He repeats the same act five times and if he gets the even numbers with ventral positions up, the cause of the illness is confirmed. He repeats the act again thinking about actual cause until he gets even number of shells on five consecutive times with ventral position up. This procedure sometimes may take hours together to arrive at a correct diagnosis of the problem. The expert relies on the blessings of his tutelary deity for his success.

The third method is symptomatic diagnosis. The specialists who rely on this method are herbalists. Internal and external symptoms are considered in diagnosing an illness. The internal signs are pain, burning sensation, loss of taste, thirst, loss of appetite, movement of an ant or frog inside the body. The common external symptoms are swelling, colour of eyes/urine etc. wounds, blisters, vomiting, coughing, patches on the skin, itching, facial expression etc. The herbalist examines these symptoms in association with each other and arrives at the diagnosis. The herbalist is known as *maddu koduvavaru* (medicine giver). They are part-time practitioners. The knowledge is generally passed on family lines. Herbalists collect their medicines alone on auspicious days like Sundays, Tuesdays and new-moon days. There is no fixed payment for the services of the herbalist.

Identification of the spirit is another form of diagnostic procedure. The exorcists are known as *peede kadeyuvavaru*. This specialization is also generally passed on family lines. The exorcist is consulted on Sundays and Tuesdays to identify the spirit and expel it. Three types of spirits (*gali*) are identified by the commoners as well as the exorcists. They are *sannagali* (small spirit), doddagali (big spirit) and *valadagali*. Sannagali is the spirit of an individual who dies without fulfilling his desires. It can be driven out after satisfying his desires. Generally, these spirits ask for a particular type of food.

Doddagali refers to the spirits of individuals who had unnatural death like suicide, accident or murder. The spirits of the dead bodies, which did not undergo proper death rituals, also belong to this category. The third category of spirits are those of psychotic patients who met with unnatural deaths. The exorcist find it difficult to expel the third category of spirits since they do not obey the orders of the exorcist.

The last method of diagnosis known as *kempu neeru* (reddish water) is used to diagnose a culture-specific illness called *soku*. This illness generally affects children. An elderly woman does this diagnosis by putting turmeric and lime on water contained in a small plate. The plate is waved in front by the patient and a piece of burning charcoal is put on it. If the water turns to red, the illness is confirmed as *soku*. Children generally suffer from *soku*. This is marked by the symptoms such as crying, restlessness and refusal to eat food or such breast milk.

### *Treatment of Illnesses*

The pattern of treatment resorted to by the Jenu Kurubas can be categorized into two types, viz., magico-religious and herbal.

Magico-religious treatment is resorted to when the cause of illness is attributed to some 'personalistic agents' (Foster, 1978) such as sorcerer, spirit or supernatural deities like Maramma. The healing rituals are performed either by the family members (as in the case of *soku*) or by the specialist such as spirit exorcist (as in the case of peede or g*ali)* or by the sorcerer (as in the case of *datu*).

The Jenu Kurubas have a rich heritage of herbal medicines. The herbal treatment is resorted to when the cause of the illness is identified as a natural substance or phenomena. Certain foods are restricted to the patients during the treatment. The herbalists claim that they can cure most of the illnesses except cancer cholera, tuberculosis and diarrhoea. Plant medicines are used to treat headache, dysentery, sores on any part of the body, stomach ache, snake-bite, scorpion-sting, measles, eczema, body swelling, toothache, migraine, mouth sores, sprain, asthma etc.

## Conclusion

Ethnomedicines have to be interpreted in both biological and behavioural frame works. Both have substantial impact. The use of plant or material medicines may be found to influence the human physiology. Diet and medicines are not strictly separated in Jenu Kurubas ethnomedicine. Diet may be a medicine or *vice versa* at different contexts and times. Laboratory analysis is required to assess the impact of various medicines on the human body. Pharmacologic interpretations of the materia medica will advance the knowledge of ethnomedicine of Jenu Kuruba.

The behavioural interpretations of ethnomedicine show that Jenu Kuruba society and culture is having a unique theme of socio-cultural integration. This theme revolves around suspicion and distrust. The traditional ecological and economic conditions of the tribe promoted this kind of integration of the society. The Jenu Kurubas who lived in the dense forest always struggled for their livelihood, which consisted of honey and various kinds of tubers, leaves and animals. The struggle for the limited resources made them to suspect each other. The scarce and difficult conditions of forest life seem to have contributed to the development of ideas related to sorcery and other magical practices. Jenu Kuruba ethnomedicine (a little tradition) is also linked to the Ayurvedic tradition (a great tradition) as illustrated in these concepts of three humours.

## REFERENCES

Foster, G.M. and B.G. Anderson (1978), *Medical Anthropology*, New York: Wiley.

Lock, M. and N. Scheper Hughes (1990), A critical-interpretive approach in medical anthropology: rituals and routines of discipline and dissent. In *Medical Anthropology: Contemporary Theory and Method.* Ed. by T.M. Johnson and C.F. Sargent New York: Praeger.

Misra, P.K. (2003), *Primitive tribes in the Southern Region: A Case study in Eastern Anthropologist*, Vol. 56 Nos. 2-4.

Misra, P.K. (1969), The Jenu Kuruba, *Bulletin*, Anthropological Survey of India, Calcutta.

Rhodes, L.A. (1990), Studying biomedicine as a cultural system In *Medical Anthropology: Contemporary Theory and Method.* Ed. by T.M.Johnson and C.F. Sargent, New York: Praeger.

Ruebel, A.J. and M.R. Hass (1990), Ethnomedicine (ch. 6) In *Medical Anthropology: Contemporary Theory and Method ed.*, by T.M. Johnson and C.F. Sargent. New York: Praeger.

Vijayendra, B.R. (1997), 'Ethnomedical study among the selected tribal communities of Southern Karnataka'. Unpublished Ph.D. thesis submitted to University of Mysore.

# PART V

# POLICY ASPECTS IN TRIBAL HEALTH AND MEDICINES

# 27

# Issues in Tribal Health and Medicines

P.C. JOSHI

The tribal systems of medicines connote diversity of cultural practices, traditional knowledge and social organizations. Therefore, there can not be any one tribal system of medicines. What we may have would be systems of medicines, knowledge of herbs, ritualistic practices, explanatory models, amulets and charms, humoral ideology, bone setters, midwives and myriad other ecologically meaningful and culturally appropriate ideas, beliefs, practices and personnel. We may also find broad regional patterns as medical knowledge is known to be especially suited to diffusion and assimilation. Thus, the medical systems in the Himalayan tribes would show similarity across cultures in contradistinction to the tribes inhabiting middle India or for that matter the north-eastern or Andaman Islands. Regional similarities albeit, there will however be pan-Indian patterns in use of herbs, conceptualization of supernatural world, child birth practices, exorcism, divination, the text of incantations and above all in assimilation of Allopathic system of medicines.

The tribal areas in general are marked by poor coverage in health care, specific patterning of bio-genetic diseases, high concentration of infectious diseases, lack of health education and cultural practices adversely affecting the health. Special provisions in the health care programmes have made some impact but in many remote areas which are far off from the road and rail link, the impact of new knowledge and technology is a distant dream. There are currently two contradictory objectives that need to be simultaneously met in respect of tribal health and medicines. At one extreme is the need to look after the burden of childhood diarrhoea, acute respiratory infections, chicken pox, measles, night blindness, tuberculosis, marasmus, kwashiorkor, skin infections, orthopedic fractures, high risk pregnancies, malaria, etc. which require health education and awareness regarding good diet, hygienic living, sanitation besides immunization. The burden of non-communicable diseases such as psychiatric and neurological diseases along with burden of alcoholism and drug addiction is also considerable. The latter would require special clinical programmes like community psychiatry or community neurology.

The PHC approach, which definitely has great advantages, has not been able to cover the entire tribal belt. As a result, many areas in the tribal hinterland are still awaiting scientific knowledge and interventions. Consequently, mobility in coverage of health care by means of road, rail and even air routes has to be thought of if we are serious about the health care of our tribal areas. So far the trend has been to send the frustrated and rejected clinical staff to the tribal area in the form of punishment postings. The time has come when we should think of sending the best cadre, highly motivated and open hearted doctors to expose people to the real fruits of new knowledge. Therefore, the strategy should not only be geared towards upgrading and modernizing clinical infrastructure but also towards improvement of human resources.

The other major issue in the area of tribal medicines consists of gainful utilization of the tribal medicinal heritage. Since time immemorial, the tribal communities have been using herbs, minerals and other substances in treating their sick patients. They also have physiotherapeutic knowledge used in treatment of fractures, sprains, spasms and other internal conditions besides immense knowledge of child birth and gynecology. The entire medicinal heritage of tribal can also be seen as alternative system of therapy. The challenge on this front is two-fold. The first concern examination of therapeutic efficacy of tribal medicines and its re-introduction back in the system for health promotion, prevention and curative purposes. Anthropologists and botanists have amassed vast amount of data on ethnomedicines. The tribal claims of their medicines have to be verified. The intellectual property rights of the tribal medicines and propagation of therapeutic heritage beyond, of course, after ascertaining it benevolent properties is the second major challenge confronting us today. It has to be carefully seen that the fruits of intellectual property return back to its rightful custodians. This will require interdisciplinary efforts by anthropologists, biotechnologist, lawyers, pharmacologists, social activists and above all the alert and aware tribal.

The tribal systems of medicine have been characterized as magico-religious for the simple reason that the element of magic and religion greatly influences the nosology, etiology and therapeutics in these systems of medicines. The disease causation theory in tribal system of medicine takes its main inspiration from the culturally postulated supernatural forces and agents which are believed to be intricately linked to the human world. Some supernatural forces are part of religious world, largely benevolent, requiring good conduct, appeasement and regular offerings from the human beings. In event of mistakes and forgetfulness on parts of the people, the protective supernatural beings show their anger and frustration in the form of misfortunes such as disease and sufferings to the people. The individual disease of a person thus, may be conceptualized as merely a projection of the wrath of supernatural and therefore, the intervention of medicines may not be considered necessary and desirable by the people.

Another set of supernatural agencies consist mainly of obnoxious and malevolent forces wandering in the atmosphere waiting for an opportunity to harm human beings. This is the magical world of supernatural forces consisting of thirsty spirits, ghost, demons, witches and powers that intrude in the human body and affect the health and peace of people. These forces are to be driven out, banished and at times punished.

The shaman, sorcerers, priests, bhagats, bhopas, guniyas, bharra are the human agents having the capacity to intervene and mediate in the events of supernatural encounters. Some of them are also feared for they have the capacity to domesticate these nefarious forces and thus are considered capable of inducing harm through these agencies.

In any concrete situation, the names of the agencies may differ but the interrelationship between human beings and the supernatural world would show great similarity. The issue before us is what should be done if the tribal subscribe to the magico-religious world view. Should we act as social reformers and teach them that their beliefs and practices are all hocus-pocus and they should stop believing in them. In order to do this, we will first have to make sure that we provide them with effective and guaranteed alternative. The problem does not end here. We will also have to know the clinical and social importance of the tribal magico-religious practices. The psychotherapeutic significance of magico-religious practices, that have been so much talked about needs to be contextualized. The significance of magico-religious practices in reduction of anxiety, neurosis, phobias, stress and other psychopathological conditions have to be clinically evaluated. Beyond all this, the contribution of magico-religious ritual which often involve a large group and have mass therapeutic effect through public singing, trance and catharsis should also be ascertained.

One of the great strength of tribal systems of medicine is the involvement of group in therapy. The role and responsibilities of kins, affines, lineage-mates and the villagers who form the therapy management group in health seeking and helping in therapeutic outcomes is a remarkable property of these systems. It is the lack of social milieu that has made hospitals and health centres alien places where the approach is individualistic and atomistic. The social support network in health seeking process participates, shares, suggests, admonishes and above all exhibits concern and gives re-assurance to the patient and his immediate dependents. The therapy therefore becomes a group concern. If the patient suffers and cries in pain, the entire group shares the agony. The experience of sickness thereby becomes a shared experience. In such a scenario, the rehabilitation of the patient is never a problem and stigma of disease is a non-entity.

The importance of social milieu becomes extremely relevant in event of severe mental illness and disability. The tribal world is generally tolerant to such extreme debilitating cases. The psychiatric patients are not discarded and isolated but are assimilated and given a gainful place in the society. In matters of social support the other world has so much to learn from the tribal systems.

The impact of organized efforts in improving the health status of the people in the tribal areas has resulted in partial improvements. The situation is alarming in some areas. The overall impact of economic development, modernization, globalization and political enlightenment of the tribal have ruptured the protective sheathe. Migration of tribal people to cities, towns, industrial areas, tea estates and myriad other places for employment and education along with arrival of outsiders into the tribal area have adversely affected the natural immunity of the tribal. New patterns of morbidity, in the form of tuberculosis, nutritional deficiencies, sexually transmitted diseases, reproductive tract infections, malaria, dengue and myriad other maladies, is troubling the tribal with added vigour. The need of the hour is to think beyond and evolve strategies to save the tribal communities from unwanted mortality. There are many primitive tribal communities whose number is fast depleting due to new pattern of morbidity. Vertical approach alone will not be sufficient and area–specific strategy for health improvement would be required. Increased immunization, people's participation, dietary intervention, hygiene and sanitation improvement and prevention of infections would therefore have to be the added focus in health care delivery.

# 28

# Tribal Health and Medicine

RAMESH CHANDRA

In India there are 664 tribes, some of them living in more than one state, notified as scheduled tribes under Article 342 of the Constitution. As per 1991 Census the Scheduled Tribe population of the country is 67.8 million constituting 8.08 per cent of the total population. These Scheduled Tribes are spread over different states and union territories but for Chandigarh, Delhi, Haryana, Pondicherry and Punjab. They have large concentration of their population in Central Indian states and the north-eastern region. Largest number of scheduled tribes are in Orissa with 62 scheduled tribe communities. As per the Indian Constitution, a number of tribes needed safeguard for their welfare and development; and in this account first order regarding notification of scheduled tribes under article 342 of the Constitution was passed in the year 1950. The Article 342 explicitly recognizes those tribal communities who have been declared as such by the President through an initial Public Notification, as Scheduled Tribes. The list of Scheduled tribes is state specific; necessarily a Scheduled Tribe thus notified in one state may not have the same status in another state. To notify any community as scheduled tribe, characteristics considered are (i) primitive traits, (ii) distinctive culture, (iii) shyness of contact with public at large, (iv) geographical isolation and (v) social and economic backwardness. Of the 664 tribal communities, 75 such tribal communities are identified as Primitive Tribal Groups (PTGs). It is a matter of concern that while the scheduled tribe population as such lags behind the rest of the Indian society on account of their socio-economic backwardness, the condition of the Primitive Tribal Groups (PTG) is still worse than the rest of the tribal communities for their being at a level of preagricultural stage and technology, low level of literacy and demographically being a stagnant or even declining population.

Nearly three-fourth of the tribal population of India is spread in eight states of the country viz. Andhra Pradesh, Bihar, Gujarat, Madhya Pradesh, Orissa, Rajasthan, Maharashtra and Himachal Pradesh. Their larger concentration can be seen in the plains of India and seven north-eastern states.

It is a matter of concern that though tribal people usually live close to nature and in and around healthy surroundings of natural environment and they apparently appear to be normally healthy persons but majority of them need health care of one kind or the other on account of abject poverty, malnutrition, lack of safe drinking water, poor environment, sanitation and hygienic condition, etc.

Lack of awareness and socio-cultural barriers and apathy to prefer available health services in whatever form and extent these are also causes adversely on the health status of the tribal people. In wake of opening of tribal areas, highways and changes occurring on account of industrialization, modernization and communication facilties, health problems and diseases too affect the tribal people. Endemics, viz. Malaria, vulnerability to diseases like deficiency of G6PD, venereal diseases and AIDS are not untouched in the pockets of tribal populations all over the country. However, lack of safe drinking water and malnutrition are two well-recognized major health hazards. It is rather difficult to establish that tribals have a satisfactory dietary pattern in view of deficiency of calcium, vitamin A, vitamin C, riboflavin and animal protein is usually found in their diets. Malnutrition and undernutrition are common observance in case of primitive tribal groups who largely depend upon food either gathered or cultivated by them using simple methods. Instances of such precarious conditions are known in the country from one region or the other on a similar pattern. The nutritional status of tribal women directly influences their reproductive performances and infants' health status crucial for his survival, growth and development.

A comparative picture with regard to the health and child care facilities available to the tribal areas can be seen in the table given in Table 28.1:

**Table 28.1:** State-wise health and child care facilities available in the tribal areas

| *States/Union Territories* | *Health and Child Care* | | | | | |
|---|---|---|---|---|---|---|
| | *Primary Health Centres (1996)* | | *Health Sub-Centres (1996)* | | *ICDS Projects (1998-99)* | |
| | *Total* | *STs* | *Total* | *STs* | *Total* | *STs* |
| India | 21853 | 3258 (14.9%) | 132778 | 20355 (15.3%) | 4200 | 750 (17.8%) |
| States | | | | | | |
| Andhra Pradesh | 1283 | 115 | 7894 | 824 | 209 | 29 |
| Arunachal Pradesh | 47 | 42 | 223 | 236 | 45 | 39 |
| Assam | 619 | 74 | 5280 | 445 | 107 | 23 |
| Bihar | 2209 | 208 | 14799 | 1824 | 323 | 93 |
| Goa | 21 | NA | 175 | NA | 11 | Nil |
| Gujarat | 957 | 227 | 7284 | 1929 | 203 | 34 |
| Haryana | 397 | Nil | 2299 | Nil | 114 | Nil |
| Himachal Pradesh | 245 | 17 | 1954 | 99 | 72 | 8 |
| Jammu & Kashmir | 335 | NA | 1700 | NA | 113 | 3 |
| Karnataka | 1459 | 307 | 7993 | 1850 | 185 | 7 |
| Kerala | 959 | 62 | 5094 | 268 | 120 | 1 |
| Madhya Pradesh | 1376 | 633 | 11937 | 4959 | 355 | 129 |
| Maharashtra | 1695 | 353 | 9725 | 1873 | 271 | 50 |
| Manipur | 72 | 35 | 420 | 221 | 32 | 20 |
| Meghalaya | 88 | 88 | 337 | 355 | 30 | 29 |
| Mizoram | 38 | 56 | 261 | 261 | 21 | 19 |
| Nagaland | 33 | 65 | 244 | 213 | 41 | 41 |
| Orissa | 1056 | 349 | 5927 | 485 | 279 | 126 |
| Punjab | 484 | Nil | 2852 | Nil | 110 | Nil |

*(Contd.)*

**Table 28.1** *(Contd.)*

| *States/Union Territories* | *Health and Child Care* | | | | | |
|---|---|---|---|---|---|---|
| | *Primary Health Centres (1996)* | | *Health Sub-Centres (1996)* | | *ICDS Projects (1998-99)* | |
| | *Total* | *STs* | *Total* | *STs* | *Total* | *STs* |
| Rajasthan | 1572 | 171 | 8692 | 934 | 191 | 30 |
| Sikkim | 24 | 3 | 147 | 19 | 5 | NA |
| Tamil Nadu | 1436 | 15 | 8681 | 111 | 432 | 3 |
| Tripura | 63 | 28 | 536 | 250 | 31 | 6 |
| Uttar Pradesh | 3761 | 189 | 20153 | 1376 | 560 | 10 |
| West bengal | 1556 | 205 | 7873 | 738 | 294 | 46 |
| Union Territories | | | | | | |
| A&N Islands | 17 | 3 | 96 | 29 | 5 | 2 |
| Chandigarh | 0 | Nil | 12 | Nil | 3 | Nil |
| Dadra & Nagar Haveli | 6 | 6 | 34 | 34 | 1 | 1 |
| Daman & Diu | 4 | 0 | 21 | 9 | 2 | Nil |
| Delhi | 8 | Nil | 42 | Nil | 29 | Nil |
| Lakshadweep | 7 | 7 | 14 | 14 | 1 | 1 |
| Pondicherry | 26 | Nil | 79 | Nil | 5 | Nil |

Infant mortality rate per thousand life birth = 84.2

Child mortality rate per thousand population = 46.3

Tribes in India are considered to be socially and economically backward. They have their own way of living within given social and cultural moorings, purely governed on the basis of local conditions and ethos. Lack of proper health care and age-old traditional practices with regard to cure and ailments, irrational belief system are some factors said to be aggravating the health and nutritional problems of these people; which need special attention primarily for two reasons (i) many of the tribal communities are backward and thus need special attention and (ii) the growth of tribal population is rather uneven; even few tribal communities are known as declining in their population; even some have threat to their existence. The decline in their population though only connote low level of fertility to the understanding but indeed it is a matter of concern for probe and research as post-natal and infant mortality surpassing the survival on account of balanced nutrition, healthy environment and hygienic conditions remains a serious impediment in this area.

General scene with regard to tribal health portrays a common picture that tribals suffer from many chronic diseases of which vector and water borne diseases take heavy toll than any other disease. Contaminated water is also source for intestinal and skin diseases. Diarrhoea, dysentery, cholera are some common diseases needing attention on medical account to keep the tribals away from these diseases. Similarly on nutritional side, deficiency of certain minerals and other elements is also taking the tribal populations within their clutches. It is a common knowledge that iodine deficiency causing goiter is widely spread in the Himalayan ranges and terai areas. G6PD syndrome and variety of fevers among the tribes of Gujarat, Madhya Pradesh and parts of Rajasthan have become common knowledge. Atleast six types of fevers relating to malaria have been reported in a study conducted by Centre for Social Studies, Surat. Intensification of nutritional deficiency resulting in tuberculosis and deficiency based diseases among expectant and lactating mothers in the tribal population poses another constant worry. Intense of venereal diseases has attained heights in certain Himalayan dwelling tribes in Himachal Pradesh, Uttaranchal and in the north-eastern states; besides, tribes living in plains in Madhya Pradesh, Bihar, Orissa and Andhra Pradesh. Recent blow of instance of AIDS can also not be ruled out especially for the tribes living along the roadside settlements on highways connecting one state to another. Some studies done in the tribal health sector have indicated that diseases like goiter, yaws and cholera were endemic in tribal pockets. Occurrence of tapeworm and guineaworms in some tribal areas has aggravated the situation. Sickle cell disease among the Adiyan tribes of Kerala as reported by Basu, 1991 (cited from Naidu, T.S., 2002) and other physical anthropologists like Negi, Shastri, Gulati and others have similar stories about tribal health to tell.

There is a good understanding among the anthropologists about the healthy nexus and co-existence of tribals with the nature for the tribes living in healthy natural surroundings like that of Andaman and Nicobar Islands; and often arguments have been put forward in favour of good standard of tribal health from these illustrations. However, on account of nutritional status of these tribes, the Regional Medical Research Centre (ICMR), Port Blair has carried out studies among Great Andamanese, Onges and Shompens. These studies based on diet survey, nutritional anthropometry survey, clinical examination, measurement of Hb concentration and stool examination have revealed that the intake of green leafy vegetables, other vegetables, milk and milk products are much less than the respective recommended dietary allowances (RDA). Their average daily consumption of fats and pulses is two to four times more than RDA. Average consumption per Consumption Unit (CU) of all the nutrients except Iron, Vitamin A and Vitamin C are above the recommended levels and that malnutrition is common among the tribal children. 57 per cent of Great Andamanese children, aged 6 years and less, have moderate to severe degree of malnutrition and another 28.6 per cent have mild degree of malnutrition, making the prevalence of undernourishment among pre-school children 85.6 per cent. On the other hand, 85 per cent of the Onges children in this age group have mild to moderate degree of malnutrition and 10 per cent have severe degree of malnutrition, making the prevalence of undernourishment among pre-school children 95 per cent.

Anaemia is very common among all the three tribes. 94 per cent Great Andamanese, 86.6 per cent Onges and 85.5 per cent Shompens are found anaemic as per WHO definition of anaemia. (Rao *et al.*, 2002).

A study done by Dave *et al.* in Panch Mahal, Gujarat to assess nutritional status of tribal children revealed that more than 83 per cent children suffered from malnutrition (cited from Patnakar, M., 1994).

## II

After taking a glimpse into scenario concerning tribal population it may be worth pondering over that the situation is so gloomy and what can be attempted to restore their normal health standards even by accepting a few generous traditionally upheld system of curing healing practice of tribals based on their vast experience of natural resources and manipulation of the same to their advantage. It is widely held that in the direction of the health and medical facilities there are some four features which may be held responsible as the shortfall in the field of medical attendance (i) the need for the correct approach, (ii) lack of faith and trust among the people both tribal patients and the medical practitioners, inadequacy of the infrastructure in terms of personnel, resources and access, (iii) lack of awareness and positive approach towards the western medicine system and (iv) it is a common finding of many anthropological studies that in interior areas the tribal people hesitate to come forward to accept medical treatment and prefer their own system of diagnosis and cure including herbal medicines on one side and faith healing on the other. Many of the tribal people are carried away by the notion that diseases are caused by evil spirits or on account of violation of social code of conduct in terms of taboo. In such situation more often than not the tribal people prefer their own witch doctor, shamons and faith healers etc. and surrendering to the western medicine system remains only the last resort for these people.

It is rather accepted fact that considering the vast area of spread of these people that too in sporadic and scattered manner, shortage of medical personnels and qualified medical and para medical personnels remains far away from being sufficient besides an unwilling approach of the professional qualified medical personnels to serve in the remote tribal areas. Logistically they may be right on their own stand since the minimum supporting system in terms of infrastructure to have some minimum basic standard of life from the viewpoint of these qualified medical personnels remain totally absent or quite inadequate.

As a proactive approach to the issue of tribal health the importance of folk medicines including herbal medicines have been recognized. Many tribal communities have built up good resource of health and medical knowledge using psychosomatic line of treatment as well as herbal medicines collected from the forests on the basis of a deep-rooted knowledge about the use of each part of the plant. It may be mentioned that nearly 6650 folk claims from the tribal areas have been documented and nearly 4000 such claims have been standardized as database. Due weightage is being given to the research in Unani medicine, Siddha and Ayurveda to help develop a medical system having roots in nature and cure in its essence (Ministry of Health, 2004).

The health and medical problems of the tribal people cannot be overcome merely by providing all necessary facilities, be it supply of medicine, establishing primary health centres and hospitals, flocking of qualified medical personnels and para medical forces. In order to win over the crisis of tribal health and nutritional deficiencies the effort is to be too prompt while on one side the facilities are important on the other necessary awareness raising confidence building and raising trust level is equally significant while extending the medical facilities, already existing knowledge of ayurveda, siddha way of treatment should not loose sight of as it has been helping the people in their simple way of lifestyle, albeit under limited conditions has proved its worth more than desired level of expectation. The encouragement to dovetail this traditional wisdom with modern medical system can serve as a proactive approach to help the tribal people to build up a strong base for warding off health disasters and keep diseases at bay specially in a situation when modern medicine is reaching tribal world slowly but consistently.

## REFERENCES

Ministry of Tribal Affairs, Government of India (2001). *Report of the Working Group for empowering the Scheduled Tribes during the 10th Five Year Plan (2002-2007).*

Naidu, T.S. (2002). *Woman and Child Health among the primitive tribes of Tamil Nadu.* Pondicherry: Pondicherry Central University, p. 297.

Patnakar, M. (1994). Diet and Nutritional status of tribals in India with special reference to children. In: Mahanti, N. (Ed.). *Tribal Economy Health and Wasteland Development.* N. Delhi: M.C. Mittal, Inter-India Publications, pp. 152-57.

Planning Commission (BC&TD Dev.), Government of India (2000). *Tribes in India: Empowering the Tribals of India (A Data sheet).*

Planning Commission, Government of India (2001). *Report of the Steering Committee on Empowering the Scheduled Tribes for the 10th Five Year Plan (2002-2007).*

Rao, V.G. *et al.* (2002). Nutritional Status of some tribes of Andaman and Nicobar Islands. *Tribal Health Bulletin.* July 2002. Vol. 8(2). Jabalpur: Regional Medical Research Centre for Tribals, pp. 13-18.

# 29

# State and Tribal Health Care Programmes: Strategies for Fifty Years

K.K. GANGULY

Almost sixty-eight million people in this country are tribe. There are 437 different groups of tribe in this country. The population of tribe in this country is almost eight per cent of India's total population (Government of India Census 2001). Nearly six hundred and thirty-five tribes are located in five different parts of India. And three-forth of tribals are located in five states of the country. However the north-east and Jharkhand provinces are dominated by the tribes only. And the tribal occupy fifteen per cent of the land mass of this country. Though these figures remained more or less same since independence. According to projected estimate by the Census of India it was reported that the population of the tribe will touch 83 million by 2001.

The common beliefs, customs, traditions, values and practices associated with health and disease in the tribal world is not merely connected with treatment of the individual per se but the individual is taken as an integral identity of the tribal world view. In other words he is not merely an entity to be looked in isolation but as a part of a larger system. In most tribal communities, there is wealth of folklore associated with health beliefs. Knowledge of folklore of different socio-cultural systems of tribal may have positive impact which could provide the appropriate and sustainable health practices in a given eco-system.

This paper is an endavour to understand the tribal and their health status in the light of the various development concept administered by the government since independence besides, the role of state and existing status of health care machinery and other social apparatus as well as role of international organizations to deliver health in the present century.

It is an irony that even after five decades of independence progressive growth curve in terms of population is not visible in cases of tribes, i.e. Great Andamanese, Onge, Jarwa, the Birhors and Chola Naiken. Contrarily, these people have also faced the axe of population control in the decades of sixties, seventies and eighties like any other non-tribal population, as the officials were interested in achievement of targets not actual control. They never thought, whom to control, why and how? Compounded by the misery of depleting natural resources and vagaries of nature, they migrated from their soil for a better pasture and shifted their mode of living and earning in a very unskilful manner. Many of them have shifted to non-agricultural activities from traditional agricultural practices as well as hunting and food gathering. These types of shifts have been observed through the studies carried out by Anthropological Survey of India, by the studies conducted by various other non-governmental organisations as well as department of Anthropology of various universities (Ganguly, 2003).

These people are spread over various ecological and geo-climatic regions resulting into non-accessibility of various facilities and apparent isolation from the main stream. Misery for them is getting aggravated by gradual ecological degradation combined with various miscalculated politico-economic decisions in the name of planned growth. This type of situation warrants immediate tribal area specific population policy and tribal specific plans.

The misery gets compounded when the social scientist in general and anthropologist in specific easily purchase more than half century old (since independence) gimmicks, the tribes are poor so they are illiterate having high maternal and infant mortality combined with low actual growth of the population. Moreover, they are disease prone as they live in hostile terrain and do not get good sanitary and hygienic condition to live and potable water to drink combined with their blind belief in their traditional practices and apathy towards modern medicine and health care services. These arguments are inherently capable of misleading the thinkers to take effective steps to undo the wrong doings of so many decades, contrary it helps sustain a sense of complacency among the thinkers and doers alike, that the malady is in the tribal practices and beliefs and not in the lackadaisical planned programmes.

But the problem still remains complex and unresolved due to all round under-developed status of the tribe in this country. This paper has tried to look into the abysmal health status of the tribe in the country and the various factors responsible for such lack luster performance of the state to redress the poor health status of the tribes as well as role of experts in taking various decisions for the tribal health care in this country.

## Tribal Medicine: An Anthropological Perspective

Ethnographic accounts of medical cultural data are found in writings of James Frazer and E.B. Tylor. As early as in the sixteenth century, anthropologists made contribution on the socio-cultural aspects of illness and curing. From a holistic point of view, anthropology seems to have combined in one discipline, the approaches of biological science, social science and humanities. Knowingly or unknowingly many of our social scientists as well as our planners have concentrated too much on one of the dimensions of the said three. Thus, it resulted into a one-sided understanding of the total issue. This kind of situation did more harm than good to the body of knowledge of medical anthropology in general and understanding of tribal medicine and health care in specific.

However, it is necessary to reiterate the concepts and postulates designed and delivered by various gurus of tribal medicine and health care. They not only hold out distinctly different views of tribal medicine but also tries to prove at times that the whole domain of tribal medicine need to be understood from different perspectives, i.e. the magico-religious, psycho-cultural and many other plains as well. At the same time the non-tribal medicine (modern) is considered to be a practice of medical care through understanding of cause and effect related interpretation of disease and it is diametrically opposite to tribal interpretation of ailment or disease.

In 1952 Whiting and Child used cross-cultural material from seventy-five societies to test their hypothesis that child socialization practices are related to adult conception of the causes of the disease. They based the analysis of explanation of illness on five factors:

(a) The agency causing the illness.
(b) The degree of patients responsibility of illness.
(c) The act or the failure to act of the patient.

(d) The material which have to do with production of illness, and finally,

(e) The means by which such material have an effect—where they are ingested: brought into external contact with the body or used in ritual etc.

Turner in 1966 while studying Ndembu society and their illness interpreted their illness as "illness generally points cleavage in the societal solidarity. Consequently, the therapeutic activities, in such situation are primarily oriented towards cementing the social ties". In other words etiology of illness in these societies are explained as breach of societal norm by breach of taboo and hence the divine punishment. Divination has special role in traditional and tribal system of medicine. Diviners are ascribed with the role of go between, culturally postulated super human on one hand and the society on the other. And these diviners are the selected few and they are the one who are born to be diviners.

Not withstanding some extremely sophisticated semantic treatment of concepts of health, illness and disease by the anthropology or sociology fraternity, it will be more rationale to strike a balance between the definition of health postulated by WHO on one and the socio-cultural and psychological interpretation of the various health care and ill health practices of the tribes made by different groups social scientist at different point of time.

To understand the tribal health and its care process, we have to digress a bit from the understanding of conventional tribal health care in terms of magico-religious healing, shamanism or for that matter ethno medicine and hard core tribal medicinal practices. As I understand here, the time is ripe enough to understand the tribal health care in the context of over all government health policy *vis-a-vis* the development stances taken by the government particularly in the social sectors.

Though it is true no specific policy was adopted for the tribal to get good health care but it also true that they have to face the ills of the government policy since the inception of five-year plan as a part of larger society.

## Domains of Developmental Maladies in Social Sector

Almost 400 million men, women and children in this country go hungry to bed every night. In stark contradiction to China, where only 4 per cent of the population face this kind of situation (Malcom S. Adiseshiah). Half of our six lakh villages have no roads, or electricity, nearly fifty per cent of the people do not have access to safe drinking water (though the fifty per cent who are getting the potable water, to what extent their supply is worth taking is a big question in itself, with massive degradation of water quality due to bad state of rivers, ponds and pools in this country) and one-third of the children are not enrolled in primary schools, and two-third of the enrolled dropout from the school every year. And sixty per cent of the adults are illiterate (with about 20 to 25 per cent more in case of women and Scheduled Tribes and caste adults).

It is necessary in this situation to look into two basic planks of social sectors which has a large impact on our everyday life, including that of healthy living. Before health status of the tribal is understood in the present scenario, it was felt necessary to appraise the status of primary education in this country with special emphasis on the tribes and their. educational status. The primary education was thought essential by the United Nation as late as 1990 and after this realization a declaration was made in Jomotin, Thailand.

The Jomotin declaration of Thailand, under the aegis of UN, in the year of 1990, "education for all by 2000" came into vogue. As a signatory to this UN resolution India also embarked upon implementation of this resolution by taking a soft loan package of US$ 400 million from the World Bank, to implement countrywide primary education in all states, the emphasis was primarily on the tribal and girl child of this country. However, this venture also got technical and financial assistance from DFID and European Union. This loan was given for a period of five years to start with in order to do a good deal of capacity building in the field of primary education. Though, in spite early ratification of the programme by Government of India, the programme could start in right earnest in the year 1994, (District Primary Education Programme, Guidelines,1995).

This programme got extended for another five years up to 2003 as per a recent MOU signed between the Government of India and the World Bank. The World Bank again pumped in nearly same amount of money for the extension of the programme. The tribal child in general and girl child in specific were also to be covered extensively in this programme for the second phase as well, as the first phase did not show distinct change in their educational status. The components they stressed in order to cater the tribal were environment building, making the social factors more amenable to make the situation worthy, gender sensitization of the village and the teacher community, etc. In spite of such ambitious endeavour, the problem of the tribal child and enrollment and retention remained as low as ever, as the programme never ensured active participation of any social scientist, the tribal educated people and pundits of tribal affairs at the implementation level, however the tribal experts joined their western brothers at the level of policy formulation and draft document preparation to tell the government that the western intervention in implementation of primary education is a must.

Even, after ten years of its implementation the tribal child are yet to find their right place in the main stream education. The most plausible reasons for such lack luster performance of the decade can be attributed to the following factors:

- Inadequate curriculum (non-specific) for the tribal child combined with a the kind of medium of teaching and communication which is rid of tribal dialect and expressions.
- The tribal were wooed to join school by tempting them with monetary incentives and mid day meals with out realizing the fact that such gestures will not allow the child to remain with the family for larger duration as the parents get greater premium in their child's company at home to accomplish their daily chores.
- The policy never ensured any short term benefit for the school educated child in terms of job or gainful employment.

We started our development on the basis of received wisdom, treating development as trade off between the ideology based on both the analytic stance of the sociology of knowledge and the concept of social theorizing. It was part of the concept of progress borrowed from the method of natural sciences. Development for us was the Harrod Domar model of economic growth (the first five year plan was based on the said model).

Subsequently, the Keynesian model of mixed economy and strong over tone of Rostow and Mahalanobis in terms of command area development as the background of over all health care in general and tribal health care in specific shaped the health care across the board i.e. primary, secondary as well as tertiary, almost over four decades.

Poverty, illiteracy and political will are the primary correlates of low health status. It is also true that allied correlates, socio-cultural parameters combined with ecological factors are to a large extent components of great value for determination of health status among the tribe. There is no denial of the fact that health is not guaranteed by economic development, as countries with low GNP, i.e. Cuba, enjoys a very good health status in comparison to countries of higher GNP, i.e. Indonesia, Malaysia, Thailand, etc.

The economic theory has gone profound modification in the last two to three decades. It is no longer an article of faith that social progress should be result of economic growth and investment of savings. Changes of economic factors are casually interrelated with what happens to all other factors in social change.

Development has to be health focused not disease and equity based not GNP or GDP oriented (as health cannot be equated with any other commodity in the market). It is necessarily rooted in the natural and cultural environment of the population concerned, more so when it is a matter of tribal health. The rich dividend in the health field can be accrued by cautious trading (keeping the said factors in mind) combined with retaining the locus of control and management at the grassroots level.

These can be achieved by a commitment from the planners, managers and the social scientist, their desire to work for the upliftment of people's health in general and tribes in particular. The growth of health sector could never be sustained as the premium for the investor in this area was always low and it remained non-profitable proposition.

## Factors Need to be Considered in Health Services

Health is not a blanket phenomena, to be understood and assessed by given set of formula or by a particular system as and when need arises. It is understood differently by different people in different ways, according to ones culture, history and environment, social and economic organization. That understanding also evolves within dynamic context of their society and expressed through their health seeking behaviour. General indicators, such as infant mortality, life expectancy, literacy may not have the same meaning for all. Some less easily quantifiable indicators, such as sustainability of development, rate of political participation, position of women in the society, cultural survival are also informative and relevant (Borrini).

Health status of disadvantaged group is an index of socio-economic development of a country in modern times, more so when most of the countries signed the UN resolution in Alma Ata (including India). Moreover, welfare of tribal, is one of the special responsibilities of the Government of India. This needs political will to be supported by moral commitments of the elites particularly of those in power, commensurate with meaningful actions of those people.

Response by increasing number of institutions, councils, commissions and health centres is not enough, they constitute an item of statistics of national progress. It is great deal more difficult to make them work and contribute adequately and appropriately for health in the community. So long as we are unable to bridge the gap between what we think is the need (top down) and what is actual need at the grassroots level (felt need), the brain storming pedagogic exercise combined with cosmetic action plan is no way meaningful and effective to redress the health care problem of both the tribal and marginal group of this country.

Historically many countries, whenever they have decided to solve problems of communities, mainly of socially and economically deprived of resources and those who are less known, have made special arrangements to run programmes or to monitor them or both. India is no exception. The Council for Tribal and Rural development is an instance in that direction. However, in the present day scenario one is bound to ask, in spite of conception of a good deal of such state run bodies (which have come up in last couple of decades), programmes specifically designed to empower these people could not yield much desired result.

This essentially titillates one to think that where and how the steps taken in the name of betterment and welfare of these people have gone wrong. This also prods one to think, are we trying to find solution of a long drawn complicated problem in too much easy and straight jacket manner. Does the state and the planner of the policies need to do certain amount of philosophical and ideological introspection of the situation.

Tribal epidemiology, tribal demography and tribal health are not only connected with tribal economy but with globalisation and economic reforms, through its structural adjustment it is most likely to effect the health care status. The "health funds" need to be evolved by the royalty of the herbs and plants being used by the state from the tribal area. This kind of move will not only give real stake holdership into the whole process but also ensure steady flow of fund for the tribal health expenses.

This may also transform health services, which is languishing in the recent times, in the tribal areas through economic benefits in direct manner from private and state profits. In this connection one may also keenly observe the issue of "patent rights" and "Intellectual Property Right" (IPR). Particularly for the tribal medicinal plants. of high economic value being used by the tribal in their day to day care and cure. The knowledge of such plant and herb or shrub can only be given to a pharmaceutical multinational by taking adequate compensation from the deal. This compensation in turn can help make the part of the health fund. This warrants an organized state supported mechanism to bring forth so far unattended resource of knowledge and know how. The tribal need to have self-esteem and feel proud of their own resources so that the era of SAP or globalisation does not prove to be real nemesis for the tribal.

## Tribal Health Care and Structural Adjustment Policy

It will be easy to understand the Structural Adjustment Policy and Globalisation in the field of health care, if, the maxim of present day market players and international funding agency is understood in the following manner. Public Health and preventive services is for public good which may be funded by public funds, and curative health care as private good which may financed by private funds. This creates new roles for the government as the provider of "public health and preventive services" and the subsidizer and guardian of contracted curative health service. This type of situation leaves the tribal population of India in absolute limbo. To understand the status of tribal health in the twenty-first century in India it is essential to understand the whole issue against the backdrop of structural adjustment and globalisation.

Notwithstanding the anomalies in the present health situation, the country appears to be poised for its preparation under the SAP. The World Bank has defined the agenda for reforming (as done in case of primary education) the health sector in the developing countries. This primarily encourages cuts in public spending in health services and shifts to strengthen population control; shifting curative care to the private sector: introduction of cost recovery mechanisms in private hospital as well as sources of financing, such as user fees, insurance and self/community financing defining essential clinical and public health packages, and tackling poverty through the SAP, education and women's employment (World Bank, 1993).The SAP will essentially bring them on the cross roads of confusion and calamity.

The role anthropologist and social scientists in understanding the health and health care policy of the tribal for last two decades need to be vetted from the close quarter for a better and meaningful alternative health policy and care for the marginalized of the land.

The ensuing short-sighted images of health maintenance in general and particularly that of the tribes and associated exercises in inter-cultural information translations achieved by medical anthropological or anyother behavioural sciences research appear to have succeeded in achieving a symbiosis at the level of integration of professional/ politco-economic interests with those of dominant institutional domains of health care and cure and most often those are guided by the extrinsic forces. The role of state itself or the international funding agencies which has time and again mended the policies in the field of health care in general and tribal in particular. The quinquennial frame of reference for countries governance has seen lot of twist and turn since the beginning both at the policy formulation as well as at the implementation levels, as the donors desired. Latest in the series of changes is SAP and Globalisation, willy-nilly adopted at the behest of WB/IMF.

However, the usefulness of such myopic imagery, not withstanding its pure academic value in comprehending health related scenario nor has it been successful in augmenting the health status of social policies and social sectors. Neither it has looked into the development needs whether economic, educational, social or for that matter of health in right perspectives. Even almost sixty years after independence it is a conundrum that development for whom, how much, etc.

The continuing disarticulation of concerns between medical anthropology/sociology and real health related needs of our tribal population and all-round development warrants immediate expression of concern for both the academics and policy planners. The persistent effort of anthropologists, the planners and both the internal and international funders need to do lot of brain storming to make the rules of structural adjustment policy, new primary health care and globalisation more user friendly and really concerned for tribal and their health. To understand the nuances of globalisation in the field of health care it is necessary to quote Kuivesalo, M. (2001), who explained the issue of globalisation very aptly, and I, quote: "Globalisation is often presented as a one way track without any exit and it often offers very ideological arguments. It tends to right size the government and shift the burden of risks and cost to individuals rather than to governments or employers. It is of crucial importance to demystify the ideological arguments presented in the garb of competitive necessities and discuss and analyse the implications of different international policy choices being thrust upon the public sector and ultimately upon the health and social security of people around the world."

This type of discourse is essential to analyse the issues of human health in a true developmentalist mode in contrast to prevalent thinking in terms of arbitrary indicators of health, i.e. prevent preventable diseases only, levy user fees, the notion of disease and illness as objective bio-technology and therefore, reposing the responsibility of the care on techno savvy health care institution.

Health Development is usually measured in terms of:

(a) Hospital population ratio
(b) Doctor and Nurse population ratio
(c) Per capita consumption of calorie
(d) Birth and death rate
(e) Perinatal and maternal mortality
(f) Life expectancy at birth
(g) Morbidity due to communicable diseases
(h) Safe drinking water and safe disposal of human waste etc.

Structural Adjustment Programme (SAP) are not simple instrument for rectifying macro economic imbalances through the imposition of policies, such as currency devaluation, privatization, trade liberlisation and cuts in government spending, as proclaimed. They may be viewed instead as carefully engineered projects for generating social and economic transformation in the interests of the countries of the North. The main arbiters are International Monetary Fund (IMF) and World Bank (WB). The third world countries are told that in order to pay off loans and be eligible for more, they must implement "structural adjustment" reforms, accompanied by conditional ties as set by the leaders based in the North. The cycle never ends. Often the same conditional ties are imposed on every recipient country regardless of the kind of economic or social crises experienced or consideration of the context in which they are applied.

While the economic problems that WB/IMF endeavoured to lift remain intact, the impact of the conditional ties, such as drastic cuts in social expenditure, especially health and education, has been devastating. These conditional ties are contingent to the economic assault on the living standards of the poor by cutting consumer subsidies and raising producer prices for agricultural goods, charging user fees for social services such as health and education, all for regulating privatization to create incentives to attract foreign capital, and allow the MNC to flourish.

According to UNICEF report at least six million children under the age of five have died each year since 1982. About 1.3 billion people in the South now live in poverty out of which 260 million are living in India which is twice the number ten years ago. This is result of plummeting wages, often to levels half as low as that at the beginning of the eighties (Haq, 1997).

World Health Organisation driven New Public Health (NPH) policy is so selective and SAP compatible can be evinced from the statements given in the New NPII, i.e.

> In NPH the role of the state becomes so insignificant that it is forced to seek partners in the private, corporate and NGO sector. NPH is only concerned with health status not the means to achieve that status through the state policy and advocacy. The policy stresses very specifically on prevention of preventablé only. One of the most prominent component in NPH is focus on "lifecycle". Increasingly, the emphasis of the lifecycle approach is on the reproductive phase of the life of women. While the market is allowed to occupy the empty spaces created by a receding public sector in health, the latter influenced by the truncated vision of life cycle depends entirely on reproductive health strategy to control fertility.

Technology based disease control programmes replace social strategy based programmes of public distribution systems or food and drinking water.

As Werner *et al.* in 1996 summed up the SAP as,

- Sharp cuts in public spending on health education and other sectors.
- The removal of subsidies and lifting of price controls on staple foods and other basic commodities.
- Freezing of wages.

- A shift from production of foods and goods for domestic consumption to production for the export.
- Liberalisation of the trade polices (through tariff elimination and restriction on import).
- Efforts to attract foreign investors by providing them incentives, such as tax regulation and tax breaks.
- Privatisation of public services and state enterprises.
- Devaluation of the local currency.

With the said preambles as standard of health one is forced to think in greater details regarding the status of tribal health and its future in this country. The hospital, nurse doctor will be available with implementation of the newer policy to those clients who can afford, certainly declining social security status the tribal would in the bottom of the rung. Per capita consumption calorie is dwindling with declining purchasing power of the poor and the marginal/tribal. As a corollary to this state of affairs perinatal as well as neonatal health of the tribal child is in a state of fix at this juncture as he can not pay to get the services as and when required. Life expectancy at birth for many of the tribal declined, i e. those living in Andaman islands. The quality of life of these people is bad and appalling even if they manage to survive after a certain age, as no policy has been framed to see that they live at least up to the same age as the non tribal live. Guarantee to the tribal for living up to 64/65 years of age means the policy would need special amendment and efforts to be made to ensure the implementation of those policies.

## REFERENCES

Ackerknecht, E.H. (1942), Problems of Primitive Medicine, *Bulletin of History of Medicine* XI: 503-21.

Adiseshiah, Malcom S. (1970), *Let my Country Awake*, UNESCO deliberation, Paris.

Aristotle (1976), *Nicomachean Ethics*, Penguin. Middlesex, UK.

Banerji, D. (1982), *Poverty Class and Health Culture,* Prachi Publication, New Delhi.

Basu, S.K. (1986), "Genetic Socio—Cultural and Health Care Among Tribal Groups of Jagdalpur and Konta Tehsil of Bastar District", *Anthropology Development and Nation Building* (ed). A.K. Kalla and S.K. Singh; Concept Publishing Co., New Delhi.

Borrini Grazia, "*Health Through People's Empowerment*", Ifda Dossier; 55, 9-12.

Census of India (2001), Registrar General of India, Govt. of India. New Delhi.

District Primary Education Programme, Guideline (1995), Dept. of Education, Ministry of Human Resource, GOI. New Delhi.

Gangully, K.K. (2002), *Health and Culture of a Metropolitan Resettlement; Issues and Challenges*, Rajat Publication; New Delhi.

Gurumurty, K.G. (1990), *Anthropology and Management of Health and Hygiene: An Indian Case Study*, Studies in Medical Anthropology; Reliance Publication

Haq, M. (1997), *Human Development in South Asia*, Published for the HDC Centre, New Delhi, Oxford University Press.

Hodge J. (1995), *Heidegger and Ethics*, Routledge, London.

Horwitz Abraham, "Changing Concepts of Health Services: New Opportunities for Nutrition Promotion", *Bull PAHO* 17(1) 61-76.

Joshi, P.C. and Anil Mahajan (1990), *Medical Anthropology an Overview. Studies in Medical Anthropology,* Reliance Publication

Kakar, D.N. (1990), *Anthropology in Medicine A Review*, Studies in Medical Anthropology; Reliance Publication.

Koivusala, M. (2001), *Changes in Health Care Systems in Europe: Focus on Finland Public Health and the Poverty of Reforms,* The South Asian Predicament. Sage Publications.

McBeath, Grahm and Webb, Stephen A. (2002), *Virtue Ethics and Social Work: Being Lucky Realistic and not doing one's Duty,* British Jr. of Social Work, OUP, UK.

Qadeer, I. (2001), *Impact of structural adjustment programmes on concepts in public health*, "Public health and the poverty of reforms; The south Asian predicament". Sage Publications.

Rostow, W.W. (1966), *Stages of Economic Growth*, Cambridge University Press. UK.

Sen, K. (2001), *Health reforms and developing countries–A Critique.* "Public health and the poverty of reforms"; The South Asian Predicament. Sage Publications.

Turner, V.W. (1964), *An Ndembu Doctor and Practice; In Magic, Faith and Healing,* Ari Kiev, Ed. New York. The Free Press.

Werner, D.; Sanders D.; Weston J.; Babb, S. and Roudriguez, B. (1996), *Questioning the Solution: The Politics of Primary Health Care and Child Survival.* Pal Alto: Health Rights.

Whiting, J. and Child, I. (1952), *Child Training and Personality Development: A Cross Cultural Survey,* New Haven: Yale University Press.

*World Bank Report* (1993), Washington, USA.

# 30

# Public-Private Partnership: A Strategy for Improvement of Health in Scheduled Tribe

RAJESH KHANNA and A.K. KAPOOR

## Public-Private Partnership (PPP): A Concept

"Public-Private Partnership" (PPP) is defined as collaborative programme between the public sector and the not-for-profit/for-profit private sector. It is a contractual arrangement between the public and private sectors, with clear agreement on shared objectives, for the delivery of an asset or service that would otherwise have been provided through traditional public sector procurement.

It is important to recognize that the terms "public" and "private" is used in loose and ambiguous ways. For some, term 'private' is used as the opposite of 'public' to refer to all non-state organizations whether profit-seeking or not. Elsewhere the term is used to refer to that set of non-state organizations that seeks profit.

(a) *Private Sector*: The private sector comprises of those organizations controlled and financed through non-government or private bodies.

(b) *Public Sector*: The public sector comprises of those organizations controlled and financed through government.

Public-Private Partnership (PPP) allows for the best of public and private sector management skills to work together in the delivery of services for the benefit of the public. The essence of a PPP project is that the private sector will do one or more of the activities like provide private finance to fund the project; to enter into a long term service contract; enter into a joint venture arrangement with the public sector to provide a service or asset etc.

The public private partnership allows considerable leveraging of each partners resources and unique strengths and results are often attained in less time, at lower cost, and with greater sustainability than efforts by any single partner.

The most important aspect of PPP between two sectors is "Partnership". Partnership implies to a commitment to a common goal through the joint provision of complementary resources and expertise, and the joint sharing of the risks involved. Partnership means more than just understanding a piece of work together. It also means existing together, growing together and sharing with one another experiences. It connotes commitment and trust and shared interests, decisions and responsibilities throughout the implementation of project or phase. It is important to establish co-operation between two partnering agencies.

It is reported that Public Private Partnerships form a cooperation of the state and the private sector. They are based on the insight that business not only creates shareholder value but also invests in stake holder value, such as human resource development, environmental sustainability, social development and health development. Hence, Public Private Partnerships contribute to developmental goals and simultaneously meet the interest for long-term economic growth of private companies.

## Need for Public-Private Partnership in Health Sector

In India, the Ministry of Health and Family Welfare have the objectives of delivering efficient and good quality health care services, ensuring equity in access to health care and sustainable financing of health care. However, due to various constraints and limitations, public sector is unable to address the health care needs of the society, in general and tribal communities in particular, effectively and efficiently.

The crisis in the health sector has induced governments in many developing countries to review the relationship between the public and private sectors. A Public-Private Partnership has become increasingly more significant in the coming years as policy makers explore options for promoting complementary involvement of the private sector. The level of spending per capita on health is low in absolute terms, the health sector's contribution to national income in India is higher than in more developing countries at similar levels of per capita income. Despite the historical emphasis on the government's role in the health sector in India, expenditure data clearly indicates the dominance of non-government spending (Mckinsey & Company, 2002).

The private sector plays vital role in the provision of selected services, such as individual curative care through ambulatory services, diagnostic services etc. The private health expenditure in India is estimated to be about 4.25 per cent of the GDP. Insurance coverage mechanisms are negligible and most of this expenditure is out-of-pocket. The private health care expenditure in India has grown at the rate of 12.5 per cent per annum. For each one per cent increase in per capita income the private health care expenditure has increased by about 1.47 per cent (Bhat, 1996). The share of private sector investment in health infrastructure, e.g. hospitals, investment in medical equipments and technology etc. is quite significant. The data suggest that at present about 80 per cent of 3,90,000 qualified allopathic doctors registered with medical councils in India and 6,50,000 providers from other systems of medicine are working in the private sector. Approximately 57 per cent of hospitals and 32 per cent of hospital-beds are in the private sector. Further, most qualified doctors work in private sector. The dependence on private sector is, therefore, considerable. Utilisation studies also show that 1/3rd of in-patient cases and 3/4th of out-patients utilise the private health care facilities (Duggal and Amin, 1989; Yesudian, 1990; Visaria and Gumber, 1994).

The Public Private Partnership in health sector begins when funding agencies decides to take on the catalyst role and bring public and private organizations together to tackle a specific health problem. The catalyst investment makes it possible for public and private organization to join forces and apply their strengths to achieve health goals.

A Public-Private Partnership in health sector is an approach to addressing public health issues through the joint efforts of public, private, and development organizations. (Policy for Private Investment in Medical Institutions, 1996). Each partner makes a contribution in its area of special competence, bringing in expertise. The partners in a Public-Private Partnership (PPP) assemble around a common cause, while at the same time pursuing some of their own organizational/individual objectives. The main challenges with regard to Public-Private Partnership (PPP) in health sector include:

(a) Enhancing the scope and importance of the private sector, while improving the quality of health services;
(b) Encouraging private sector involvement in preventive and curative aspects of health care rather than solely in individual curative care;
(c) Promoting partnership between the public, private and voluntary sectors;
(d) Increasing efficiency through contracting out of the services; and
(e) Improving the existing arrangement for regulating health care.

The public-private partnership in health sector can be tried in two broad areas: i.e. Clinical (Speciality care; Reaching vulnerable and target groups of population; Addressing problems of access in remote area where public health services cannot reach) and Non-Clinical (Contracting out the services like diet, catering, laundry, security etc.; and Community based projects) (Bhatia and Mills, 1997). One of the biggest incentives for companies, private foundations and other non-government organisations to commit themselves to partnership is having the confidence that the public is serious about developing the appropriate infrastructure and capacities necessary to use partnership outputs for enhancing health (Cross, 1998).

There is no time-tested model for public-private sector partnership in India. Some efforts have been made sporadically in some places, but they are very specific to certain socio-economic conditions and not replicable to other places. The model of handing over the management of Primary Health Centre (PHC) to SEWA-Rural at Jagadhia in Gujarat, or the model of involving Non-Government Organisations (NGOs) in providing non-clinical services in one or two hospitals in Himachal Pradesh (Khanna, 2003), or the model of partnership under Andhra Pradesh Urban Slum Healthcare Project (Rao, 1997) are successful to some extent in their respective area and social conditions. None of them is proven as scalable on larger area.

The private sector and relevance of public-private partnership policies in the health care services are perhaps the least studied areas in our country. Notwithstanding all statements made in our plan and the policy documents, it is evident that in health care, it is not the public sector but the private sector which occupies a predominant place. This is clear from the fact that over 78 per cent of the health care expenditure in country is accounted for by the private sector (World

Bank, 1997). The private sector is conspicuous by its absence in plan documents.

The public-private partnership is not even tried out at a smaller scale to understand their relevance. Not only that, certain public private partnership methods used in health care, like contracting out in building construction, involvement of private doctors in the disease control programme, occasional philanthropic donations for public health institutions etc. have not been studied and their efficiency compared with the public provision of health care especially for the tribal areas.

### Health Need Status Among Scheduled Tribes

In context of scheduled tribal health, the tribesmen consider diseases as manifestation of evil spirit or to the wrath of certain society are that disease is caused by the breach of some taboo or by hostile spirit of dead. Sickness is the routine punishment for every lapse and crime meted out to them by these spirits (Basu ed., 1994, Kshatriya *et al.*, 1994, Mann, 1993).

The maternal care in tribal community is largely neglected and the expectant mother to a great extent is not inoculated against tetanus. The consumption of iron, calcium and vitamins during pregnancy is poor. From the inception of pregnancy to its termination, no specific nutritious diet is consumed by a woman. Vaccination and immunization of infant and children are inadequate. In addition, extremes of magico-religious beliefs and taboos tend to aggravate the problems which influence high mortality, (Kantikar, 1979; Kar, 1993). It is being reported in various studies that birth rate and death rate in tribal population are very high as compared with general population. High death rate is directly linked with high birth rate. For this cause, health services and birth control devices are much required for these tribal people. (Kshastriya, 2000; Rajpramukh, 1998; Rajyalakshmi and Geervani, 1992).

Among family planning acceptors, the percentage of males is very low as compared with females. It is reported that population density, female literacy rate, growth rate, achievement of maternal and child health care, etc. in the population of tribal area are very low as compared with the population of non-tribal area (Chaudhary, 1986; Pandey and Saxena 1988; Pandey Roy and Tiwary, 2001). It is being reported that users of contraceptive devices are quite low. Though fertility is a biological phenomenon there are a number of other factors influencing the levels and differentials of fertility among tribals. One of the realisation of modern social and life science is to intensify the interdisciplinary approach in understanding the tribal situation (Kapoor, 1996).

For more than a quarter century, Non-Government Organizations and private organizations have played a key role in the provision of health services in tribal areas. (Kapoor and Singh, 1997). The Department of Health and Family Welfare assumed an increasingly important role in the direct provision of services. In Government of India's Health programme, in any districts, the Primary Health Centre provide health services to 30,000 population for plain areas and 20,000 for tribal and hilly region. Whereas sub-centres cater to the population of 5,000 in plain areas and 3,000 population in tribal and hill region.

NGOs, for which national/international donors had been the largest source of financial support, face increasing hardship, as did the profit-seeking organisations. Notwithstanding the NGOs and profit-making organisations have continued to seek opportunities to rationalise health services delivery, reduce the cost burden on the population and improve the quality of care (Tandon, 1989).

Whereas the public health institutions lack professional approach and commitment, the profit-seeking private health organizations fail to reach the poorest of the poor because of their high cost of service and unwillingness to work in the remote areas. The non-profit secking voluntary organizations have the dedication and willingness to work for the poor in the remote areas but most of them lack professional training, financial and technical support from government.

There is general agreement that measures of health development for the tribal and their delivery system cannot be same for general population and there have to be variation even in the inter-intra-tribal situation depending upon the health status and consequent health needs of various groups. In order to improve the health situation of Scheduled Tribes, appropriate solution heave to be found by planning and understanding their health needs, associated with many other socio-cultural and developmental indices. Hence, there is a need for developing a mechanism of partnership among the public and private sectors (for-profit and not-for-profit) to supplement the strengths of each other in tribal areas.

## Proposed Public-Private Partnership Mechanism for Health Care Among Scheduled Tribes

NGOs have been engaged in several activities related to health and family planning programmes in tribal areas. These include service programme, field experimentation, community organisation and mobilisation, health education and demand creation, advocacy, community-based research, training, documentation, policy formulation and partnership with government. While some of these activities such as implementation of service programme, field experimentation, community—organisation and demand creation are undertaken by grassroots NGOs, other activities such as community-based research, advocacy, training, documentation and policy formulation are more often on the agendas of support groups intermediary NGOs (Kapoor, 1998).

A good number of Non-Government Organizations (NGOs) are trying to develop and implementing various models for providing quality healthcare to the Scheduled Tribes at a low cost. However, none of these models can be considered as perfect and universally replicable. This is truer in case of partnership with profit seeking private health sector. In fact, no model has been implemented in India where profit-seeking private organisations have truly entered into partnership with public sector for providing health services, particularly clinical health services, for the Scheduled Tribes.

## *Approach*

The following steps may be taken for involving the private/NGO sector in Health programme in tribal areas.

### *Need Assessment*

Before taking up any project, the need for the particular project should be assessed in the target area and among target population.

### *Project Identification*

Partnership with NGOs can be developed for implementing each identified project in the target area. The partnership strategy may vary depending on the need and outcome of the project.

### *Deciding on Partnership Mechanism*

Based on the project that is to be implemented in a particular area, the partnership mechanism has to be selected from a number of options and fine tuned as per the condition of the local area. The most models which seem suitable for the local condition and the project may be adopted and adapted as per the needs.

*Developing Terms of Reference (ToR) for NGOs/Private Parties*

The ToRs outlining the partnership arrangements should be worked out before hand. These may include (a) objectives of the partnership arrangements, (b) tasks required to be carried out by the NGO/private parties, (c) time schedule for completion of preparatory tasks such as recruitment of staff and household survey for identification of eligible couples, (d) facilities that would be provided by the Government, (e) reports required to be submitted by the NGO/private parties and (f) review mechanism that would govern funds flow.

*Inviting NGOs/Private Parties to Participate*

Based on the partnership arrangements and the ToR, the NGOs/private parties should be invited to participate in the project. The invitation to the private parties may be open or limited as suggested in the partnership model.

*Implementation Through Private Participation*

The NGO/private parties for a particular project should be selected based on certain selection criteria developed by Health Department, and the project will be implemented as per the partnership mechanism.

The state government can take initiative in developing a model of public-private partnership in tribal areas with financial assistance from international funding agencies. A large number of NGOs are institution-based, running dispensaries/hospitals for the poor and backward classes and providing curative and preventive services to the tribals. State government should take initiative to promote, strengthen and bring efficiency among the NGOs in forming collaboration in Family Welfare Programme. The Health Department may develop grant-in-aid schemes for NGOs, invite their participation, fund the activities, monitor or organize monitoring them and provide for/or arrange technical support.

***Role of State Government***

In this mechanism, the state government can play the important roles of:

(a) Promoting collaboration of NGOs by maintaining continuous dialogue with NGOs;
(b) Facilitate the identification of grant-in-aid schemes which would meet the objectives of both state government and NGOs and invite proposals for schemes from NGOs and fund them;
(c) Strengthening functioning of NGOs by monitoring their programme activities;
(d) Providing technical assistance in pre-project, project and post-project phases and training manpower of NGOs;
(e) Co-ordinating NGOs work with government by bringing collaboration with the work of government machinery and avoiding duplication of efforts; and
(f) Facilitating exchange of experiences among NGOs and mutual learning between governmental agencies and NGOs in the health and family welfare field.

### *General Issues Involved in Public-Private Partnership for Tribal Areas*

The Public-Private Partnership should be based on mutual trust and sense of complement, where both sides admit, understand and appreciate each other's strengths and limitations. General issues involved in public private partnership are

(a) Transparency and impartiality in the process of identification and selection of the NGOs for funding. An independent selection forum of experts of wide representation, including from NGOs can be created to assist state government in identification and selection process. Standard rating mechanism should be adopted for identification and selection of NGOs.
(b) The partnership duration should not be less than two years, as the first year will be required to complete the formalities, understand the mechanism, start the work and evaluate the performance, and the second year will be the year of taking corrective measures and improving performance.
(c) The tribal area/villages handed over to the Non-Government Organisation can be part (one or more sub-centres) or whole of a PHC, or equivalent area; the NGO can be fully involved

in the choice of the area, the size being determined by the ability of the NGO to handle work load.

(d) All levels of personnel in the government hierarchy who are likely to come in contact with the work of the NGO from time to time be specifically informed about the special importance of the partnership venture and encouraged to minimize impediments and maximize positive response in dealing with the NGO. This may mean inter-sectoral meetings at high levels that can then percolate such positive attitudes in the hierarchy down to the grassroots levels.

(e) In the interest of voluntarism and independence of the NGO, it may be desirable to limit funding to less than 100 per cent of the estimated cost of the project.

(f) While specific measures to help the NGOs cope with various elaborate and cumbersome procedure of the government need to be instituted, it would be a useful practice to provide for deputation of various levels of technical and non-technical staff with the working of the government system, and are interested in helping such NGOs. This has, of course, to be done with mutual consent and should provide a welcome break to sincere and committed officers in the government, while being of immense benefit to the NGOs. Such deputations should naturally be non-transferable for at least the period of the partnership projects.

As mentioned above, necessary technical and non-technical government staff can be placed on deputation to the NGO for the period of the project. Besides health workers and administrative personnel, doctors and anthropologists from various relevant departments would be extremely valuable. This, of course, should be done with complete acceptance of all parties concerned.

While deputation may fill some requirements of the NGOs, it is likely that in other cases, there may be no candidates for some posts fulfilling all the criteria for qualifying for government job. It would be desirable under these circumstances to permit recruitment of less qualified staff by the NGOs, with appropriate relaxation of recruitment criteria. The staff employed or deputed would be totally answerable and responsible to NGO alone for the period of the project.

When staffs are employed by the NGO, their basic training for the job, as for example for health workers, may need to be arranged at government or government-approved training centres, with acceptance of appropriate relaxation.

The system for monitoring the partnership project should be separate and independent of the system that monitors other PHCs. This may be the single most important measure to ensure successful completion of the project.

An apex committee may be constituted by experts, NGO representatives, and government officers familiar with simplified accounting procedures etc. The committee can be empowered to deal with virtually all aspects of the partnership, beginning from identification of the NGO, through finalizing the terms of the project, to ongoing monitoring of all aspects of the progress.

In general, reporting should be simplified as far as possible. State Government should help the NGOs with reporting procedures where required, by giving timely inputs and anticipating problems, if necessary by deputing appropriate accounts officers for the purpose.

The NGO's should be permitted considerable freedom as regards recording procedures. This should be to encourage simplified procedures that should work in the atmosphere of trust that is expected in an NGO.

The release of the grant should be from state to avoid bottlenecks from the bureaucracy at lower levels, which can be very upsetting to the work of an NGO unwilling to compromise on basic values.

### *Areas of Activities for Public Private Partnership*

The Public-Private Partnership (PPP) may be developed in the following areas of activities in tribal areas:

(a) Campaigns, advocacy and lobbying both at central and state levels evolving new policies aimed at improving the health status of tribal people.

(b) Organizing formal and non-formal training programmes and doing follow-up to strengthen capacity building of voluntary agencies and their members in tribal areas.

(c) Strengthening grassroots-level health care delivery by equipping village health workers with training and communication materials.

(d) Implementing effective communication strategies through various audio-visual and folk mediums.
(e) Managing the complete health activities of Primary Health Centre or Sub-Centre.
(f) Dissemination of information on various health issues among the tribals at various level.

In Public-Private Partnership, privatization of public health facilities is another tricky issue, which needs policy decision at government level. The implementation of Public-Private Partnership mechanism depends on government's willingness to accept private sector as partner in health service provision.

The NGO sector should be supported to undertake a broad range of activities to strengthen the health and family welfare programme in tribal areas. However, the heterogeneous nature of the NGO sector should be kept in view while determining the role of NGOs in these programmes. Consequently, although the NGO sector as a whole could assume varied role, the role of individual NGOs would necessarily depend on their particular motivations, interest, capacities and commitment to specific activities. The public-private partnership process for primary care services would have the particular success, helping to avoid duplication in geographical distribution of the government heath centres and thus having the potential to reduce the overall cost of care in areas. However, certain structural problems can be faced by the private sector in the health care system and the economic environment inhibit its ability to sustain quality services; among these—High cost of medical technology and pharmaceuticals; High cost of equipment maintenance; Weakness in administrative and financial management and subjective competition (accumulation of surplus equipment in one geographic area) and problems pertinent to the NGOs could be sharp decline of donor assistance, resulting in an inability to cover operational expenses and expertise overflow (i.e., transfer of qualified physicians and nurses from NGOs to Ministries or for profit facilities)

**Conclusion**

The concepts of private-public mix in its true spirit, which is recognized by the top functionaries of the particular programme percolate down to programme managers and officers. The private-public partnerships would aim at complementing the Government's programme in a highly localized manner. It is time for the Government to try to overcome the apathy in the private sector to give it a sense of involvement. There has to be an attitudinal change in approaching, initiating and evolving methods for joint planning and implementation. The programme has to recognize the autonomous nature of private practice and formulate its approach accordingly, taking into account that there is no real incentive for the private practitioners except to appeal to their sense of community and social responsibility. In fact, there has to be a specific training and orientation towards this within the particular programme itself before inviting partnerships. The partnership between the public and private sectors in the provision of health services would have both positive effects (Improved access to health facilities, More affordable health care, Institutionalization of individual responsibility for own health) and negative effects. (Discrimination, consumer to demand unreasonable and exaggerated outcomes). Involvement of non-regulated private sector in health care leads to serious quality problems. As the private sector is largely motivated by profit or the pursuit of individual earnings, an inherent feature of unregulated private provision is that providers will provide care to those whose willingness and ability to pay allows providers to make a profit.

## REFERENCES

Basu, S.K. (ed.) (1993), *Tribal Health in India*, New Delhi, Manak Publishers

Basu, S.K.; Jindal, A. and Kshatriya, G.K. (1994), 'Perception of Health and Pattern of Health Seeking Behaviour among the Selected Tribal Population Groups of Madhya Pradesh and Orissa, (In) *Tribal Health in India* Ed. S.K. Basu. Published by New Delhi Manak Publication Ltd.

Bennett, Sara and V.R. Muraleedharan (1998), 'Reforming the Role of Government in Tamil Nadu Health Sector,' Paper No. 28, Development Administration Group, University of Birmingham.

Bhat, Ramesh and S. Sharma, (1997), 'Current issues in the implementation of user fees in public facilities in West Bengal,' DFID Report prepared for Strategic Planning Cell, West Bengal Health Sector Development Programme, Health and Family Welfare Department, Government of West Bengal.

Bhat, Ramesh, (1996), 'Regulation of the Private Health Sector in India,' *International Journal of Health Planning and Management*, Vol. 11: 253-274.

Bhatia, M. and Anne Mills (1997), 'Contracting out of dietary services by public hospitals in Bombay,' (In) *Private Health Providers in Developing Countries* (eds.) Sara Bennett, Barbara McPake and Anne Mills, Zed Books

Chaudhary, B (1986), *Tribal Health*, New Delhi, Sunil Printers

Cross, C. (1998), 'Partnerships between non-governmental development organizations'. *Annals of Tropical Medicine & Parasitology*. 92 Suppl 1: S155-6, Apr.

Duggal, Ravi and Suchetha Amin (1989), 'Cost of Health Care: A Household Survey in an Indian District', Bombay, The Foundation for Research in Community Health.

Kantikar, T. (1979), 'Development of Maternal and Child Health Services in India' (In) *Child in India*, Ed. K. Srinivasan, P.C Saxena and Tara Kantikar. New Delhi, Himalaya Publishing House.

Kapoor, A.K. (1998), 'Role of NGO's in Human Development: A Domain of Anthropology', *J.Ind. Anthrop. Soc.*, 33:283:300.

Kapoor, A.K. (1996), 'Tribe, Anthropology and Future', pp 07-80 (In) *Tribes of India: Ongoing Challenges* by R.S. Mann (Ed) Delhi, M.D. Publication.

Kapoor, A.K. and D. Singh (1997), *Rural Development through NGOs*, Jaipur, Rawat Publications.

Kar, R.K. (1993), 'Health Behaviour among the tribes of North-East India: A profile', *Journal of Indian Anthropologist*, Vol. 28 (2), pp. 115-24.

Khanna, R. (1998), 'Mina Tribe Development: Problem, Perspective and the People', M.Sc Unpublished Dissertation.

Khanna, R. (2001), 'Study on ICDS's Health Supply and Service Delivery System', *report prepared for CARE*, India.

Khanna, R (2003), 'Framework for Public Private Partnership, networking of NGOs and their Effective Participation in Service Delivery of Primary Health Care', *report prepared for Sector Investment Programme Office* (EC).

Khanna, R. and A.K. Kapoor (2000), 'Ethnographic Profile of Kinnauris' pp. 51-59, In *Tribal in India* by P.C. Mehta (ed), Udaipur, Shiv Publication.

Kshastriya, G.K. (2000), 'Ecology and health with special reference to Indian tribes,' In M.K. Bhasin and V. Bhasin (Eds), *Man-Environment Relationship*. Delhi: Kamla-Raj Publications.

Mann, R.S. (1993), *Culture and Integration of Indian Tribes*, Delhi, MD Publication.

Mckinsey & Company (2002), 'Health Care in India: The Road Ahead', Delhi, CII.

Nandraj, Sunil (1994), 'Beyond the Law and the Lord: Quality of Private Health Care,' *Economic and Political Weekly*, July 2.

Pandey, G.D., and Saxena, B.N. (1988), 'District Level Planning for Health and Family Welfare for Tribals. *Demography in India*, 17(2):216.

Pandey, G.D.; Roy, J. and Tiwary, R.S. (2001), 'Socio-Cultural Aspects and Health Care in Pando Tribe of Madhya Pradesh,' *J. Hum. Ecol.*, 12(5):391-394.

Policy for Private Investment in Medical Institutions, (1996) Medical and Health Department, Department of Health and Family Welfare, Government of Rajasthan.

Prüss, A. and Mariotti S.P. (2000), 'Preventing trachoma through environmental sanitation' *WHO Bulletin*, 78, (2), 258.

Rajpramukh, K.E. (1998), 'Tribal health in Visakhapatnam District of Andhra Pradesh', *Journal of Human Ecology*, Vol. 9(2), pp. 191-93.

Rajyalakshmi, P. and Geervani, P. (1992), 'Food Nutrition and Morbidity: Some Observations among four Tribal Groups of South India'. *J. Hum. Ecol.*, 3 (2):115-214.

Rao, K. Sujatha, (1997), 'Financing of Primary Health Care in Andhra Pradesh,' *Report prepared for World Health Organisation.*

Rao, M.G. and Tapas Sen, (1993), 'Government Expenditure in India: Level, Growth and Composition', National Institute of Public Finance and Policy.

Tandon, Rajesh (1989), 'NGO-Government Relations: A Source of Life or a Kiss of Death,' *Consultation Report*, New Delhi: Participatory Research in Asia (PRIA).

Tulasidhar, V.B. (1993), 'Expenditure Compression and Health Sector Outlays,' *Economic and Political Weekly*, November 6.

Visaria, P. and A. Gumber (1994), 'Utilisation of and Expenditure on Health Care in India: 1986-87,' Gujarat, Gujarat Institute of Development Research.

W.H.O. (1998), 'Health For All in the Twenty-First Century,' *World Health Organisation Document* A51/5 Geneva.

Whyatt, Sylvia and Ramesh Bhat (1997), 'Options for improving the relationship between public, private and other healthcare providers in West Bengal,' *DFID Report* prepared for Strategic Planning Cell, West Bengal Health Sector Development Programme, Health and Family Welfare Department, Government of West Bengal.

World Bank (1997), 'India New Directions in Health Sector Development at the State Level: An Operational Perspective,' Population and Human Resource Division, South Asia Country Department II.

World Bank (1997), 'India, Andhra Pradesh: Agenda for Economic Reform,' *Report No. 15901-IN*, 1997.

World Health Organisation (1996), 'Guidelines for drug donations,' Geneva: World Health Organisation. *WHO/DAP/96.2.*

Yesudian, C.A.K. (1990), 'Utilisation Pattern of Health Services and its Implications for Urban Health Policy,' Takemi Programme in International Health, Harvard School of Public Health.

Yesudian, C.A.K. (1994), 'The Nature of Private Sector Health Services in Bombay,' Health Policy and Planning, 9(1).

# INDEX